AF564855

RURAL HEALTH EDUCATION

BOOKS BY THE SAME AUTHOR

1. Advanced Public Administration
2. Public Administration: Theory and Practice
3. Public Financial Administration
4. Public Health Policy and Administration
5. Public Personnel Administration: Theory and Practice
6. Administration and Management of NGOs: Text and Case Studies
7. Panchayati Raj in India: Theory and Practice
8. Urban Development and Management
9. Management Techniques: Principles and Practices
10. Encyclopaedia of Disaster Management (Set in 3 Vols.)
11. Management of Hospitals: Hospital Administration in the 21st Century (Set in 4 Vols.)
12. Hospital Core Services
13. Hospital Managerial Services
14. Hospital Preventive and Promotive Services
15. Hospital Supportive Services
16. Health Care System and Management (Set in 4 Vols.)
17. Health Care Management and Administration
18. Primary Health Care Management
19. Health Care Organisation and Structure
20. Health Care, Policies and Programmes
21. Nursing Services: Management and Administration
22. Distance Education in 21st Century
23. Encyclopaedia of Higher Education in 21st Century
24. Human Values and Education
25. Stress Management
26. Population Policy and Family Welfare Administration
27. International Administration
28. International Civil Service : Principles, Practice and Prospects
29. Social Welfare Administration (2 Volumes)
30. Family Planning Programme and Beyond
31. Education Policy and Administration
32. Human Resource Development in 21st Century
33. Disaster Management
34. Slum Improvement through Participatory Urban Based Community Structures
35. Development Planning and Administration
36. Public Health Administration
37. Hospital Administration: Theory and Practice
38. Principles, Problems and Prospects of Co-operative Administration
39. Personnel Administration in Co-operatives
40. Public Personnel Administration and Management
41. Right to Information and Good Governance
42. Health Education: Theory and Practice
43. School Health Education
44. Good Governance: An Integral Approach
45. Disaster Administration and Management

IN PRESS

46. Education of Lifestyle and Lifetime Diseases
47. Health Education of Communicable and Non-Communicable Disease
48. Health Education Administration : From International Level to Village Level
49. Education for Healthy Urban Cities
50. Environment and Value Education
51. Women Health Education
52. Rural Health Education

RURAL HEALTH EDUCATION

DR. S.L. GOEL
Editor, The Indian Journal of Public Administration, New Delhi
Former Vice-President, Executive Council,
Indian Institute of Public Administration, New Delhi
Professor of Public Administration (Retd.)
Panjab University, Chandigarh
Emeritus Fellow, University Grants Commission
Director, State Bank of India (Local Board), Chandigarh
Director, National Horticulture Board, Ministry of Horticulture,
Government of India, New Delhi
Formerly Member UGC, Member Distance Education Council
and Member All India Board of Management, AICTE

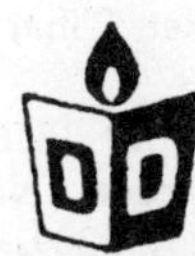

DEEP & DEEP PUBLICATIONS PVT. LTD.
F-159, Rajouri Garden, New Delhi-110027

RURAL HEALTH EDUCATION

ISBN 978-81-8450-115-5

Typeset by S.S. COMPOSERS,
3190, Mohindra Park, Shakur Basti, Delhi-110034.

Printed in India at MAYUR ENTERPRISES,
WZ Plot No. 3, Gujjar Market, Tihar Village, New Delhi-110018.

Published by DEEP & DEEP PUBLICATIONS PVT. LTD.,
F-159, Rajouri Garden, New Delhi-110027.
Phones: 25435369, 25440916
E-mail: ddpbooks@yahoo.co.in • ddpubs@gmail.com
Showroom:
2/13, Ansari Road, Daryaganj, New Delhi-110002 • Telefax: 23245122

Contents

Preface

"Just as the whole universe is contained in the self, so is India contained in the villages."

—*Mahatma Gandhi*

People in rural areas generally remain unhealthy inspite of the fact that nature has provided them with good facilities—pure air, natural environment and good life style. However because of their poverty and lack of general education and especially health education they are prone to many diseases for which they rush to health facilities in the cities. Health education in the rural areas can do miracles if the people in rural areas understand that their health is in their hands and their own responsibility. For this, they have to make their village or area healthy which include—

(a) Removal of poverty through a large number of anti-poverty alleviation programmes. In these programmes, the villagers through their panchayati raj system must participate. Poverty is responsible for most of the problems in the villages.
(b) Health education about the knowledge of health infrastructure so that they can utilize health services provided for them.
(c) Health education for the use of potable drinking water supply as large number of diseases emerge from polluted water.
(d) Education for sanitation of the house and the village which would take care of the health of the people.
(e) The villagers must participate in all the programmes of making their villages healthy so that they understand their responsibility.
(f) Education for making the village beautiful through plantation, cleaning and meeting which would have positive impact on their health.
(g) Ensuring the sustainable development of their village through conservation of resources.
(h) Provide health education about infectious diseases so that timely action is taken.

Health and education are the most important factors influencing the overall quality of life enjoyed by the people in an area, region or country.

The mere presence of natural resources doesn't guarantee riches for an area, unless the human element steps in with technology, innovation and enterprise. Therefore, more and more resources need to be invested in social infrastructure rather than economic infrastructure, for ensuring long-term sustainable development.

In the light of 73rd and 74th Amendment to the constitution, wherein the local self-governments have been institutionalized in rural and urban areas respectively, the prospects of the successful Community Healthcare have substantially brightened. It is envisaged that the locally elected representatives would have a better understanding of the problems and felt needs of the people. With adequate administrative and financial decentralization of powers and resources from the State to the local bodies, the promotion of health could be invigorated. It would be easier to evoke people participation in the administration of health, which can make the entire process, sustainable and rewarding.

The Health development is the process of continuous progressive improvement of the health status of the population. Its outcome is the rising level of human well-being, not only by reduction in the burden of the disease but also by the attainment of positive, physical and mental health related to satisfactory economic functioning and social integration. Health is both an input and output and is linked with development. Inspite of this realization, the people, especially those in rural areas, are not getting facilities of modern medicine. The state of hopelessness and frustration among people is not because of lack of professional knowledge or competence, but due to poor administration of health services."

Based on the recommendations of expert committees, Alma Ata Declaration and the National Health Policy, a Primary Healthcare system was developed and diversified to make health services accessible and available to people near their living places. As a result of these developments, by March 2001, there were established 1,37,311 sub-centres, 22,842 PHCs and 3043 CHCs in the country. However, these institutions of Primary Healthcare are not being utilized by the people as anticipated. This is also evident from the fact that the improvement in health status has not been commensurate with the expansion of health services infrastructure and functions. The population growth rate continues to be high, morbidity rates for women and children are distressingly high, nutritional status is low, infant mortality rate is high, communicable diseases and non-communicable diseases are still to be controlled, negligible population have access to safe-drinking water and basic sanitation facilities. Further, diseases like blindness, leprosy, TB, diarrhoea, etc. continue to have high incidence, lowering the health status of the people.

We must empower the community to plan and execute the health programmes in their areas as per local needs, aspirations and socio-cultural practices. Health committees at sub-centre, PHC, CHC levels can be set-up. Government must understand that concretization of the people and their active participation in the development process, on one hand, and asserting their rights, on the other, does not weaken the authority of the State but is the symptom of true and mature democracy. A partnership between government and community will foster a participatory relationship to encourage more effective programme implementation and facilitate local problem solving, thus becoming more sustainable in the process and promote self-reliance. The failure of community health efforts can be attributed to inadequate matching of the perceptions of health needs and priorities between the local people and the health services staff, as a result of inadequate communication and the lack of a continuing dialogue.

The structure of the Primary Healthcare Services provided by the government is impressive. However, the government has not been able to provide and maintain critical infrastructure, adequate resources in terms of manpower, finances and equipment, a sound administrative set-up, accountability and responsiveness of the system and commitment of the Health Department. This half-hearted approach fails to satisfy the people and cannot provide job satisfaction to the providers of Community Healthcare. All these problems also emanate from the fact that Government has been rapidly expanding the number of health institutions without focusing on improving the Physical facilities in the existing institutions. There is a need to consolidate existing infrastructure to ensure proper facilities in the existing institutions.

The functioning of Rural Healthcare System is not doing well. Even the Ninth Five Year Plan (1997-2002) has admitted it and enlisted a number of factors responsible for inefficient functioning:

1. Persistent gaps in manpower and infrastructure especially at the primary healthcare level.
2. Sub-optimal functioning of the infrastructure; poor referral services.
3. Plethora of hospitals not having appropriate manpower, diagnostic and therapeutic services and drugs, in Government voluntary and private sector.
4. Massive interstate/interdistrict differences in performance as assessed by health and demography indices; availability and utilisation of services are poorest in the most needy states/districts.
5. Sub-optimal intersectoral coordination.
6. Increasing dual disease burden of communicable and non-communicable diseases because of ongoing demographic, lifestyle and environmental transitions.
7. Technological advances which widen the spectrum of possible interventions.
8. Increasing awareness and expectations of the population regarding healthcare services.
9. Escalating costs of healthcare, ever widening gaps between what is possible and what the individual or the country can afford.

At the time of Independence, Healthcare Services were mainly urban-centered and hospital-based. Realising the importance of creating a functional Primary Healthcare infrastructure, national norms for the primary healthcare infrastructure were drawn up. These take into account the population, population density and terrain. At the national level the total number of functional Sub-Centres and the PHCs nearly meets the set norms. However, there are marked disparities at the State and District level. It is a matter of concern that many of the districts with poor health indices do not have adequate health infrastructure. There is considerable backlog in terms of construction of the buildings for sub-centres and PHCs. Some States have adopted innovative measures including mobilisation of local resources to clear this backlog. Taking cognizance of the widening disparities among the States in the availability of Basic Minimum Service (BMS), the Conference of the Chief Ministers in July 1996, recommended that Additional Central Assistance (ACA) may be provided to the states for correcting the existing gaps in the provision of seven Basic Minimum Services (BMS). The modalities of implementation of the programme are discussed in detail in the section on Basic Minimum Services. Of these, access to primary healthcare, safe drinking water and primary education were given higher priority with the mandate that universal access to these services is to be achieved by 2000 A.D. There is an urgent need to encourage involvement of the people's representatives, voluntary organisations and the people themselves in these activities.

The term "primary" has acquired a variety of connotations, some of them technical (referring to the first contact with the health system, or the first level of care, or simple treatments that could be delivered by relatively untrained providers, or interventions acting on primary causes of disease) and some political (depending on multi-sectoral implications for policy) help explain why there is no one model of primary care, and why it has been difficult to follow the successful examples of the countries or states that provided the first evidence that a substantial improvement in health could be achieved at affordable cost. There was a substantial effort in many countries to train and use community health workers who could deliver basic, cost-effective services in simple rural facilities to populations that previously had little or no access to modern care. In India, for example, such workers were trained and placed in over 1,000,000 health posts, intended to serve nearly two-thirds of the population.

Despite these efforts, many such programmes were eventually considered at least partial failures. Funding was inadequate, the workers had little time to spend on prevention and community out-reach; their training and equipment were insufficient for the problems they confronted; and quality of care was often so poor as to be characterised as "primitive" rather than "primary", particularly when primary care was limited to the poor and to only the simplest services. Referral systems, which are unique to health services and necessary to their proper performance, have proved particularly difficult to operate adequately. Lower level services were often poorly utilized, and patients who could do so commonly bypassed the lower levels of the system to go directly to hospitals. Partly in consequence, countries continued to invest in tertiary, urban-based centres.

We must attend to all the areas which can make our village healthy, vibrant, happy and equal partners.

In this volume "Rural Health Education" we have attempted to make rural India healthy through Health Education Inter-sectoral, Co-ordination, People's Participation, etc. We are sure that this would be useful to all concerned with rural India.

S.L. GOEL

Note: In this volume we are using Rural Health Services and Primary Healthcare as one and the same.

CHAPTER I

HEALTH EDUCATION AND RURAL HEALTH INFRASTRUCTURE

> Health is Wealth
> Health is not only basic to lead a happy life for an individual but also necessary for all productive activities in the Society.
>
> —*Author*

Health Education and Rural Health Infrastructure

SIGNIFICANCE OF HEALTH

Health is the topmost priority in every individual's life. Its importance is evident in old saying, "Health is Wealth." Health is not only basic to lead a happy life for an individual, but also necessary for all productive activities in the society. The whole development cycle of a person depends upon his intellectual caliber, curiosity and constructive thinking, but all these qualities depend upon his good health. Therefore, to meet this very important need of the healthy citizens of a healthy society, health services are *sine-qua-non* for the Government.

Phisek Ponrattana Wanarom, in his Article "Health is Development", rightly says: "Good health is a prerequisite to human productivity and the development process." It is essential to economic and technological development. A healthy community is the infrastructure upon which to build an economically viable society. The progress of society greatly depends on the quality of its people. Unhealthy people can hardly be expected to make any valid contribution towards developmental programmes. Health is man's greatest possession, for it lays a solid foundation for his happiness."[1] Charaka, the renowned Ayurvedic Physician, is known to have said: "Health is vital for ethical, artistic, material and spiritual development of man."[2] Ramesh Kanbargi, in his Article, "Health and Development in India: Trends and Prospects", has rightly said that one of the basic objectives of the national and international initiatives in health sector is the conviction based on the experience of several decades that good health of a population promotes economic and social development.[3]

"Health is a function of the overall integrated development of the society and the health status is one of the indicators of the quality of life."[4]

Buddha has said that, of all the gains, the gains of health are the highest and the best. Health is not only basic to leading a happy life for an individual but it is also necessary for all productive activities in the society. Who would deny that a soldier who is not keeping good health cannot be expected to defend the frontiers of his country, even when he is provided with the latest sophisticated weapons? Similarly, who would deny that unhealthy farmer with the best possible technological know-how, would not succeed in producing the best that can be expected of him? Obviously, what is true of an unhealthy soldier or an unhealthy farmer, is also true of other categories of workers. Thus, no industry can expect the optimum output, if it does not employ healthy workers or does not make and provide adequate facilities for proper maintenance of their health. Undoubtedly, professional efficiency, good health and productivity are interrelated. Yet, health cannot be bestowed upon people if they themselves do not make any effort to maintain a proper balance between their external and internal environments.

K.S. Dodzie, United Nations Director-General for Development and International Economic Co-operation has rightly said: "The promotion and protection of the health of the people is essential to sustained economic and social development and contributes to a better quality of life and to world peace."[5]

Dr. E.J. Thiersy, in his article, "laying the Foundations", succinctly remarked that, "Health is man's most precious possession; it influences all his activities, it shapes the destinies of people. Without it, there can be no solid Introduction 3 foundation for man's happiness. Nevertheless, all too often, social planners, forget this simple truth and leave health out of account. Integration of health schemes in overall development plans are of paramount importance."[6]

It has been accepted by the World Health Assembly that good health is a fundamental human right. World Health Organisation defines health as "a state of complete physical, mental, social and spiritual well-being and not merely the absence of disease or physical infirmity." This is a holistic concept of health. As stated in the First Five Year Plan, "Health is a state of positive well-being in which harmonious development of mental and physical capacities of the individuals leads to the enjoyment of a rich and full life. It implies adjustment of the individual to his total environment—Physical and Social."[7]

The Health development is the process of continuous progressive improvement of the health status of the population. Its product is rising level of human well-being not only by reduction in the burden of the disease but also by the attainment of positive, physical and mental health related to satisfactory economic functioning and social integration.[8]

P. Durgaprasad and N.V. Madhuri in their article, "Partnership and Networking for Health Development" in *Kuruksehtra Journals*, Jan. 2004 clearly mention that towards rural society, the breaking of the vicious cycle of malnutrition and ill-health necessitates formulation of a set of distinct but mutually related strategies to combat the inextricably linked socio-political and economic factors and cause ill-health, and adversely affect the livelihood. Therefore, critical public policy-making and strategic programming, cast in partnership and network mode, can alone bring about overall health development of communities and individuals. The bottom line of all prosperity and health in future should be a development process and outcome that is essentially facilitated by development partnerships and networks, which nurture as well as further the goals of health and human development with focus on 'putting health into the hands of the people'.

The 'dependency syndrome' generated essentially by the governments and some NGOs and inefficient and ineffective investments of public health programme has been the root cause of getting the health development priorities wrong in the last five decades of planned development. While capital investment, in health development are important, people's knowledge and indigenous skills have not been regarded as a major source that people possess. It is this knowledge and inherent skill of people, what needs to be made a basis of the new paradigm shift.

While the major strengths of partnerships and networking include groups action for individual and community benefits, democratization of knowledge, demystification of technology, horizontal networking, transparency, accountability and sustainability among others, the weaknesses may arise from inadequacies in Human Resource Development, politicization and negative assertions. However, the opportunities that the partnerships and networking endeavours promise in terms of group action, consolidation, carrying the 'instruments of change' with the 'groups at stake', capacity building, achievement orientation and empowerment, should outweigh the anticipated threats, and dilute the weaknesses. The bottom line of all (health) development endeavours should be 'putting the instruments of (health) development into the hands of the people and their organizations.'

Jatanthi Paulraj in his article, "Nutrition for All" in *Yojna,* Sept. 2004, signifies the role of nutrition for all community:

- The Nutrition Policy recognizes that "nutrition affects development as much as development affects nutrition." The principal challenge of the future would be to put in place an effective sustainable approach that is capable of fostering a healthy childhood.
- Vigorous awareness campaigns on malnutrition to make nutrition a talking point in the villages; direct interventions in districts with high malnutrition particularly for 0-2 years old, adolescent girls, pregnant and lactating mothers and establishing nutrition surveillance in the states in a phased manner are the three major components of the proposed Nutrition Mission.
- A balanced diet should have a proportionate amount of

proteins, fats, carbohydrates, minerals, salts, water, vitamins and non-digestible 'roughage'.

- The adoption of National Nutrition Policy (NNP) by the Government under the aegis of the Deptt. of Women and Child Development in 1993 has been one of the significant achievements on the nutrition scene in the country. The Nutrition Policy recognized that "Nutrition affects development as much as development effects nutrition." Integration of nutritional concerns in various developmental policies and programmes was recognized as an important food tool for maximizing the nutritional outcome of developmental measures. The Policy advocates a series of actions in different spheres like food production, food distribution, education, health and family welfare, people with special needs and nutritional surveillance. The direct and indirect instruments of nutrition policy were recommended to be institutionalized through inter-sectoral co-ordination mechanism between Centre and the States.

NATURE OF RURAL HEALTHCARE (PRIMARY HEALTH CENTRE)

The WHO has defined Primary Healthcare as "essential healthcare made universally accessible to individuals and families in the community by means acceptable to them through their full participation and at a cost that the community and country can afford. It forms an integral part of both the country's health system of which it is the nucleus and of the overall social and economic development of the community."[9]

The first International Conference of Primary Healthcare defined it as "essential healthcare based on scientifically sound and socially acceptable methods and technology, made universally acceptable to individuals and families in the community through their full participation and at a cost that the community and country can afford to maintain at every stage of their development in a spirit of self-reliance and self-determination."[10] There are many different ways of defining primary healthcare. The 29th World Health Assembly accepted the working definition of primary healthcare. According to this definition, primary healthcare is taken to mean. A health approach which integrates at the community level all the elements necessary to make an impact upon the state of health of the people. Such an approach should be an integral part of the national healthcare system. It is an expression or response to the fundamental human needs of how a person can know of and be assisted in the actions required to live a healthy life and where a person can go if he or she gets no relief from pain or suffering. A response to such needs must be a series of simple and effective measures in terms of cost, technique and organisation which are easily accessible to the people in need and which assist in improving the living conditions of individuals, families and communities. These include preventive, promotive, curative and rehabilitative health measures and community development.[11]

RATIONALE AND BASIS OF RURAL HEALTHCARE AND HEALTH EDUCATION

(i) Union and State Governments

Government of India has shown its concern for Public Health, both during Britsih and in-post-independence era. The health of the nation (British India), reviewed by Bhore Committee, under the Chairmanship of Sir Joseph Bhore (GOI, 1946), observed that no individual shall fail to secure adequate medical care because of inability to pay for it. After independence, a number of research studies were carried out to meet the growing challenges of public health under the Welfare State. Prominent among the specialized studies are the reports of Health Survey and Planning Committee-Chairman Laxman Swami Mudaliar (GOI, 1962), Group of Medical Education and Support Manpower—Chairman, J.B. Srivastava (GOI, 1975), Five Year Plan documents, Central Council of health reports, etc. The relevant plan documents have also indicated emerging issues and reviews of the prevailing health system in the Union and State Governments.

In the twilight period between the Sixth and Seventh Plan, it was realised that the country had no health policy. This shortcoming was removed by the approval of Health Policy by the Rajya Sabha on August 4, 1983 and the Lok Sabha on December 22, 1983, which reflected philosophy, approach, strategies and targets to achieve the objectives of Alma-Ata Declaration-Health For All by 2000 AD. Since the genesis, evolution, growth and diversification of Primary Healthcare System in India is the outcome of these expert committees, it would be quite useful and fruitful to analyse the recommendations of these committees.

I. Bhore Committee (1943-46)

Taking into consideration the findings of interim report of National Planning Committee on Health (1940) and being dissatisfied with the then healthcare system in meeting the health problems of the community, particularly of rural population, in 1943, the then British Government appointed the "Health Survey and Development Committee" with Sir Joseph Bhore as Chairman, to make a survey of the existing health conditions and health organisations and to make recommendations for future development.

The recommendations and guidance provided by the Bhore Committee formed the basis for organisation of Basic Health Services in India. The report was submitted to Government in 1946.

The Bhore Committee made two types of recommendations:

(a) A comprehensive blue print for the distant future (20 to 40 years)—the smallest service unit was to be Primary Health Unit, serving a population of 10,000 to 20,000; and
(b) A short-term scheme covering 2 to 5 years period—the emphasis

would be on setting up 30 bedded hospitals, one for every two Primary Health Units.

The country-side was the focal point of these recommendations. Other recommendations were:

(i) Formation of Village Health Committee to secure active cooperation and support in the development of health programme.
(ii) Provision for Doctor of future who should be a "Social Doctor" combining both curative and preventive measures.
(iii) Formation of a District Health Board for each district comprising of district health officials and representatives of the public.
(iv) To ensure suitable housing, sanitary surroundings, safe drinking water supply, elimination of unemployment and to IAY special emphasis on preventive work.
(v) Intersectoral approach to health services development.

II. Mudaliar Committee (1959-61)

The Government of India, in the Ministry of Health, set-up a Committee on the 12th June, 1959, under the Chairmanship of Dr. A. Lakshmanswami Mudaliar.

Detailed recommendations on these aspects were submitted in 1961. Their salient features were:

(a) Upgrading and strengthening of PHUs.
(b) Strengthening of District Hospitals.
(c) Mobile Service teams for Rural Areas.
(d) Levying of small fee for availing hospital facilities.
(e) Long range health insurance policy for all citizens.
(f) Formation of Central Health Cadre.
(g) Extension of the functions of the University Grants Commission to education in the fields of the Medicine, Engineering, Agriculture and Veterinary Sciences.
(h) Institution of National Programmes for eradication of Malaria, Small Pox, Cholera, Leprosy, Tuberculosis and Filariasis.
(i) Making the Central Council of Health more effective.
(j) Director General of Health Services should enjoy the Status of an Additional Secretary.

III. Chadha Committee (1963)

In April 1963, a special Committee was constituted by the Government of India under the Chairmanship of Director General of Health Services, Dr. M.S. Chadha, to go into the details of the requirements of primary health centres, their planning, the necessary priority required according to the 'needs of the maintenance phase of Malaria Eradication

Programme' and also for other health activities and the manner in which the technical and supervisory staff of the NMEP organisation should be utilised after malaria eradication has been achieved. The committee considered that the maintenance was the responsibility of the general health services, which should be adequately strengthened, particularly the rural health services. Vigilance through medical institutions (government or non-government) must be developed. Multi--purpose domiciliary health services should be developed for all health programmes, including malaria, small-pox, control of other communicable diseases, health education, etc.

IV. Mukherjee Committee (1966)

The Central Council of Health, at its meeting on the 31st December 1965, in Madras, appointed a Committee under the Chairmanship of Union Health Secretary to undertake the review of Family Planning Programme and its strategy. The Committee recommended strengthening of the administrative set-up at all levels from the Primary Health Units to the State Headquarters. It also recommended delinking of malaria maintenance activities from Family Planning Programme, so that the latter could receive undivided attention of its staff and could be carried through as a crash mass programme.

V. Singh Committee (1972-73)

In pursuance of the recommendations made by the Executive Committee of the Central Family Planning Council, the Government of India constituted a committee in October 1972, which recommended that:

(a) Multi-purpose workers for the delivery of health, family planning and nutrition services to the rural communities are both feasible and desirable.
(b) To begin with, one Male Health Worker (Multi-purpose) should be available for a population of six to seven thousands.
(c) Atleast one Female Health Worker (ANM) should be available for a population of ten to twelve thousands.
(d) Each PHC should ultimately serve 50,000 population and should have 16 sub-centres spread over its area.
(e) Training for all workers engaged in the field of health, family planning and nutrition should be integrated.

VI. Shrivastava Committee (1974-75)

The Government of India, in 1974, formed a Committee on 'Medical Education and Support Manpower' under the Chairmanship of Dr. J.B. Srivastava. The Committee submitted its detailed report in 1975 and made specific recommendations for the initiation of the following major programmes for immediate action:

(a) Organisation of the basic health services (including nutrition, health education and family planning) within the community itself and training the personnel needed for the purpose.

(b) Organisation of an economic and efficient programme or health services to bridge the community with the first level referral centre, viz., the PHC (including the strengthening of the PHC itself).

(c) The creation of a National Referral Services Complex by the development of proper linkages between the PHC and higher level referral and service centres.

(d) To create the necessary administrative and financial machinery for the re-organisation of the entire programme of medical and health education from the point of view of the objectives and needs of the proposed programme of national health services.

VII. National Health Policy Document (1983)

The major directions laid down in the Seventh National Health Policy Document (1983) are:

- Provision of universal and comprehensive primary healthcare services with special emphasis on the preventive, promotive and rehabilitative aspects.
- Securing small family norms through efforts and moving towards the goal of population stabilisation and enunciation of a national population policy.
- To formulate a National Medical and Health Education Policy for health manpower development and to ensure that personnel at all levels are socially motivated to adopt community health approach.
- To decentralise the primary healthcare system by restructuring the healthcare services to promote community participation and linking it with a systematic back up support of referral services at secondary and tertiary levels.
- Integrally linking the health education and extension activities with primary healthcare services.
- Transferring simple healthcare knowledge, skills and appropriate technology to community, so that majority of common health actions could be handled effectively by the community.
- Mobilizing untapped health resources and encouraging investment by private sector, NCOs, and voluntary bodies to establish curative services, wherein all affluent sectors could be looked after by paying for the services.
- To remove the existing regional imbalances and to provide services within the reach of all, whether residing in the rural or the urban areas.
- Assist in the enlargement of the services being provided by private voluntary organisations active in the health field, specially those which seek to serve the needs of the rural areas and the urban slums.

- The entire approach to health manpower development should ensure their functioning as a "Health Team."
- To integrate the services of ISM practitioners at the appropriate levels, within specified areas of responsibility and functioning in the over-all healthcare delivery system, specially with regard to the preventive, promotive and public healthcare aspects.

VIII. National Health Policy, 2002

The main objective of the policy is to achieve an acceptable standard of good health amongst the general population of the country and increase access to the decentralized public health system by establishing new infrastructure in deficient areas, and by upgrading the infrastructure in the existing institutions. Salient features of the policy are as follows:

(i) Increase health sector expenditure to 6 per cent of COP with 2 per cent of COP being contributed as public health investment by the year 2010.

(ii) Increased allocation of 55 per cent of the total public health investment for the primary health sector; the secondary and tertiary health sectors being targeted for 35 per cent and 19 per cent respectively.

(iii) Key role for the Central Government in designing national programmes with the active participation of the State Governments. The Policy ensures the provisioning of financial resources in addition to technical support, monitoring and evaluation at the national level by the Centre.

(iv) Apart from the exclusive staff in a vertical structure for the disease control programmes, all rural health staff would be available for the entire gamut of public health activities at the decentralized level.

(v) Revival of the Primary Health System by providing some essential drugs under Central Government funding through the decentralized health system. Provisioning of essential drugs at the public health service centre would create a demand for other professional services also from the local population.

(vi) More frequent in service training of public health medical personnel at the level of medical officers as well as paramedics.

(vii) Expand the pool of medical practitioners to include a cadre of licentiates of medical practice, as also practitioners of Indian systems of Medicine and Homoeopathy.

(viii) Implementation of public health programmes through local self-government institutions and decentralize the implementation of the programmes to such institutions by 2005.

(ix) Minimal statutory norms for the deployment of doctors and nurses in medical institutions.

(x) Setting up of a Medical Grants Commission for funding new

Government Medical and Dental Colleges in different parts of the country.

(xi) Modify the existing curriculum.

(xii) Enable fresh graduates to contribute effectively to the providing of primary health services as the physician of first contact.

(xiii) Raise the proportion of post-graduate seats in public health and family medicine discipline in medical training institutions to 114th of the earmarked seats.

(xiv) Improvement in the ratio of nurses *vis-a-vis* doctors/beds.

(xv) Improving the skill-level of nurses and increasing the ratio of degree holding nurses *vis-a-vis* diploma holding nurses.

(xvi) Need for basing treatment regimens, in both the public and private domain on a limited number of essential drugs of a generic nature.

(xvii) At least 50% of the requirement of vaccines/sera to be sourced from public sector institutions to ensure uninterrupted supply of vaccines at an affordable price.

(xviii) Setting up of an organized urban primary healthcare structure.

(xix) Funding for the urban primary health system to be jointly borne by the local self-government institutions and State and Central Governments.

(xx) Established of fully-equipped 'hub-spoke' trauma care networks in large urban agglomerations to reduce accident mortality.

(xxi) Inter-personal communication of information and folk and other traditional media to bring about behavioural change.

(xxii) Association of PRIs/NGOs/Trusts in IEC activities.

(xxiii) Increase in government-funded health research to a level of per cent of the total health spending by 2005; and thereafter, up to 2 per cent by 2010.

(xxiv) Enactment of suitable legislation for regulating minimum infrastructure and quality standards in clinical establishments/ medical institutions by 2003.

(xxv) Encourage setting up of private insurance instruments for increasing the scope of the coverage of the secondary and tertiary sector under private health insurance packages.

(xxvi) Disease control programmes should earmark at least 10% of the budget in respect of identified programme components, to be exclusively implemented through NGOs.

Rural Healthcare Infrastructure

The entire Health and Family Welfare Programme in rural areas is being implemented through Primary Healthcare System. The Primary Healthcare Infrastructure has been developed as a three-tier system and is based on the following population norms:

Rural Healthcare System in India

CHC
A 30 bed Hospital/Referral Unit for 4 PHCs with Specialised Services

↓

PHC
A Referral Unit for 6 Sub-Centres
4-6 bed manned with a Medical Officer In-charge and 14 subordinate paramedical staff

↓

SUB-CENTRE
Most peripheral contact point between Primary Health Care System and Community manned with one MPW(F)/ANM and One MPW(M)

Community Health Centre

WHO defines Community Health Centre as the Reference Health Centre. "The reference health centre differs from the generic health centre in that it is a functional concept that can be realized by strengthening one or more health centres to improve referral within the health system in rural areas. Thus, in addition to its generic health centre functions, it provides essential surgical, maternity and medical care, as well as carrying out preventive and promotive activities in the neighbourhood it serves. The reference health centre lightens the burden of the first-referral hospital by taking over certain routine interventions, at the same time bringing appropriate care closer to the population at only a fraction of the cost of similar operations performed in local hospitals. Health centres, including reference health centres and hospitals, are components of a healthcare system, each playing a different but complementary role.[12]

In Karnataka, there were 252 Community Health Centres by the end of March 1999. A Community Health Centre is established for a population of about one lakh. Out of four Primary Health Centres, one community health centre has been created with 30 beds in rural areas and 50 beds at taluk level to serve as referral hospital for the rural population. The purpose is to provide second tier referral services near their place and with better facilities, so that their unnecessary approaching district hospitals may be avoided to save cost and provide better services to the rural population. Facilities required for 30 bedded/80 bedded hospitals have been provided in the Primary Health Centres upgraded in terms of infrastructure, personnel, equipment, etc., so that these institutions can handle cases coming to them directly or referred from Primary Health Centres.

These centres offer considerable advantages to both patients and society. From the point of view of society, hospitalization both protects the

Centre	Population Norms	
	Plain Area	Hilly/Tribal/ Difficult Desert Areas
Sub-centre	5000	3000
PHC	30000	30000
CHC	120000	80000

family from many of the disruptive effects of caring for the ill in the home and operates as a means of guiding the sick and injured in medically supervised institutions, where their problems are less disruptive for society as a whole.[13] To quote Perry, the success with which a hospital contributes towards meeting the patients needs can be measured by the fullness of the life he is able to lead on leaving it."[14]

A comprehensive definition of Hospital has been given by WHO. Hospital is an integral part of a social and medical organization, the function of which is to provide for the population complete healthcare—both curative and preventive and whose out-patients services reach out to the family and its home environment; the hospital is also a centre for training of health workers and for bio-social research.[15]

CHCs are being established and maintained by the State Government under MNP/BMS. It is manned by four medical specialists, i.e. Surgeon, Physician, Gynaecologist and Paediatrician supported by 21 paramedical and other staff. It has 30 in-door beds with one OT, X-Ray, Labour Room and Laboratory facilities. It serves as a referral centre for 4 PHCs. There are 3043 CHCs functioning in the country. Under RCH Programme, CHCs are entitled to hire services of private anaesthetists for conducting emergency operations. To promote institutional deliveries, provision has been made under the current RCH Programme to give additional honorarium to the staff to encourage round the clock delivery services at PHCs and CHCs.

Primary Health Centres

Rationale and Philosophy

WHO has defined the health centre as that which covers all health facilities other than hospitals. It is usually the facility at the first contact level and has a unique potential, as well as responsibility, for increasing people's ability to solve their own problems with confidence. It provides a full range of health promotion and preventive services, as well as curative care limited mainly to ambulatory patients. It has multi-disciplinary team capabale of providing the range of services mentioned above.[16]

The concept of the PHC as an institution to provide both curative and preventive services can be traced to the report of the consultative council on Medical and Allied Services, held in 1920, in England, under the chairmanship of Lord Dawson of Penn. In this region, the PHC was

CHART I

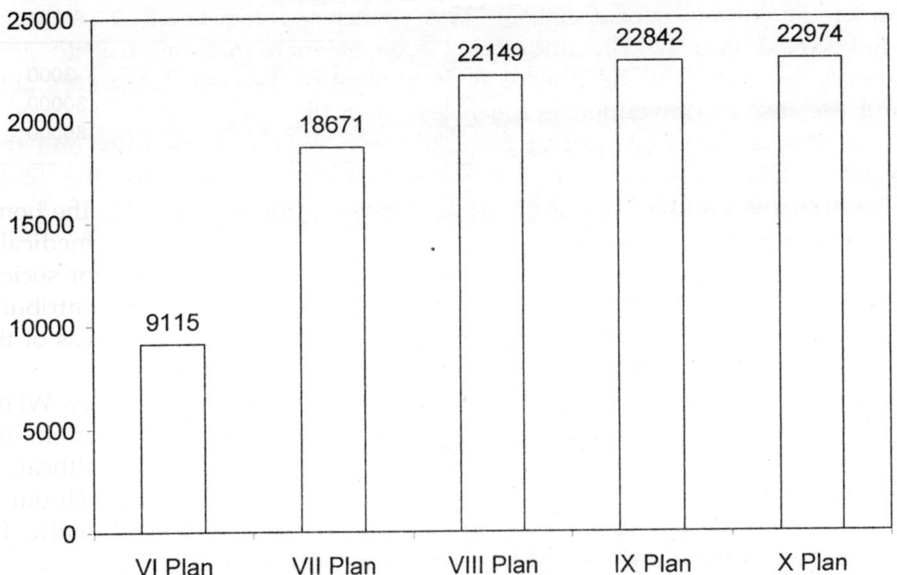

established at Kalutura, Ceylon, in 1926 with the assistance of Rockefeller Foundation.[17] Provision of Rural Health Services through Rural Health Centres was recommended by the European Conference on Rural Hygiene of Geneva, in 1931 under the Health Organisation of League of Nations. It defined the "Rural Health Centres" as:

"An institution for the promotion of the health and welfare of the people in a given (rural) area, which seeks to achieve its purpose by grouping under one roof or coordinating in some other manner, under the direction of a health officer, all the health work of that area, together with such welfare and relief organizations as may be related to the general public health work."[18]

A working group on the role and functions of Health Centres in District Health System met in Geneva from 12 to 16 July 1993 with participants from Dominica, Indonesia, Nigeria, Philippines and Senegal, who defined the concept as "The Generic Health Centre is a self-contained segment of the national health system guided by the district health service, of which it is a part. It comprises a variety of inter-related components that contribute to health in homes, schools, work-places and the community, including support for self-care administered at home. These components are supported by a professional staff, together with appropriate diagnostic, laboratory and logistical services and co-ordinated in a dedicated management structure."[19]

The concept gathered momentum in socialist countries. The inter-governmental Conference for Eastern countries, convened at Bandung under the auspices of League of Nations, recommended the integration of preventive and curative services in preference to curative services. Similar developments took place in Eastern European countries that have come under the influence of socialism. This concept spread to other countries after World War II. The underlying idea of such thinking was to give priority to preventive healthcare as 75 percent of diseases are preventable and the cost of prevention is much less than the cost for curative care.

PHC is the first contact point between village community and the Medical Officer. These are established and maintained by the State Governments under the Minimum Needs Programme (MNP)/Basic Minimum Services Programme.[20]

A PHC is manned by a Medical Officer supported by 14 paramedical and other staff. It acts as a referral unit for 6 Sub-centres. It has 4-6 beds for patients. The activities of PHC involve curative, preventive, promotive and Family Welfare Services. There are 22,842 PHCs are functioning in the country. Appointment of PHN/Staff Nurse on contract basis in PHCs of selected districts is being done.

Sub-Centres

A sub-centre is established on the basis of one centre for every 5,000 population in plain areas and for 3,000 population in hilly and tribal areas. Till the end of the 7th Plan 1.4.1990, 1,30,336 sub-centres were functioning. Their number rose to 142, 611 by the end of March, 2001.[20]

The MPW scheme aims at providing a package of health services to the rural population at their doorsteps. The main objective of this scheme is to ensure a minimum availability of public health facilities, which include preventive medicine, family welfare, nutrition and curative and referral services. The launching of this scheme marked the merger of the vertical programmes into an integrated health delivery system, thus lending additional strength to the Primary Health Centres. In Karnataka, there were 1676 PHCs and 8143 Sub-Centres till March 1998. As per the norms, each Sub-Centre is required to be manned by a trained Female Health Worker (ANM) and a trained Male Health Worker known as Multi-purpose Worker (Male). There were 9554 multi-purpose workers (Female) and 666 multi-purpose workers (Male) in Karnataka by the end of March 1998. However, there are many sub-centres where only female worker is posted. Such centres need to be staffed by male workers to cope up with the work. 950 posts of female workers and 813 posts of male workers were vacant as on March 1998. The Government of India had initiated a scheme of training and thereby converting the uni-purpose workers under various programmes to multi-purpose workers. However, because of the shortage of MPW's (Male) at Sub-Centre level, a scheme of basic training for MPW (Male) was initiated during the 7th Plan period. Under this scheme, 10th pass candidates are selected and trained for one year, before they are inducted into service.[21]

CHART 2

Growth of Sub-Centres

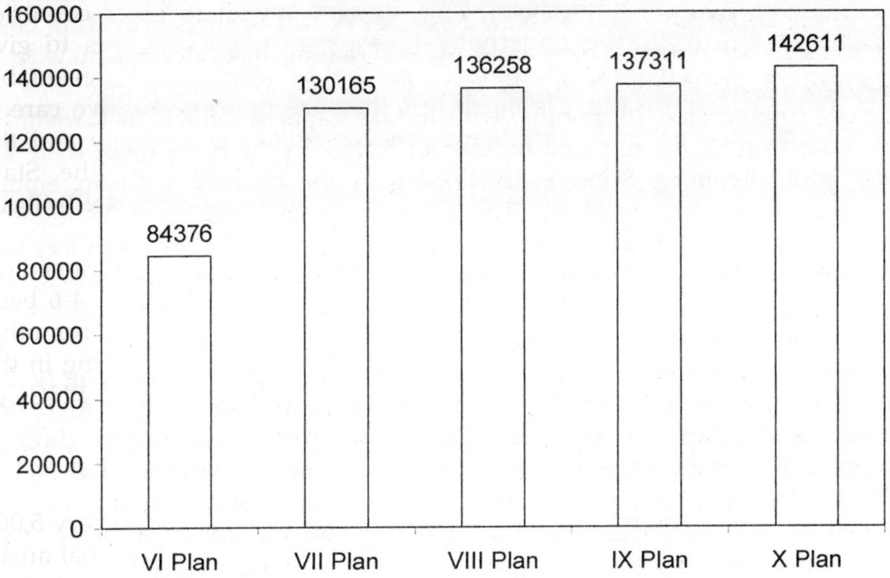

160000
140000
120000
100000
80000
60000
40000
20000
0
84376
130165
136258
137311
142611
VI Plan
VII Plan
VIII Plan
IX Plan
X Plan

The Basic Training of MPW (M) was initiated in 47 Health and Family Welfare Training Centres throughout the country as 100% Centrally Sponsored Scheme. During 7th Plan (1985-90), it was observed that the

CHART 3

Growth of Community Health Centres

3500
3000
2500
2000
1500
1000
500
0
761
1910
2623
3043
3215
VI Plan
VII Plan
VIII Plan
IX Plan
X Plan

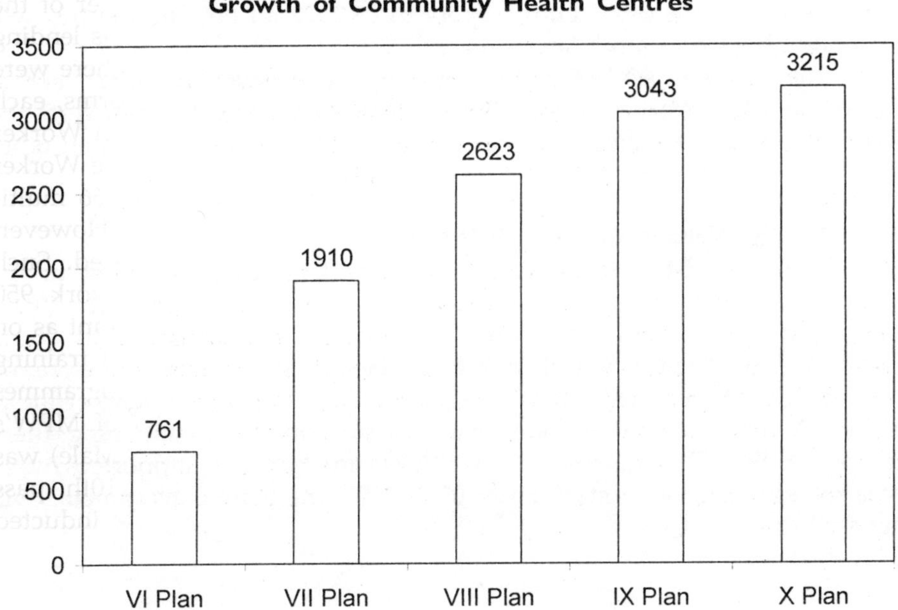

training capacity was not enough to train the required number of MPW (M) in all the Sub-Centres and hence the financial sanction to establish 50 New MPW (M) Basic Schools was given by the Government of India.[21] At present, there are 28 HfWfCs and 37 New Basic MPW (M) Schools providing basic training to MPW (M). There are 4 MPW Training Institutes for male (pre-service, 12 months) with in take capacity of 240, 19 training institutes for female (pre-service, 18 months) with in take capacity of 570, in Karnataka. In order to train the required number of ANMs in the rural areas, there are 464 ANM Training Schools functioning in the country with an annual admission capacity of 20,312. The duration of the training is 18 months. 10th pass girls preferably from the local villages, where their services will be utilised later at the Sub-Centres and Primary Health Centres, are admitted for the basic course. These are utilised for providing continuing education/training programmes for ANMs, besides providing the basic training programme of 18 months duration. The purpose of training is that these workers should develop vision, initiative and desire to achieve the goals of Health for all with dedication and perseverance through professional knowledge and behavioural techniques. Jawahar Lal Nehru has rightly said: "No one can really do first class work without a sense of function, without a measure of a crusading spirit, I am doing this, I have to achieve this as a part of great movement in a big cause."[22]

It is the most peripheral contact point between the Primary Healthcare System and the community. It is manned by one Multi-Purpose Worker (Male) and one M.P.W. (Female)/ANM and one LHV is entrusted with six Sub-Centres. Only 97,757 Sub-Centres are funded by Department of Family Welfare under Centrally Sponsored Scheme, out of a total number of 1,37,311 Sub-Centres functioning in the country. The State Governments fund the rest of the Sub-Centres. From 01.04.2002 all the Sub-Centres will be funded by the Central Government.

The salary of ANM/LHV is borne by Government of India whereas that of the Male Worker is borne by the State Government. Apart from the committed salary funding, the norms revised by the Government on other costs with effect from 07.02.2001 are as under:

Rural Family Welfare Centres (RFWCs)

There are 5435 Rural Family Welfare Centres functioning in the country. These Centres were established at all the block level PHCs sanctioned upto 1 April, 1980. Most of the states have integrated the Rural Family Welfare Centres into their Primary Healthcare System. Therefore, no separate identity for these FRWCs existing today. The Government of India, however, continues to provide financial support for maintaining these centres. A FRWC is manned by one Assistant Surgeon supported by 11 para medical and other staff. From 01.04.2002, the State Governments will fund all the RFWCs.

Items	*Expenditure per annum for the existing Sub-Centres (in rupees)*	
	As per existing norms	*As per revised norms*
Rent	1000	3000
Medicines	2000	To be supplied under RCH programme
Contingency	600	2000
Voluntary Worker	60 (honorarium)	1200 (Honorarium)

TRAINING AND DEVELOPMENT

Village Health Guides (VHG) Scheme

The Village Health Guide Scheme was initially started as Community Health Workers' Scheme on 2nd October, 1977 in all the States except Arunachal Pradesh, J & K, Kerala and Tamil Nadu. The Scheme was renamed as Village Health Guide Scheme in 1981 when it was made 100% centrally sponsored scheme under Family Welfare Programme. At present about 3.23 lakh VHGs are reported to be working. Each VHG is paid an honorarium of Rs. 501 per month. The Scheme has been reviewed by a committee of experts. Its recommendations were examined and a decision has been taken to stop Central Government participation in the Scheme w.e.f. 01.04.2002. The States have been directed to pursue the scheme [present or amended] as per their requirements and out of their own funds, if deemed necessary.

Basic Training of Female Health Workers ANM IMPW (F)

ANMs/LHVs play a vital role in MCH and Family Welfare Service in the rural areas. It is, therefore, essential that the proper training to be given to them so that quality services be provided to the rural population. For this purpose 478 ANM and 42 LHV training schools with an admission capacity of approximately 16445 and 2596 respectively are established in the country. These include training centres run by Voluntary Organisations with their own resources. These training institutions are imparting training to prepare required number of ANMs and LHVs to man the sub-centres, Primary Health Centres, Community Health Centres, Aural Family Welfare Centres and Health posts in the country. The duration of training programme of ANM is one and half years and minimum qualification in this course is 10th pass. Female Health Assistant (LHV) provides supportive supervision and technical guidance to the ANMs in sub-centres. Senior ANM with five years of experience is given six months' promotional training to become LHV/Family Health Assistant. There are 42 LHV Promotional Training Centers in the country.

The financial pattern of assistance has been revised w.e.f. 7.2.2001. Other approved costs besides salary to staff are stipend to trainee, contingency and rent. The stipend has increased from Rs. 125 to 500 per month, the contingency grant from the existing Rs. 5000 to Rs. 10000 per annum and rent admissible from 25000 to Rs. 60000 per annum. The total allocation for this scheme during this financial year is Rs. 60 crores.

Basic Training for Multi-purpose Health Worker (Male)

The basic training of MPW (M) scheme was approved during 6th Five-Year Plan and taken up since 1984, as a 100% centrally sponsored scheme. The training is of one-year duration and on successful completion of the training, the Male Health Worker is posted at the sub-centre along with Health Worker (Female). There are 30 Health and Family Welfare Training Centres and 28 new basic MPW(M) training schools imparting training.

The financial norms for this scheme have been revised w.e.f. 7.2.2001. Under the scheme the salary of the staff, rent for school and hostel, stipend, educational aids and training material, hiring for bus and contingency are supported. The total allocation for this scheme during this financial year is Rs. 10 crores. The financial norms has been revised as follows:

Maintenance and Strengthening of Health and Family Welfare Training Center (HFWTC)

In order to improve the quality and efficiency of the Family Planning Programme and to bring the changes in the attitude of the personnel engaged in the delivery of health services through in service training programmes, 47 Health and Family Welfare Training centres have been established in the country. These training centres provide in service training in Reproductive and Child Health Programmes. Various National Programmes as well as training to the Male Multi-purpose Health Workers.

Apart from the salary of the staff of the training centres, other assistance under the scheme includes contingency for purchase of educational material, rent for training centres and payment to guest faculty. The total allocation for this scheme is Rs. 13 crores in 2001-02. The financial norms revised since 7.2.2001 are as follows:

Item	*Old norm*	*Existing norm*
Rent (for new schools)	Rs. 5,000 per month	Rs. 10,000 per month
Rent for hostel (for new schools)	Rs. 125 per month per candidate	Rs. 250 per month per candidate
Stipend	Rs. 125 per month per candidate	Rs. 300 per month per candidate
Educational Aids and Training Material	Rs. 5,000 per annum	Rs. 15,000 per annum
Transportation (for hiring bus)	Rs. 15,000 per annum	Rs. 50,000 per annum
Contingency	Rs. 15,000 per annum	Rs. 30,000 per annum

Rent payable in respect of such centres that are functioning from rented, buildings.

Item	*Old norm*	*Existing norms*
Contingency	Rs. 6,000 per annum	Rs. 15,000 per annum
Rent	Rs. 18,000 per annum	Rs. 40,000 per annum
Payment to guest faculty	Rs. 15,000 per annum	Rs. 50,000 per annum

Rural Health Training Centre, Najafgarh

RHTC, Najafgarh was established as a Najafgarh Health Institute with the assistance of Rockfeller Foundation in 1937 and merged as a Rural Health Training Centre in 1969. It has been rendering various services to the rural community training to medical and para-medical health workers and nursing personnel from different Nursing Training Schools of Delhi, orientation training to Public Health Students and ANMs, training of ANMs (10 + 2) Vocational Course under Central Board of Secondary Education.

Family Welfare Training and Research Centre, Mumbai

Family Welfare Training and Research Centre (FWTRC), Mumbai was the first Family Planning Training Centre, established in June 1957 and was made responsible for the training needs of State and District-level categories of health personnel from Western Zone. This centre has been recognised as an institution for training of central health service officers in the areas of National Family Welfare Programme and National Health Policy. FWT&RC is also conducting community-based Research Projects in the field of Health and Family Welfare. The institute also conducts a one year diploma in health education (DHE).

Gandhi Gram Institute of Rural Health and Family Welfare Trust (IGIRHFWT) Gandhi Gram, Tamil Nadu

To train the teachers of ANM/LHV Training Schools and Public Health nurses during the Sixth Plan Period, Government of India established training institutions at Tamil Nadu (Gandhi Gram). The Gandhi Gram institution is also functioning as one of the Central Training Institutions in India to provide training to functionaries of Health and Family Welfare of Kerala, Karnataka, Pondicherry, A&N Islands as well as Tamil Nadu. The institute also conducts regular Diploma in Health Education Course (DHE) of one year.

Strengthening of Infrastructure under Reproductive and Child Health Programme

With a view of improving facilities in the existing rural health infrastructure under Reproductive and Child Health Programme, the Government of India is assisting all the states in improving/constructing labour room, operation theatre and providing water/electricity supply in CHCs/PHCs, etc. so that essential and emergency obstetric services are improved. Under Minor Civil Works Scheme, an amount of Rs. 10 lakhs per district has been provided. Under Major Civil Works Scheme an amount of Rs. 10 lakhs per CHC/District Hospital is being provided.

Prime Minister Gramodaya Yojana (PMGY)

1. The PMGY is an initiative to expand outreach and coverage in the provisioning for basic minimum services in rural areas, with a view to improving the quality of lives that people lead.
2. The Planning Commission of India has allocated an Additional Central Assistance, 2001-02, of Rs. 2800 crores for six sectors viz. Rural Electrification, Primary Health, Primary Education, Shelter, Drinking Water and Nutrition. A state-wise allocation, for each sector, is appended to these Guidelines.
   The Planning Commission has conveyed that during 2001-02, the mandatory earmarking for all components except nutrition will be limited to 10% of the ACA allocation of a State/UT as against a ceiling of 15% during the previous year, 2000-01. While the States and UTs must allocate 65% of their total ACA towards the six sectors, the allocation of the remaining 35% of the ACA would be determined by the States/UTs on the basis of their own priorities.
3. Funds under the PMGY may be utilized to further the goals and objectives of primary healthcare as per the following guidelines:
   (i) 50% towards strengthening the functioning of the existing primary healthcare facilities by provisioning for:
      A. Procurement of drugs (other than those supplied under the National Disease Control, Family Welfare Programme, Externally Aided Projects, etc.) as well as essential consumables, including disposable delivery kits, reagents, X-ray films, etc. for diagnostic and therapeutic procedures. 2% of the funds allocated to the Primary Health Sector under PMGY are to be earmarked for purchase of the ISM&H Drugs. Guidelines for the same will be issued by the ISM & H Deptt.
      B. Contingencies for meeting travel costs of the ANMs, maintenance of installed equipments and fixtures, inclusive of bed linen, repair of essential, repairs/replacement of furniture and movables like beds and bed-equipment, fixtures and furnishings for operation theatres, and generators.

   (ii) 50% towards strengthening, repair and maintenance of the infrastructure in Sub-centres, Primary Health Centres and in Community Health Centres, inclusive of staff quarters. Priority may be accorded to ensuring potable water supply, adequate toilet facilities, and waste management at district hospitals and in facilities below district hospitals.

4. Paras 3(i) and (ii) above refers to the entire allocation towards Primary Healthcare under PMGY, i.e. the 10% earmarked for this sector, plus the additional allocation made at the discretion of the state governments from the 35% unallocated funds.
5. PMGY funds will be released in half yearly instalments upon receipt of Statements of Expenditure from state governments. Utilization Certificates/Audited Statement will be due from state governments at the end of each financial year.
6. As a rule of thumb, about 40% of the PMGY funds provided to the States should be allocated towards strengthening the existing infrastructure so that it steadily becomes fully functional. To begin with, it is suggested that attention may be paid to the bottom 20% districts, so identified in terms of their infant mortality rate (IMR)/crude birth rate (CBR) as per Census 2001.
7. Available data from facility survey conducted by the Department of Family Welfare and the facility surveys carried out by states may be utilized to identify geographical areas and specific primary health facilities that need strengthening, and therefore become eligible to be assigned the PMGY funds under the items (i) and (ii).
8. Caution may be exercised to avoid duplication. Any facility being strengthened under any other ongoing project/programme should ordinarily be excluded from additional funding.
9. State Govts./UTs are not required to seek prior approval of Deptt. of Family Welfare/Ministry of Health and Family Welfare, GOI, before incurring expenditures under the PMGY if these expenditures are in accordance with the scheme outlined in para 3 above.[24]

ISSUES AND RECOMMENDATIONS

The various studies bring out the fact that presently the healthcare system has been functioning under following constraints:

(a) The inability of the healthcare system to make available the services required to meet the demands of those in need, who are usually too poor or geographically or socially remote to benefit from such facilities.
(b) There are wide differences in distribution of resources and services and there is a multiplicity of institutions, which are unrelated, and do not function as a system.
(c) The curative aspect of healthcare has been stressed with insufficient priority to preventive, promotive and rehabilitative care. This has resulted in fragmentation of healthcare provided to the individual.

(d) Training of health personnel is directed primarily towards medical and institutional care, and largely irrelevant to the tasks and functions required outside institutional settings.

(e) The education and training of health professionals accentuates the social distance between health professionals and the population. This results in the providers of health services being unable to identify with the beneficiaries.

(f) The people have rarely been given the opportunity to play an active role in deciding the types of activities they want. Community interest and resources have too often been inadequately expressed and activated because there has been a failure to recognize that people will be most interested in and responsive to, activities related to their own priority concerns.

We present here various recommendations, which are vital to make the Community healthcare system efficient, effective and economical and ensure decent healthcare to the people as a matter of right.

I. Infrastructural Facilities

(a) Proper Construction and Maintenance of Buildings

The study shows that buildings are not sufficient to accommodate all activities and are not well maintained. Buildings are not regularly white washed, broken glasses not removed, repairs not done, making it impossible for Healthcare functionaries to carry out their activities in a dignified way. Efforts should be made to institutionalize maintenance contracts to renovate these buildings and ensure cleanliness.

(b) Adequate Public Health Facilities

The study indicates absence of proper lavatory facilities, resulting in foul smell in the area, causing difficulties both for the health staff and the patients. Urinating near Health Centres can result in serious infections. Lavatory services should be provided adequately and well maintained.

(c) Availability of Adequate Furniture

Health personnel as well as the patients were unhappy with the quantity and quality of furniture provided. Even simple examination tables, beds in the wards, trolleys were non-functional. Most of the chairs were broken. Health department must ensure the availability of good quality furniture and other facilities at health centres to make them functional. Financial powers to repair or repaint furniture items should be exercisable by PHC doctor.

(d) Availability of Good Residential Accommodation

Health personnel travel long distances from nearby cities, as there is no arrangement for good residential accommodation in the vicinity of

PHCs. There is a need to give priority to this to make the Health team available 24 hours a day and build good rapport with the rural people.

(e) Transport Facilities for Multi-purpose Workers

Health workers waste a lot of time in commuting to different villages to provide preventive and curative services. This unproductive time can be saved by providing transport facilities in a planned way to different centres, which can result in economy and efficiency. The vehicles should be made available to health staff as per a fixed time schedule of village visits.

2. Health Personnel for Primary Healthcare

(a) Health Manpower Planning

The Health Department must ensure the availability of health personnel and fill up all vacant posts at the earliest. In our study, we found a CHC working with one staff Nurse against the sanctioned strength of six, thereby adversely affecting the in-patient services.

(b) Mismatching of Health Personnel

The staff in CHCs and PHCs have to function as teams and absence of one category of personnel would affect the overall efficacy of the organisation. There are instances when more than one doctor of same specialisation is posted to a CHC, to suit the convenience of that specialist. We have conducted analysis of manpower management applying Human Resources Accounting and Human Resource Auditing, which indicated that Health Department is underutilizing technical manpower resources and there is mismatch between the needs and availability of specialists.

(c) Indiscipline among Health Personnel

The study shows that health personnel are not punctual and generally remain absent. It is a very serious problem affecting the delivery of Primary healthcare services. The Health personnel take their job lightly and do not perform their role with full devotion. The DHO should ensure punctuality and attendance through strict supervision and control. Exemplary punishments can pave the way to good discipline, vital for good primary healthcare services.

(d) Medical Staff Lacks Administrative Competence

The Health functionaries tend to consider themselves exclusively as technicians and even their training in medical colleges emphasizes this role. Consequently, they analyse problems and work out solutions exclusively from a technical point of view. However, in reality, many of their problems are more administrative or managerial than technical. The studies show that the top personnel and even other staff lacked administrative competence. Administration of Health Institutions is a complex proposition and requires administrative capability to balance all socio-economic factors, gain the confidence of the community and approval of the health staff, in order to provide optimum care to patients. The top personnel should be imparted managerial training to learn and apply the latest techniques and tools for optimum utilisation of health resources at their disposal.

(e) Lady Doctors must in PHCs

At present, many PHCs have no Lady doctors. Since Women, especially in villages, prefer to be examined by lady doctors, it is essential that women Doctors are posted to gain the confidence of local women and provide leadership to the family-based healthcare activities. They are also essential to have better supervision of other female workers in PHC and sub-centres.

(f) Morale and Motivation of Health Personnel

The study suggested that the State Health Department and District health officers do not attach importance to health institutions in the villages and do not provide them with all facilities, i.e., medical equipment, medicines, right manpower. The health personnel in CHC, PHC and sub-centres feel alienated and do not take their work seriously. The Government must supply them all the essential facilities, so that they can take their work seriously and with keen interest. This would also encourage them and build their morale and motivation.

(g) Inculcate Team Values in Health Personnel

The study brings out absence of harmonious relationship amongst different categories of health personnel. The PHC/CHC should be conceived as a team or group of people, so related that the efforts of each duly contribute to the best patient care with utmost action. Unfortunately, this aspect has been neglected all along. Delivery of health services is essentially a team function, involving a large number of different categories of workers, each of which has its own unique role, responsibility and function. Moreover, the quality of health services depends upon its personnel, their general education, job specific training, dedication to the profession and commitment to the people.

3. Equipment, Medicine and Laboratory Facilities

(a) Availability of Essential Equipment

Personal observation and discussions revealed that 50 percent of the equipment required at various levels is not available, causing hardships to patients. The patients are forced to make use of private services, which are costly and time consuming. The essential equipment for all health institutions should be provided at the earliest.

(b) Repair Non-functional Equipment

Even Ordinary blood pressure measuring instruments are out of order. X-ray machines mostly remain out of order. This forces the technical personnel to remain idle and poor people have to pay heavily to private agencies. These may be got repaired and should be kept functional, else condemned and replaced with new equipment.

(c) Upkeep and Handling of Equipment

The available equipment in health institutions is not handled properly and there is no concept of preventive maintenance. Hence the wear and tear is faster and the functional life of the equipment gets shortened. 'Preventive maintenance' is systematic maintenance procedure, wherein the condition of the equipment is constantly watched through a systematic inspection programme and preventive action taken to reduce the incidence of breakdown.

The salient advantages of such a system would be:

(a) Reduction in idle time and continuous availability of equipment.
(b) Increased life of the equipment.
(c) Continued service.
(d) Timely replacement of spares.
(e) Optimal operational costs.
(f) Satisfactory quality of services.
(g) Safety of operation.

(d) Ensure Availability of Medicines

Doctors as well as patients complain of the short supply of drugs. Besides, patients feel that the quality of drugs is sub-standard. Success of Medicare of in-patients or ambulatory patients largely depends upon the quality of drugs being used or provided to patients. The doctors must ensure that each drug reaching the patient is effective and acceptable.

(e) Classification of Drugs

It was gathered during discussion with CHC staff that they have not classified the drugs into categories based on vital, essential and desirable. We have observed that medicines are not even stored properly. There is a need to impress upon the person in charge of dispensary the need and importance of proper inventory management of drugs.

4. Financial Resources

(a) Adequate Financial Allocation

Public health expenditure is about 5 percent of the state budget and 1.48 percent of GDP in Karnataka. These allocations are inadequate to provide essential Primary healthcare with a basic package of preventive and clinical/curative services. Recognising the link between basic public health provisions and poverty alleviation, there is a need to step up the allocation progressively.

(b) Prioritisation of Resources

The health programmes should be prioritized systematically with reference to problem-solving, so that an allied problem-oriented issue will be to decide as to what are priority health financing needs of today. Some of the issues which go against prioritization of resources are as following:

(a) Disproportionate concentration of expenditure on health services in urban areas compared with expenditure on rural areas.
(b) Heavy concentration of expenditure on Secondary and tertiary care services compared with expenditure on primary care services.
(c) Heavy concentration of expenditure on curative services compared with expenditure on preventive services.
(d) Inadequate concentration on indigenous system of system as compared to allopathic services.

(c) Emphasis on Disadvantaged Groups

The mal-distribution of health finance is sometimes linked with inadequacy of health resources. However, it is also an independent problem by itself in developing countries. The mal-distribution is related to geographical areas as well as population and various income and occupational groups. The public finances for healthcare should be allocated to disadvantaged population groups or areas, rather than raising the issue of absolute or relative inadequacy of funds.

(d) Low Cost Health Technology

Rising health costs is currently a serious health financing problem. Developing and developed countries and all population groups equally face this. This problem arises out of various situations like rapidly rising cost of living. Also it is a byproduct of rising rates of healthcare utilisation and expansion of social security measures by welfare governments in developing countries. The medical technologies have also contributed to the rising cost of healthcare. The solution lies in the measures through appropriate technologies and interventions.

(e) Efficient Utilisation of Resources

Inefficiency in spending the existing resources is noticed in general. The lack of coordination and lack of efficiency in spending the available finances are the two sides of the same problem. This problem in financing of healthcare speaks of duplications, wastages and also according wrong priorities based on non-economic and non-technical criteria of allocations and utilisation of finances. We can also promote efficiency in spending through the adoption of performance and zero-based budgeting as well as adopting performance audit and performance accounting. Since about 80 per cent of the expenditure relates to salary, there is a need to adopt human resource accounting and human resource auditing to optimize human resources.

5. Community Participation

We have interviewed the people to know their reactions about health services in their area. They are very critical of health services and feel alienated from the government and the health system, creating a wide 'credibility gap'. The government should ensure provision of quality healthcare services to ensure that local people utilize and own up the local health services, thus providing meaningful community participation. 'Quality assurance' means delivery of relevant and effective medical care in a professionally acceptable manner. Community participation is possible only by winning over the confidence of the community through good healthcare services.

(a) Empower People

We must empower the community to plan and execute the health programmes in their areas as per local needs, aspirations and socio-cultural practices. Health committees at Sub-centre, PHC, CHC levels can be set-up. Government must understand that concretization of the people and their actively participation in the development process, on one hand, and asserting their rights, on the other, does not weaken the authority of the State but is the symptom of true and mature democracy. A partnership between government and community will foster a participatory relationship to encourage more effective programme implementation and facilitate local problem-solving, thus becoming more sustainable in the process and promote self-reliance. The failure of community health efforts can be attributed to inadequate matching of the perceptions of health needs and priorities between the local people and the health services staff, as a result of inadequate communication and the lack of a continuing dialogue.

(b) Reorient Bureaucratic Mindset

Partnerships with the community involve attitudinal changes and a new approach to health development. Healthcare providers need to be convinced that the problems affecting the poor are best understood by the poor; and therefore, the community must be involved in conceptualizing, planning, implementing, monitoring and evaluating healthcare. Inspite of the accepted general principle of Primary Healthcare, i.e. Community participation, the traditional bureaucratic machinery often stands in the way of their translation into concrete actions. There is unwillingness to decentralize, that is why the community is involved only to the level of curiosity and enthusiasm. Sustained efforts need to be made to ensure community participation through creation of appropriate forums.

(c) Involve PRIs

The State has 5640 elected Gram Panchayats, which at present have 35,153 elected women members, constituting 43.60% of the total elected members. The Karnataka Panchayati Raj Act, 1993 has specifically included implementation of programmes relating to family welfare and women as functions to be performed by the Gram Panchayats. The elected members constitute a vast reservoir of potential leaders, who are available at the village level to support interventions for improving the health status of their community.

(d) NGOs and Primary Healthcare

NGO participation in healthcare at all levels, especially at the level of public health and first referral, needs to be supported and encouraged, with a special focus on the backward and remote regions. The Government has already taken initiative to enlist the participation of NGOs. In the remote tribal area of Mysore district "Swami Vivekananda Youth Movement" has been requested to run the Community Health Centre in Titmatti Village. Since these organizations are concerned with the total process of development—social as well as economic, they would provide effective intersectoral integration and co-ordination as well.

6. Referral System

The analysis of PHCs and CHCs reveals that there is no proper referral system in vogue, making all the institutions function in isolation. The purpose of creating Primary Health is to provide graded healthcare, i.e., providing patients in access to levels of care that are appropriate to their health needs, with a minimum of inconvenience and delay. However, the community is often not satisfied with the referral services being provided at the primary and secondary levels and they bypass the local facilities, causing overcrowding at referral centers. This can be attributed to lack of physical facilities, back-up support and supervision; lack of mobility of health personnel; lack of communication and transport for emergency cases; lack of effective logistic and supply system, lack of flexibility, etc. We suggest the following steps to make referral system effective:

(1) Norms of services to be provided at each level should be clearly defined;
(2) Quality of services should be maintained at each level, to inspire confidence among patients that they will be treated in an effective manner at that level;
(3) Patients and the community must have the confidence that they will be properly referred and promptly transported to higher level of healthcare in case of need;
(4) Procedures should be followed to ensure that patients do not skip the lower levels at which they could be effectively treated;
(5) Referral and feed back cards should be introduced;

(6) Referral guidelines that specify the 'what' and 'how' of implementing the referral system should be provided;
(7) An incentive system for patients who follow referral procedures should be envisaged;
(8) Linkages and communications between the first referral hospitals and primary care facilities through regular training and out reach visits should be established; and
(9) Intensive information, education and communication targeted at the providers and the community should be initiated.

The structure of the Primary Healthcare Services provided by the government is impressive. However, the government has not been able to provide and maintain critical infrastructure, adequate resources in terms of manpower, finances and equipment, a sound administrative set-up, accountability and responsiveness of the system and commitment of the Health Department. This half-hearted approach fails to satisfy the people and cannot provide job satisfaction to the providers of Community Healthcare. All these problems also emanate from the fact that Government has been rapidly expanding the number of health institutions, without focusing on improving the Physical facilities in the existing institutions. There is a need to consolidate existing infrastructure to ensure proper facilities in the existing institutions.

We hope that these suggestions would help the Policy-makers, Planners, Decision-makers as well as those engaged in the implementation of Community Healthcare, in providing effective, efficient, and decent health services to the people to realize the goal of Health for all, in an expeditious manner.

The district level structure of health services is a middle level management organisation and it is a linkage system between the state as well as regional structure on one side and the peripheral level structure at PHC and sub-centre on the other side. It receives information from the state level and transmits the same to the periphery by suitable modifications, to meet the local needs. In doing so, it adopts the functions of a manager and brings out various issues of general, organisational and administrative types in relation to the management of health services. District Health System is most convenient for healthcare delivery system. To quote WHO: "The district, which is the peripheral organizational unit of national health systems, is particularly suitable as a channel for services to communities, and as a link with more central policies and support systems.

It is at district level that the health needs of the population can best be matched with the resources to be allocated. The district health system initiative and approach were therefore designed to help countries implement their primary healthcare strategies more effectively, the district being the most appropriate level for coordinating "top-down" and "bottom up" planning, organizing community involvement in planning and implementation, supporting healthcare workers, and improving coordination between the government and private health sectors. In addition, many key development sectors are represented at this level, thereby facilitating intersectoral cooperation and management of services across a broad front."

In order to facilitate a common understanding, the WHO Global Committee, in 1986, defined the district health system based on primary healthcare as "a self-contained segment of the national health system comprised of a well-defined population living within a clearly delineated administrative and geographical area, whether urban or rural. It includes all institutions and individuals providing healthcare in the district, whether governmental, social security, non-governmental, private, or traditional. A district health system, therefore, consists of a large variety of interrelated elements that contribute to health in homes, schools, work places and communities, through the health and other related sectors. It includes self-care and all healthcare workers and facilities, upto and including the hospital at the first referral level and appropriate laboratory, other diagnostic and logistic support services. Its component elements need to be well coordinated by an officer assigned to this function in order to raw together all these elements and institutions into a fully comprehensive range of promotive, preventive, curative and rehabilitative health activities."[25]

PLANNING FOR DISTRICT HEALTH SYSTEM THROUGH DEMOCRATIC DECENTRALISATION

Planning of community health services means the careful analysis, intelligent interpretation and orderly development of these services. In accordance with modern knowledge, techniques, and experience, to meet the health needs of a nation within its resources. A health plan is a determined course of action that is firmly based on the nature and extent of health problems, from which are devised priority goals.

Decentralisation of planning can be within the Health system in a limited sense. In a broader sense, it may be political devolution of powers. Its extent may differ from state to state. So in the first place, decentralisation tries to bring about adaptability and flexibility, in order to achieve greater effectiveness and greater efficiency. It is in that sense an instrumental matter, and may be promoted from within the ministry of health itself.

Decentralization may also promote local decision-making and participation and encourage accountability by healthcare services to the people at the grassroots, who are meant to be served by them. The issue is then not efficiency, but control; not instrumental or technical questions, but political ones are central. In that case, the impulse for decentralization may not be internal to the health sector, but rise in the wider political arena. Decentralization relates to devolution of power to lower levels of the political system, such as regions, provinces or districts. While there are many cases of decentralization proceeding at a snail's pace, examples also exist of timetables that try to do too much too fast, resulting in a loss of control over the process, or in failure at the lower levels to deliver the goods.

Machinery for Democratic Decentralisation

Establishment of three-tier panchayat raj system is the first step towards decentralisation of power. It provides for a Gram Panchayat, Taluka Panchayat and Zilla Panchayat. The Zilla Panchayat or District Panchayat has authority over the entire district, except the urban areas under municipal or city or town councils. There is provision for transfer of power and functions and devolution of funds to Panchayats. Practically all the development programmes are transferred to the District Panchayat and an officer of the rank of the collector is the Chief Executive Officer of the Zilla Panchayat.

It has an elected president and vice-president from among its elected members. Elected members alone have a right to vote. There are associate members too, who are nominated and can only discuss and express their views in the meetings of Panchayat. The Chief Executive Officer, of the rank of collector, is posted to Panchayat and acts as an *ex-officio* Secretary of the Panchayat and has a pivotal role. This district panchayat functions through various committee structures and the Health Committee is one of the important committees to work for health development.

Thus PRIs are ushering in democratic decentralisation of administration. They are the active instruments of peoples' participation in the developmental process at the grass-root level. The panchayat system is taking strong roots and providing a solid base for building up and strengthening the decentralisation of the planning process. The District Planning Board (DPB) provides a forum for all sectors and organizations engaged in development work, including panchayats, to pool their efforts and assist in evolving a well coordinated and participatory approach to planning.

The Karnataka Panchayat Raj Act, 1993, which is now in force in the State, specifies the following functions to be performed by the Zilla Panchayat, in respect of Health and Family Welfare, at the district level:

(1) Management of hospital and dispensaries, excluding the District hospital and other hospitals under the direct management of Government (above 50 beds);
(2) Implementation of maternity and child health programmes;
(3) Implementation of family welfare programmes; and
(4) Implementation of immunization and vaccination programmes.

In the last decade, there have been important studies on the active participation of Panchayati Raj Institutions in the health and family welfare programme. The Gujarat and Madhya Pradesh governments have recognized the potential of these bodies and actively, involved them in the implementation of health and family welfare programme. Moreover, the role of these institutions has been visibly noticed in the successful implementation of the Pulse Polio Immunization programme at the grassroots level.

B.K. Pattanaik in his article, "Community Participation, Panchayati Raj and Rural Healthcare" in *Kurukshetra,* January 2004 clearly mention that in the last decade, there have been important studies on the active participation of Panchayati Raj Institutions in the health and family welfare programme. The Gujarat and Madhya Pradesh governments have recognized the potential of these bodies and actively involved them in the implementation of health and family welfare programmes. Moreover, the role of these institutions has been visibly noticed in the successful implementation of the Pulse Polio Immunization programme at the grassroots level.

Some of the important conclusions derived from the findings and observations in promoting community participation in upgrading health and family welfare status of the countryside population through Panchayati Raj Institutions are as follows:

1. Gender equity in the representation and balanced representation of all caste groups in the health and family welfare committees formulated at the village level would promote effective community participation.
2. The capacity building is key to community involvement. Persistent sensitization of community members through orientation trainings, Focus Group Discussions (FGDs), monthly/quarterly meetings and promoting their involvement in workshops/seminars would effectively stimulate community participation.
3. Careful management of inter and intra-community discords is very important for the smooth implementation of any rural development programme, including health and family welfare programme. The LIP, through its three step approach: (i) door to door approach; (ii) cluster approach, and (iii) village/panchayat approach have effectively managed the inter and intra-community discords through rapport-making and counselling both at individual and group levels. It is learned that while the Community Need Assessment (CNA) helps in the identification of health and family welfare needs, the Community Discords Assessment (CDA) and their management help in the effective implementation of health and family welfare programmes and projects.
4. Community contribution in cash and kind is an important requisite for community involvement and management of health and family welfare programmes. It will create a sense of community ownership and encourage community accountability

of health and family programme and will sustain the programme for a longer period. The objectives of effective community participation, sustainability and cost-effectiveness cannot be fully achieved without community contribution.

5. The health and family welfare programmes and projects launched; either by the government or by the NGOs in the countryside are required to involve these three-tier democratic institutions in the process of need assessment, planning, implementation and monitoring of their projects and programmes. Village health committees need to be formulated under the leadership of sarpanches which can be involved in the implementation of the health and health-related activities at the grass-roots.

Panchayats are the most befitting platforms in the countryside through which community participation can be effectively promoted. Promoting community participation bereft of Panchayati Raj; Institutions is half-hearted and cannot be adequately effective. The capacity building of Panchayat members and effective coordination between these Panchayati Raj (local self-government) institutions with the government development functionaries and other NGOs and village level organizations such as Mahila Mandals, youth clubs, cooperative societies, etc. will go a long way in the effective implementation of various rural development programmes and projects including the health and family welfare programmes. The panchayats are the wheels of the cart of rural development. Even though polarized, sometimes on the basis of castes and party lines, still then, they represent the voice of the community and that of the villagers.

Towards building an enduring rural society, the breaking of the vicious cycle of malnutrition and ill-health necessitates formulation of a set of distinct but mutually related strategies to combat the inextricably linked socio-political and economic factors that cause ill-health, and adversely affect the livelihoods. Therefore, critical public policy-making and strategic programming, cast in partnership and network mode, can alone bring about overall health development of communities and individuals. The bottom line of all prosperity and health in future should be a development process and outcome that is essentially facilitated by development partnerships and networks, which nurture as well as further the goals of health and human development with focus on putting health into the hands of the people. The 'dependency syndrome' generated essentially by the governments and some NGOs and inefficient and ineffective investments on public health programmes has been the root cause of getting the health development priorities wrong in the last five decades of planned development. While capital investments in health development are important, people's knowledge and indigenous skills have not been regarded as a major source that people possess. It is this knowledge and inherent skill of people, what needs to be made a basis of the new paradigm shift.

Panchayats are the most befitting platforms in the countryside through which community participation can be effectively promoted. Promoting community participation bereft of Panchayati Raj Institutions is half-hearted and cannot be adequately effective. The capacity building of Panchayat members and effective coordination between these Panchayati Raj (local self-government) institutions with the government development functionaries and other NGOs and village level organizations such as Mahila Mandals, Youth Clubs, Cooperative Societies, etc. will go a long way in the effective implementation of various rural development programmes and projects including the health and family welfare programmes. The panchayats are the wheels of the cart of rural development. Even though polarized, sometimes on the basis of castes and party lines, still then, they represent the voice of the community and that of the villages.[26]

We may conclude with the remarks that people in rural areas need more and more health education through which they can prevent large number of diseases and enjoy positive health.

Notes and References

1. Phisek Ponrattana Wanarom, "Health is Development" in *World Health,* March 1989, p. 27.
2. Quoted in S.L. Goel, Public Health Administration, Sterling, New Delhi; 1984, p. 28.
3. Ramesh Kanbargi, "Health and Development in India: Trends and Prospects in *Contours of Social and Economic Development: Policy Issues,* Editor P.V. Shenoi, Concept, New Delhi, 1997, p. 141.
4. P. Hamumantha Rayappa and T.V. Sekher, "Social Welfare Administration, Administration of Health Services" in S. Ramanathan, (ed.) Landmarks in Karnataka Administraition, New Delhi, Uppal, 1998, p. 317.
5. K.S. Dodzie, "The U.N. Answers the Challenge" in *World Health,* November, 1979, p. 6.
6. Dr. F.J. Thiersy, "laying the Foundation", in *World Health,* March 1969, p. 13.
7. Government of India, First Five Year Plan, p. 488.
8. J.F. Park and K. Park, Text Book on Preventive and Social Medicine, Jabalpur, Banarsidas, 1990, p. 33.
9. WHO: *World Health,* Primary Healthcare, May 1979, p. 488.
10. WHO: SEARO: SEA/RC Sept. 1977, p. 38.
11. WHO: World Health Assembly, Primary Healthcare, May, 1979, p. 27.
12. WHO, District Health System: Global and Regional Review Based on Experience in Various Countries, Geneva, 1995, p. 18.
13. WHOs Technical Report Series, 1968, 395, p. 6.
14. Elen, B. Perry, Ward Management, Balliere, London, 1978, p. 2.
15. WHOs Technical Report Series, 19658, 395, p. 1
16. WHO: District Health System: Global and Regional Review, based on Experience in various countries, Geneva, 1995, p. 18 (WHO/SHS/DHS/95.1)
17. England and Wales, Ministry of Health, Consultative Council on Medical and Allied Services (1920) Interim Report on the future of Medical and Allied Services, London, H.M. Stationery office.

18. W.G. Wickremesingh, The Premier Health Unit in Ceylon, Colombo, 1951.
19. League of Nations Health Organization, European Conference on Rural Hygiene (1931), Recommendations on the Principles Governing the Organization of Medical Assistance, The Public Health Services and Sanitation in Rural District of Geneva.
20. Annual Report, 1996-97, Ministry of Health and Family Welfare, Govt. of India, p. 33.
21. *Ibid.*, p. 34.
22. *Ibid.*
23. Jawarharlal Nehru and Public Administration, *IJPA*, New Delhi, 1975, p. 88.
24. Rural Health Statistics in India, March 2002, pp. 75-80.
25. WHO: District Health System: Global and Regional Review, Based on Experience in various countries, Geneva, 1995, p. 18.
26. B.K. Pattanaik, "Community Participation, Panchayati Raj and Rural Healthcare", *Kurukeshtra*, January 2004, pp. 14-18.

CHAPTER 2

HEALTH EDUCATION FOR RURAL DRINKING WATER SUPPLY

Water is critical to life, but it is also a limited resource and several interrelated factors are decreasing its availability. These factors include climate changes, increasing demand, lowered water tables and environmental degradation. There is also the growing threat of international and intercommunity disputes over water supplies. It is important, therefore that communities manage their water resources better and supply water for specific uses.

—*WHO*

Water being precious, finite and in view of growing demand, ultimately is a scarce natural endowment. Our main strategy is to optimize its availability for different purposes, and accordingly National Water Policy has defined water allocation priorities broadly for supply of water for drinking, irrigation, hydropower, ecology, agro-industries and non-agricultural industries, navigation and various other uses.

—*M.M.N. Saxena*

Health Education for Rural Drinking Water Supply

"For most people, it is not a problem to obtain the minimum amount of water necessary to sustain life. Rather, problems relate to the quantities of water required for different activities (resource allocation) and the quality of the water available (source suitability). Many places with water shortages actually receive abundant rainfall and community-based initiatives could alleviate water scarcity. Such initiatives may incorporate traditional approaches and include water management and conservation measures; sustainable rates of extraction; sustainable crop production; catchment protection; rainwater harvesting; and soil conservation."

—*WHO*

Dr. Able Wolman's Charter is one of the "father-figures" of environmental health in today's world. Professor emeritus of sanitary engineering at the Johns Hopkins School of Engineering, Baltimore, USA, he is also a former President of the American Public Health Association, and has spent the greater part of a long lifetime engaged in research into the control of the environment for the reduction of disease and the welfare of man. Here he contributes his own 20-point "Charter" for improving the world's health:

(1) Life is impossible without water. The statement is accurate. It always leads great conferences to pass resolutions to do something about providing water to impoverished people. Resolutions become opiates, because they are gratifying substitutes for action.

(2) Statistics are necessary, but they do not stir the emotions! One sick child, if it is yours, makes the world weep.

CHART 2.1

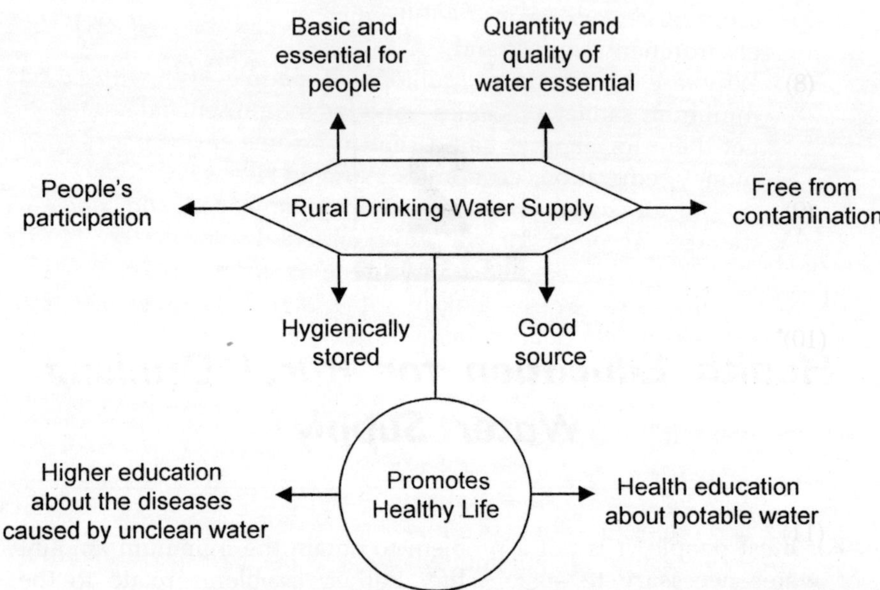

(3) How much drama is there is repeating, time and again, that more than 1,000 million people in developing countries cannot conveniently and safely drink, cook or wash with water? Astronomical numbers, of anything, are so often unintelligible. One should see people *en masse,* without these amenities, in villages or in slums, bidonvilles or favelas!

(4) Progress, of course, has been made in the last 30 years. WHO reports, in its recent survey of some 90 developing countries, that 69 per cent of urban dwellers had adequate community water supply and excreta disposal services.

(5) The situation for the rural or urban fringe dweller is dismal. For them, only 20 per cent have even reasonable access to safe water. Less than 10 per cent of these individuals have any real form of sanitary excreta disposal facilities.

(6) Viewed on a global basis, we have little to be sanguine about. The disease consequences of poor and insufficient water, of living with human excreta, and of unhygienic personal habits, are disastrous; they have been familiar for so long a time that they no longer excite even the statistician or epidemiologist. People accept their devastation, as they so often abjectly bear their real and spiritual poverty. We speak of the toll of deaths, due to environmental deficiencies, in a casual way, even though the figures mount to hundreds of millions. The communicable diseases, often the sequels of poor sanitation, are maiming and killing men, women, and children—not computer data.

(7) No "health house" can or should be built on an in-sanitary foundation. Healthcare and hospitalization, important as they are, will always be in default when structured upon a sanitary environmental quicksand.

(8) Why are hundreds of millions of people still without even minimum sanitary facilities—and, at the present rate, unlikely to get them for another half a century? Some say religion, custom, money, education, economics stand in the way.

(9) As in all social diagnoses, no single cause and non-single therapy account for all environmental disabilities. No two countries are alike and no two regions within the same country are the same. Let us look at some of the blocks to progress.

(10) It has been abundantly demonstrated that no one likes to be sick or die. Everyone (whether Moslem, Hindu, Christian, or any chosen religion) likes to wash so as to sleep at night, free from wake fullness infighting hordes of body vermin. Regardless of history or culture, people learn to protect themselves when given the opportunity and understanding.

(11) Too often, the slow pace has been blamed upon the people. The major cause for delinquent action lies in the motivation of governments. Do they really mean what their resolutions say—militantly enough to go into action? Is only lip service the main response of presidents, prime ministers, kings, and ministers?

(12) Unfortunately, the exceptions are still too few. What lessons stem from their successes? Motivation and intention, diligently and persistently pursued, remain in first place.

(13) Equally important are the desires of the people themselves, which can be met through education, understanding and participation. Much of the time these factors are missing and must be created and stimulated.

(14) This is not easy, but must be deliberately undertaken, preferably village by village, by the local "barefoot" somebody.

(15) To do this well requires the machinery and personnel of a permanent and sympathetic government, operating through regional and local units. Their nature and number will vary from country to country.

(16) Movement toward broad sanitary reform should go forward jointly or in parallel with other social and economic undertakings in the same areas. Room for exceptions must be available.

(17) It should be clear by now that maneuvering on this complex stage demands manpower, unfortunately in scarce supply in too many countries. The spectrum of manpower required runs from the highly skilled supervisor to the equally important, earthy village worker. Almost always, training on the spot is essential

(18) What about money? Strangely enough, this is not the dominant constraint. Some is needed, of course, but often, with local self-help (material, physical, and monetary), money can be found.

(19) Technology likewise is at hand. Failures lie in its abuse rather than in its unavailability. Certainly, innovation, simplicity, lower cost will all help, but progress is not retarded greatly by the inadequacy of present tools, materials or equipment.

(20) The task for the future is difficult, but possible. People should not be consigned to premature death, simply because we are less than courageous and diligent. The pace must be accelerated.[1]

Government of India in its document, "Guidelines for Implementation of Rural Water Supply Programme" observes that since independence, India has been making earnest efforts for achieving social and economic development. India has been implementing national strategies and plans through various multi-pronged development schemes and programmes. To relieve the women and young girls from the drudgery of fetching water from long distances and, to combat the scourge of water-borne diseases, the Government of India and States/Union Territories have been implementing water supply programme in the rural areas.

The importance of a country attaches to the provision of adequate and safe water supply is an index of its concern for socio-economic development of its people. The ever-increasing population in the country inevitably brings in its wake complex problems of potable water supply systems and environmental concerns in the implementation of the rural water supply programme.

India's rural water supply programme is the biggest in the world and has been remarkably successful. Around 95% of the rural habitations have access to one or more sources of drinking water. However, there are still a number of challenges to be faced in providing potable water to the remaining uncovered rural habituations. Depleting ground water, pollution, problems of quality of drinking water add to this. Developing hygiene awareness, helping people to become conscious of the relationship between safe water, sanitation, health and development and bringing about a change in the attitude and behaviour appear to be some of the difficult tasks to be carried out in the coming years.

M.M.N. Saxena in his article, "Initiatives in Promoting Water Resources in India", in *Yojna*, June 2003 clearly mentions that water being precious, finite and in view of growing demand, ultimately is a scarce natural endowment. Our main strategy is to optimize its availability for different purposes, and accordingly National Water Policy has defined water allocation priorities broadly for supply of water for drinking, irrigation, hydropower, ecology, agro-industries and non-agricultural industries, navigation and various other uses. Of equal importance are the objectives of achievements of efficiency, equity, and sustainability in the use of water.

With the existing water resources of the country, per capita availability of water varies in the range of 2000 to 13745 cubic meters (cu. m.) per year with the national annual average of per capita availability about 1829 cu. m. in 2001. By 2015 AD the country will be facing water stress conditions with annual per capita availability of water at about 1557 cu. m. The conditions will be further worsening due to continued population growth and by 2050 AD the projected annual per capita availability of 1168 cu. m. would take the country to the threshold of water scarce conditions. It is estimated that by 2050 AD 22% of the geographical areas and 17% of population of the country will be under absolute scarcity conditions having access of water availability of less than 500 cu. m. per year and 70% of the area and 76% of population will be on the verge of affected health and economic activities with access to water available of less than 100 cu. m. per year, which is identified as stress or scarcity level.

Water is life. This colourless, odourless and tasteless liquid is essential for all forms of growth and development—human, animal and plant. Water is a fundamental basic need for sustaining human economic activities. Not only does water support a wide range of activities, it also plays a central symbolic role in rituals throughout the world and is considered a divine gift by many religions.

Dr. Halfdan Mahler, WHO, former Director-General mentioned that: I am utterly convinced that the number of water taps per 1,000 population will be an infinitely more meaningful health indicator than the number of hospital beds per 1,000 population

Providing water in the desired quantity and quality; and at the right time and place, has been a constant endeavour of all civilizations. No other natural resource has had such an overwhelming influence on human history. As the human population increases, as people express their desire for a better standard of living, and as economic activities continue to expand in scale and diversity, the demands on fresh water resources will continue to grow.

While water is a renewable resource, its availability in space (at a specific location) and time (at different periods of the year) is limited, being largely determined by climatic, geographical and physical conditions, by affordable technological solutions which permit its exploitation, and by the efficiency with which water is conserved and used.

Much of the world's fresh water is consumed by the agricultural, industrial and domestic sectors. Increasing water demands and the inadequacy of these sectors to effectively manage this resource, has meant that crises situations have arisen in many parts of the world, crises over the availability of adequate, quality water.[2]

WATER FOR ALL: A HUMAN RIGHT

Water is a basic human need for health—indeed, for survival- and therefore it is not an exaggeration to call it one of the basic human rights.

Without safe water and sanitation, there is no real development. A community ravaged by diarrhoeal diseases, dracunculiasis or schistorsomiasis cannot look beyond its immediate problems towards social and economic welfare. Safe water is the doorway to health and health is the prerequisite for progress, social equity and human dignity.

Despite the achievements of the 1980s—an additional 1600 million people were served with safe water supplies—an estimated 1200 million people in developing countries still do not have proper access to safe water. They are at constant risk of contracting water and sanitation-related diseases. The upsurge of cholera since 1990 has underlined the need for clean water to protect health, particularly in the expanding shanties and slums in and around the cities of developing countries.

An adequate quantity of water, by itself, is not enough to safeguard health. Unsafe water supplies lead directly to diseases that affect hundreds of millions of people, mainly living in the tropics. This issue of *World Health* describes some of the problems and what is being done about them.

An accessible and safe water supply, improved personal and domestic hygiene, and stronger community participation are the main ways to avoid water-borne diseases. But to be really effective they must be accompanied by other measures such as pollution control and proper drainage of surface waters. Since environmental protection of fresh water source is the basic step to ensure a sustainable clean water supply, this must always be an integral component of both environment and health programmes.[3]

Water is essential to life on earth. Plant and animal life are vitally dependent on water, which is an essential ingredient and a lubricant of nature. Human existence is affected if there is too little or too much water and, if it becomes polluted, it becomes a health threat and a hindrance to economic prosperity. There is hardly any current issue that more conclusively demonstrates the integrated nature of environment and development than that of fresh water. The challenge of securing for all people the basic human need of a reliable supply of fresh water, adequate in quantity and quality, is perhaps the most fundamental development issue.[4]

IMPROVEMENTS IN WATER AND SANITATION CAN SAVE LIVES

Drinking water and sanitation improvements could reduce the overall incidence of infant and child diarrhoea by one quarter and cut total infant and child mortality by more than one-half. Country programmes are increasingly taking measures to improve water supply and sanitation within their primary healthcare programmes. Guinea-worm disease can be effectively prevented by providing safe drinking water and its global eradication is clearly possible within the next few years. As for schistosomiasis, some 60% reduction could be achieved by improving water supplies. Building latrines, giving health education and introducing selected drug therapy could reduce the prevalence even more.[5]

Water is part of a large constantly moving cycle. Simply explained, it evaporates from the surface of the earth, and turns into clouds that produce rain and snow, which fall on the earth's surface. Then through rivers and underground water tables it passes to the oceans and lakes, and thus the cycle continues.

Climatic changes caused by human activity—like cutting down forests—have reduced the water supply in many parts of the world. As temperature and rain and snow precipitation patterns change, many rivers carry less water. At times they carry too much water, resulting in floods. Trees and other vegetation help to retain water in the solid and prevent landslides. Chemical substances from industry sometimes pass into the air. One of the results is acid rain, which kills fish and vegetation in many lakes and rivers. Sometimes dangerous products from industry, agriculture and other human activities enter the rivers, lakes, oceans and underground water, and can contaminate our drinking water.

At the same time, the demand for water from villages and towns, and from industry and agriculture, is steadily increasing. Water can therefore no longer be considered an unlimited resource, which costs nothing and which can be wasted. In the next century water supplies will certainly be considered a very valued service, and each one of us will have to pay what it costs to have clean water.[6]

Safe water and improved sanitations are a necessary condition for better health, and there can be no lasting improvement of public health without them.

We all know that determined government action is needed to change the prevailing situation. We also know that clean water and sanitation will remain an unattainable objective in poor countries without development assistance.

Many countries are making efforts towards implementing the objectives of the International Drinking Water Supply and Sanitation Decade. But much still needs to be done-and can be done.[7]

The Americas: Attainable Goals—Governments in the Americas are increasingly aware that providing water and sanitation services is the single most important activity they can undertake to improve people's health and raise productivity.

Hours of personal drudgery are devoted to obtaining safe water and disposing of human wastes in a sanitary manner. When water must be carried from a source, which is five kilometers from the house, someone must spend about three hours a day in making the two trips that will be needed to carry the 30 to 40 litres of water the family will use. And this amount, which is often of dubious quality, will barely serve to quench their thirst, meet their cooking needs, and leave a little over for basic hygienic needs. Unless even this limited amount of water is properly disposed of, it can serve as the focus of a long of diseases.[8]

Millions in Need

Drinking water and sanitation are health programmes, not disease programmes. They are the essential precondition for the promotion of health, where health is under threat from communicable diseases.

A good drinking water supply is good for health. This simple fact was recognized more than a hundred years ago during one of the great cholera epidemics in London. John Snow stopped the pump on Board Street that supplied parts of the city with water from the River Thames and, by doing so, not only demonstrated that the disease was caused by infected river water but also showed that diseases like cholera cannot be permanently resisted unless people are provided with safe drinking water.

Why then are researchers today spending time and money yet again to disprove what has already been proven? Because of a misconception. They start from the premise that drinking water and environmental sanitation are interventions designed to control the diarrhoeal diseases. This is wrong. Drinking water supply and sanitation are the only permanent solutions that can prevent infant deaths from diarrhoea (and remember there are more than five million such deaths a year in the developing world). But it is wrong to assume that they should be provided merely to fight the diarrhoeal diseases. Drinking water and sanitation are health programmes; they are the essential precondition for the promotion of health, where health is threatened by a vast array of communicable diseases, and often the only permanent solution.

Moreover, drinking water and sanitation are an essential precondition for community development, and ultimately for social and economic development. Since we know this, we may ask why economists like the researchers referred to above continue to ask questions about these essential services? Is it because they prefer to invest the money in projects, which seem to offer a higher financial rate of return? Is it because they shy away from putting money down for water supply and sanitation since-admittedly-to build and maintain these services will call for more ingenuity and hard work than putting money into a bank where it will earn interest?

When delegates to the 39th World Health Assembly last May reviewed the progress made so far in the International Drinking Water Supply and Sanitation Decade, they started by saying that the case for adequate water supply and sanitation did not need to be restated. However, they noted the disparities in progress made between urban and rural areas, and between water supply and sanitation. They insisted that more should be done for water supply and sanitation in the future, and not less.

Children and women are suffering most in the present situation and they felt it was important to promote local technologies for water supply and sanitation, and to develop health education strategies aimed at increasing the awareness of communities of their role, especially in planning and maintaining their own water supply and sanitation facilities.

The delegates also stressed that improving water supply and sanitation means meeting the basic needs of millions of people; it followed, therefore, that financial resources should be made available in the light of a new and more equitable international economic order and as a contribution to the quest for peace. Everybody had to get involved, not only the health sector; the delegates concluded that inter-sectoral cooperation would be of prime importance to the attainment of the objectives during the second half of the decade.[9]

There is today just as much fresh water on the earth as there was millions of a year ago: about 40,000 cubic kilometers. But whereas there were 1,000 million people on the planet in 1820, there are 6,000 million today. Obviously this means that there is less water to go round. In addition, since the advent of the industrial era, there has been a dramatic increase in demand for water, commensurate with population growth and improved living standards. Each individual is using more fresh water every day for domestic, agricultural and industrial use, so it is all the more urgent to protect the water that is available to make the most of it and share it equally.

The International Drinking Water Supply and Sanitation Decade, is striving to bring safe water to everyone's doorstep. All too often, women and children spend hours in the drudgery of collecting water from remote and possibly polluted streams and wells. Having safe water means better health and nutrition, more time for education; it also means a better chance of a style of life that opens the way to social and economic growth. The technologies exist to bring water into every household. People must now work together to make this a reality and prove that "Happy are those who build their development on water."

Health plays a crucial role in any effort for development, and good health is closely related to the status of water supply and sanitation. Our graph on the opposite page shows the direct and indirect effects of water supply and sanitation on health. It indicates how water and health, in common with many other sectors, form a basis for development.[10]

Fresh water from inland sources can be broadly classified into, (i) Surface Water comprising rivers, lakes and ponds, and (ii) Ground Water comprising of wells and springs. A portion of the water falling on land soaks into the ground. This is stored in underground tunnels as groundwater. Groundwater is pure as it has already percolated through the solid and purified by a natural process of filtration. This is increasingly being preferred for use by people. But finding adequate groundwater sources for supplying large urban populations is difficult. Cities that do have good groundwater supplies benefit, because the cost of treatment is minimal. The treatment basically removing excessive minerals. Often the water is pure enough so that chlorine or other chemicals are not needed to make it usable, even for drinking.

Of all the water available on earth, potable or water fit for human consumption can be found only in the rainwater, inland surface water bodies like rivers, lakes, ponds and underground water from wells and handpumps.[11]

Until very recent times, most people took water for granted—as free, on nearly so, and certainly inexhaustible. But a long with the rapidly increasing population and greed of people have led to severe water shortages. And because people are spread widely over the world, water must be transported long distances to supply their needs.

Since water resources are limited, this trend of increasing use creates considerable pressure on declining water supplies. Further quality of water is also deteriorating because on increased levels of pollution and increases in salinity.[12]

The ground water is exploited by tube wells causing its level go down and hence potable water is becoming a problem. In villages and cities, water is obtained through wells, which may be shallow—(water above the first impervious layer), Deep wells (Below the first imperious layer) and tube wells run mechanically or electrically.

The order to avoid the wells or surface water from contamination, we should make wells on an elevated area at least 15-20 meters away from source of contamination and we should not urinate or put night soils near the well. The environment of wells and tube well need to protect scientifically to obtain potable water supply. There is also need of disinfecting wells frequently through chlorination and in the days of epidemics, it must be done on every night. Even chlorine tablets of 05 gram are available to make 20 litres of water clean.

Water purification is done through sedimentation, filtration, chlorination ozonation, ultraviolet irradiation, etc. The water is not completely purified because of less use of material or material of sub-standard quality.

The standards for drinking water take into account the following constituents in determining the quality and make water free of them through treatments.

- Microbiological pollutants: bacteria, viruses, etc.;
- Toxic substances: arsenic, cadmium, cyanide, lead, mercury, selenium, etc.;
- Specific substances affecting health: fluorides, nitrates, poly-nuclear aromatic hydrocarbons;
- Acceptability of water colour, odour, hardness and taste or water; and
- Radio-active substances.

No matter how it is accomplished, keeping water pure enough to be usable has become expensive. Clean water in the future will undoubtedly account for a large percentage of money, but the investment in clean water contributes greatly to public health. Clean water is a people's issue. Because of corrupt practices, clean water even in beautiful city like Chandigarh has become a remote possibility.[13]

WATER QUALITY ASSESSMENT AUTHORITY

The problem of pollution of national water resources has become a matter of serious concern in India. To circumvent the situation on the advice of Ministry of Water Resources (MoWR), the Ministry of Environment and Forests (MOEF), Constituted the "Water Quality Assessment Authority (WQAA)" with effect from 29 May 2001 for the purpose of performing the powers and functions enumerated therein to protect the quality of National Water Resources. The 12-member Authority is headed by the Secretary, Ministry of Environment and Forests as the Chairman and the Commissioner (Water Management), MoWR as the Member Secretary.[14]

Drinking water supply and Sanitation are State subjects, included in the Eleventh Schedule of the constitution among the subjects that may be entrusted to Panchayats by the States. The Government of India supplement efforts made by the States by providing financial and technical assistance under the two centrally sponsored programmes, namely, the Accelerated Rural Water Supply Programme (ARWSP) and the Central Rural Sanitation Programme (CRSP).

Substantial investment to the tune of about Rs. 50,000 crore has been made in the rural water supply sector alone by the Central and State Governments since 1st Five Year Plan in approx. 37 lakh hand Jumps and 1.45 lakh piped water supply schemes, crediting the country with one of the largest rural drinking water supply networks in the world. While significant achievement has been made in terms of providing access to potable drinking water with 5.34% rural habitations fully covered and another 28% partially covered, the sanitation coverage in rural areas continues to be a challenge, with only 22% of the rural population having access to basic sanitation, as per the 200I Census.

A national water supply and sanitation programme was introduced in the social sector in country in 1954. The Government of India provided assistance to the States to establish special investigation divisions in the Fourth Five Year Plan to many out identification of problem villages. Taking into account the magnitude of the problem, and to accelerate the pace of coverage of problem villages, the Government of India introduced the Accelerated Rural Water Supply Programme (ARWSP) in 1972-73 to assist States and Union Territories with 100% grants-in-aid to implement drinking water supply schemes in such villages. The entire programme was given a Mission approach when the Technology Mission on Drinking Water Management, called the National Drinking Water Mission (NDWM), was Introduced as one of the five Missions in social sector in 1986. NDWM was renamed as Rajiv Gandhi National Drinking Water Mission (RGNDWM) in 1991. During the International Water and Sanitation Decade in 1980s, Central Rural Sanitation Programme (CRSP) was launched in 1986 in the Ministry of Rural Development to accelerate sanitation coverage in rural areas with the objective of improving quality of life of the rural people and also to provide privacy and dignity to women.

Presently Rajiv Gandhi National Drinking Water Mission (RGNDWM), Department of Drinking Water Supply, Ministry of Rural Development administers the Centrally Sponsored programmes in Rural Drinking Water Supply and Rural Sanitation sectors.

The Xth Plan accords the highest priority to providing the Not Covered (NC) habitations with sustainable and stipulated supply of drinking water.

It is envisaged to cover all the rural habitations including those which might have been slipped back to NC/PC category by the end of Xth Plan. The Tenth Plan emphasizes the participatory approach where PRIs should be the key institutions for convergence of drinking water supply programmes at the ground level. Considerable success has been achieved in meeting drinking water needs of the rural population and 95.34% rural habitations are Fully Covered with stipulated level drinking water facilities. The Partially covered habitations are 4.28%. The Not Covered habitations are about 0.38%. As per the latest report from the States/UTs, the coverage status as on 1.11.2004 based on comprehensive Action Plan, 1999 and coverage reported by States/UTs.

Thereafter is as under:

Type of coverage	*No. of habitations*	*Percentage of total*
Not Covered (NC)	5368	0.38
Partially Covered (PC)	60884	4.28
Fully Covered (FC)	1356031	95.34
Uninhabitated migrated	381	
Total	1422664	

Statement showing State-wise coverage position is given at Annexure XL/II.

The strategy to achieve the Tenth Plan objectives can be briefly summarized as Accelerating coverage of the remaining Not Covered and Partially Covered habitations, including those slipped back from Fully Covered to Partially and Not Covered categories, with safe drinking water systems.

- To tackle problems of water quality in affected habitations and to institutionalize water quality monitoring and surveillance systems.
- To promote sustainability, both of systems and sources, to ensure continued supply of safe drinking water in covered habitations.

The quality problems of drinking water both due to geogenic factors leading to chemical contamination like excess fluoride, arsenic, iron, salinity, nitrate, etc. and anthropogenic factors resulting in bacteriological contamination, pose serious public health problems. Water Quality survey data has revealed 2,16,968 quality affected habitations, with the following break-up: excess Fluoride—31,306, excess Arsenic—5,029 excess Salinity—23,495, excess iron—1,18,088, excess Nitrate—13,958 and Multiple reasons—25,092. Water quality has to be ensured through a comprehensive surveillance process, incorporating monitoring data processing, evaluation sanitary surveys public health assessment and remedial and reventive action throughout the length and breadth of the country. Separate Sub-Mission programmes have been part of the ARWSP to address specific quality problems. The Department has finalized a Water Quality Monitoring and surveillance programme on Catchment Area approach by Utilizing the available district and sub-district level rater-testing infrastructure in educational institution and private and suitable capacity development PRIs and other villages level functionaries.

Despite respectable coverage in terms of access to drinking water proper upkeep of water supply themes has been a problem. Many factors like sources going dry increase in quality problems systems becoming defunct due to poor maintenance demand from other competing sectors like culture industry, etc. pose threat to sustainability of drinking water supply schemes. Putting in place an effective operation and maintenance system calls for huge investments. The total estimated cost of operation and maintenance of the water supply networks created so far is estimated at Rs. 6750 crore per annum whereas the total funds being utilized for O & M purposes under ARWSP are approx. 5.450 crore only. As such, as a part of the strategy to ensure sustainability of systems, reforms were introduced in 1999 with approval of the Cabinet which meant a paradigm shift from supply driven, norms based, centralized form of funding to one based on the principles of demand responsiveness, community leadership and decentralized mode of management.

Initially, the reforms were introduced in 67 pilot districts as Sector Reform Projects. Based on the experience gained, the reforms initiative was scaled throughout the country by launching Swajaldhara December 2002.

Unlike Sector Reform Projects, which had district as the unit for implementation. Swajaldhard themes can be implemented by the Beneficiary group, Gram Panchayat, Block Panchayat or District Panchayat. All the States across the country are implementing Swajaldhara schemes now. Under the Sector Reform and Swajaldhara, the individual water supply schemes are planned, designed, implemented, operated and maintained by the community through the village level committees. A major thrust of the reforms initiative in the rural water supply sector is on empowerment of Panchayati Raj system, for not only operating and maintaining drinking water schemes but also managing the entire rural water supply sector.

During the Ninth Plan period special initiative was taken to cover rural habitations with proper sanitation. The CRSP was restructured in

1999 with a provision for phasing out the allocation-based component by the end of the IXth Plan, i.e. 2001-02. The total Sanitation Campaign (TSC) under the restructured CRSP was launched with effect from 1.4.1999 following a community led and people centered approach. TSC moves away from the principle of state-wise allocation to a "demand-driven" approach. The programme gives emphasis on Information, Education and Communication (IEC) for demand generation of sanitation facilities and offering a wide range of technological choices of sanitation hardware through an effective delivery mechanism of Rural Sanitary Mart and Production Centre to meet the demand for sanitation facilities so generated. It also lays emphasis on school sanitation and hygiene education for bringing about attitudinal and behavioural changes for relevant sanitation and hygiene practices from young age.

SCHEMES OF RURAL WATER SUPPLY

I. Accelerated Rural Water Supply Programme (ARWSP)

Objectives

- To ensure coverage of all rural habitations with access to safe drinking water;
- To ensure sustainability of drinking water systems and sources;
- To tackle the problem of water quality in affected habitations; and
- To institutionalise the reform initiative in rural drinking water supply sector.

Rural water supply is a State subject. States have been taking up projects and schemes for the provision of safe drinking water from their own resources. However, recognising the importance of providing safe drinking water in rural habitations, Government of India has been providing financial assistance to State Governments under the Centrally Sponsored Scheme, "Accelerated Rural Water Supply Programme (ARWSP)."

Coverage Norms

- Ipcd of drinking water for human beings;
- 30 Ipcd of additional water for cattle in areas under the DDP;
- One handpump or standpost for every 250 persons; and
- Availability of water source in the habitation or within 1.6 km in the plains and 100 metres elevation in hilly areas.

Funding Pattern

(i) Under ARWSP, funds are provided to States for making provision of safe drinking water in rural habitations. 15% of these funds can be spent on operation and maintenance (O&M) of the existing drinking water systems and sources. State Governments should match funds released by this Department on 1 : 1 basis.

(ii) Upto 20 per cent of the funds can be utilized by the State Governments: (a) to take up projects under the Sub-Mission programme to tackle water quality problems like fluorosis, arsenic, brackishness, etc., and (b) to ensure source sustainability by conserving water, recharging aquifers, etc.

Out of this, 15% should be utilised for projects for quality and 5% for projects for sustainability of sources. Funding is done in the ratio of 3 : 1 between Central and State Governments.

(iii) 20 per cent of the annual outlay of ARWSP have been earmarked for implementation of reforms-oriented Swajaldhara and Sector Reform projects. The funding pattern for these projects is 90% from Government of India and 10% by way of community contribution.

(iv) About 5 per cent of the annual allocation is also earmarked to States covered by Desert Development Programme (DDP) under ARWSP. This is funded as 100% Central grant to the States.

(v) Further, to meet the contingencies arising due to natural calamities and emergent situation, 5% of the ARWSP allocation is earmarked. This is funded at 100% grant from the Central Government.

(vi) In pursuance of the announcement made by the then Prime Minister on 15.8.2002 three programmes viz. Installation of one lakh Hand Pumps providing drinking water facilities to one lakh rural Primary Schools and revival of one lakh traditional sources of water. The programmes will be completed in two years, 2003-04 and 2004-05.

Implementing Agencies

State Governments side the implementing agencies for the programme. The agencies may be the Public Health and Engineering Department (PHED), Rural Development Department or the Panchayati Raj Department. Implementation is also taken up by the Government Boards/ Nigams/Agencies in a few States, for example, the Gujarat Water Supply and Sewerage Board is the implementing agency in Gujarat, Uttar Pradesh Jal Nigam is the agency in Uttar Pradesh and Tamil Nadu Water and Drainage Board in Tamil Nadu.

Financial Progress

Government of India and State Governments have so far invested about Rs. 50,000 crore on rural drinking water supply schemes. The Central outlay for the Rural Water Supply Sector for 2004-05 is Rs. 2900.00 crore, which is likely to increase to Rs. 3148.00 crores through supplementary grant.

State-wise allocation of funds and releases made under ARWSP (Normal), ARWSP (DDP), Swajaldhara and three programmes of Prime Minister (as on 31.1.05) may be seen at Annexures XLIV, XLV, XLVI and XLVII respectively.

Delegation of Power

Keeping in view the concept of decentralisation of power, Government of India has delegated powers to States. All projects and schemes proposed under ARWSP are approved by the State Level Scheme Sanctioning Committee. Under Sector Reforms Pilot Projects, powers to plan and implement projects and schemes have been delegated to the community, who will also own, operate and maintain the systems. The community also has the power to choose the systems of their preferences. As per the Guidelines issued in June 2003 the District Water and Sanitation Committees are empowered to sanction projects under Swajaldhara.

Role of Panchayats

As per the 73rd Amendment to the Constitution of India, the subject of rural water supply vests with the Panchayati Raj Institutions (PRIs). The Panchayats are to play major role in providing safe drinking water and managing the systems and sources in their respective areas. They can be involved in the implementation of schemes, particularly in selecting the location of hand pumps, standposts and spot sources; in Operation and Maintenance (O&M), etc. Moreover, Government of India emphasis on empowering and capacity building of the PRIs to enable them for discharging their responsibilities in drinking water supply.

North-Eastern States: The States of the North-East have been facing problems to meet State matching share against central releases in the past.

As a result arrears of matching share has been accumulated. The Department of Drinking Water Supply has given maximum financial flexibility in the guidelines for implementation of Rural Water Supply Programme in respect of North-Eastern States in view of the fact that 10% of the total Central outlay for the programme is earmarked for the NE States. To ensure that the unutilized funds released to North-Eastern States are not lapsed, a Non-lapsable control Pool of Resources has been created. Any unutilised funds of Government of India share are credited in to this Pool under which the State Governments can take up various projects.

Sub-Mission programmes of the Government of India were launched with the objective to provide safe drinking water facilities in rural habitations affected by water quality problems like fluorosis, arsenic, brackishness, excess iron, nitrate, etc. The States undertakes these projects. For ensuring source sustainability through rainwater harvesting, artificial recharge, etc. State Governments also use funds under Sub-Mission. Quality problems in groundwater are of two types, viz chemical and biological. It is inherent in the form of contamination caused by the nature of the geological formation.

Excess fluoride, arsenic, iron or brackishness fall under this category. Groundwater pollution is also caused by human intervention (biological contamination).

It has been noticed that groundwater depletion has aggravated water quality problems due to excess fluoride arsenic and brackishness in certain areas. This gets manifested in the form of various diseases like floozies and arsenical dermatitis. This has forced the State Governments to abandon low-cost handpumps preferring costly piped water supply schemes.

Central Assistance under Sub-Mission Programme

Control assistance is extended to States for the following:

- Approved capital cost of treatment plants desalination, defluoridation, arsenic; and Iron removal;
- O&M cost of desalination plants;
- Cost of water conservation measures;
- Cost of holding awareness camps epidemiological surveys and water quality testing;
- Water testing laboratories non-recurring cost of equipment and recurring cost on technical staff, chemicals, etc., and
- Mobile water quality testing laboratories.

20 per cent of ARWSP funds are earmarked and utilized new projects under the Sub-Mission activities. However, if the States/UTs have achieved full coverage of habitations as per the national norms, they may utilise more funds to tackle quality problems subject to Government of India concurrence. Priority is given to the NC and PC habitations which are also affected by quality problems. In order to assess the ground position with regard to quality problems. water quality survey was conducted. As per the information furnished by the State Governments, the following number of habitations were affected with quality problems of drinking water shown on next page.

The Department has prepared a concept paper on tackling the water quality problem. It is estimated that Rs. 10000 crore as the Central share are required to tackle water quality problem. The project has been posed for World Bank funding.

Even though the coverage has been impressive over the last decade, various studies indicate that there is no institutionalized quality monitoring and surveillance system in the country. This is going to be critical to the entire water supply sector in the future owing to increase in pollution and

Nature or Quality problem habitations	No. or affected
Excess Fluoride	31306
Excess Arsenic	5029
Excess Salinity	23495
Excess Iron	118088
Excess Nitrate	13958
Multiple	25092
Total	216968

depletion of water sources. The National Workshop held on 7-9 August, 1997 recommended that there is a need to institutionalise water quality monitoring and surveillance systems in the country. Establishing of water quality labs could be only one of the components of the programme. A "Catchment Area Approach" would be adopted by involving various grass-root level educational and technical institutions by utilising existing resources and strengthening them by providing additional financial resources to these institutions. This may be implemented at three levels consisting of a Nodal Unit at the top level catchment like a premier technical institution, university, etc., intermediary level units like district laboratories, polytechnics, etc. and grass-root Ievel units like (+2) level education institutions, labs., etc. Activities relating to preliminary water testing, etc. could be carried out at the grass-root level itself and more complicated cases could be referred to higher levels in such a way that only focussed cases of complex nature and of value and utility at State level reach the nodal unit. The nodal units will be networked with the State headquarters (PHED). 100% funding, as per the approved norms, would be provided to the States for strengthening water quality monitoring facilities, based on projects received from the State Governments. Restructuring the State PHEDs with the required grant-in-aid support, as indicated in para 3.7, to bring in the much missed link up with the Health authorities will also be attempted as a part of institutionalising the monitoring system. Health Department officials will be increasingly involved in the surveillance activity.

A programme for water quality monitoring and surveillance system has been finalized in consultation with Ministry of Health and Family Welfare. The system will be implemented through a National Level, and State Level Referral Institutions. National Institute of Communicable Diseases (NICD) has given consent to act as National Level Water Quality Referral Institution. Manual on Catchment Area Approach has been finalised. Information on district level WQ Testing Laboratories, listing problems in their functioning and listing of alternative facilities is under compilation. Many States have already identified State Referral Institutes and matter is being pursued with the remaining.

Sustainability

This is an important Sub-Mission for the success of water supply schemes on a long-term basis. Central Ground Water Board (CGWB) and National Geophysical Research Institute (NGRI) have been engaged in the programme since the inception of the Mission. Further State Governments have been advised that up to 5 per cent of the funds released under ARWSP should be used for Sub-Mission—

- Reasons for taking up sustainability in drinking water sector:
- Fast depletion of groundwater level leading to quality problems like arsenic and fluorosis;
- Sources go dry due to deforestation, leading to reduced recharge of aquifers;
- Poor maintenance of the existing water supply systems;
- Non-participation of people in the operations and maintenance of the systems; and
- Neglect of traditional water management practices and systems.

In order to overcome these problems, Government of India aims to concentrate on: (a) control on over extraction of groundwater; (b) funds for repairs and rehabilitation; (c) emphasis on community participation; (d) promotion of water as a socio-economic good; and (e) stronger links with watershed development programmes.

Further, the following action has also been taken by the Department of Drinking Water Supply for source sustainability:

- Ministry of Urban Development has been requested to make rainwater-harvesting structures mandatory for urban constructions;
- Ministry of Water Resources has been requested to promote water-harvesting measures;
- All MPs have been requested to encourage/take up water harvesting schemes from their Local Area Development Fund;
- Technical Manual on Water Harvesting and Artificial Recharge has been finalized;
- A CD indicating different models of rainwater harvesting has been prepared and circulated to the States for wider dissemination;
- A model bill for Legislation by States to promote rainwater harvesting is being finalized in consultation with Ministry of Law; and
- For finding household, community and institution level rainwater harvesting structure, bankable schemes have been worked and are being finalised in consultation with the States.

Sector Reform

It has been realised that to strengthen the socio-economic conditions of rural India, mere administrative decentralisation or increased investment is not enough. The power of people's participation has been recognised and brought to therefore. Despite good investments, and improvement in the rural water supply and increased outlay by the Government, particularly in the last one decade, general satisfaction is rather limited at the community level. Earlier emphasis was laid on hand-pumps fitted to tube-wells and bore-wells had resulted in an impressive increase in the total rural water supply coverage. However, the availability of potable drinking water in rural areas, especially during the summer months is still not satisfactory. Though about lakh habitations are covered every year, the number of problem habitations has not declined proportionately. Hence, Government of India realized that sustainability of sources and system is key to people's satisfaction. Systems are falling idle and into disrepair. This is due to the perception of the rural people that water is a social right to be provided by the Government, free of cost.

The Government tried to drive home the principles that water is an economic and social good and should be treated as such. It should be managed at the lowest appropriate with users involved in the planning and implementation of projects. With this aim in view, Government of India has brought about policy changes by introducing reforms in the rural drinking water supply sector. ARWSP was improved in April 1999 to include proposals to mobilize community participation in rural water supply programmes, and 20 per cent of the annual outlay has been earmarked for providing funds for such projects.

This shift envisages demand-responsive approach, community participation and decentralisation of powers for implementing and operating drinking water supply schemes. To ensure people's participation, the Central Government is following three basic principles:

- Adoption of a demand-responsive and adaptable approach based on empowerment of villagers to ensure their full participation in the project through a decision-making role in the choice of scheme design control of finances and management arrangements;
- Shifting role of government from direct service delivery to that of planning policy formulation monitoring and evaluation and partial financial support; and
- Partial capital cost sharing either in cash or kind or both and 100 per cent responsibility of O & M by the users.

Accordingly, on a pilot basis, Sector Reform projects were sanctioned in 67 pilot districts across the country for implementation. Based on the demand-generated the total estimated project outlay of Sector Reform Pilot Projects was only Rs. 1328.38 crore. These pilot projects will enable the community to plan sanction partially fund, and implement, operate, maintain and replace Rural Water Supply Schemes of their choice. In order to instill a sense of ownership in the project, the community has to contribute at least 10% of the capital cost either in cash or kind (labour, land or material). The community will also shoulder the entire O & M cost.

In this new approach the government plays the role of a facilitator. Efforts are being made to create awareness through Information Education and Communication (IEC) amongst the people about the need for their effective participation in this programme. The community should be willing to be involved in the implementation of the water supply schemes for which they should have a feeling of ownership of the assets created. With the experience gained from Sector Reform pilot projects the reform process has now been extended to the entire country by launching Swajaldhara programme on 25.12.2002.

COMMUNITY PARTICIPATION

Background

Water is today perceived by the rural public as a social right to be provided free by the Government, rather than as a scarce resource which must be managed locally as a socio-economic good in order to ensure its effective use. This perception has been grown out of the fact that the present rural water supply systems are designed and executed by the Department/ Boards and, imposed on end-users. Demand preferences of the people are not taken into account while executing the schemes. In other words, rural water supply programme till now has been adopting a supply driven approach. Experience has shown that the present approach has led to the failure of a large number of water supply systems/schemes due to poor operation and maintenance.

Now that substantial investment has been made in the sector and huge infrastructure and systems built up, it is paramount that they are made functional to a great degree to achieve sustainability. There is a general recognition that a transformation from a target-based, supply-driven approach which pays little attention to the actual practices and/or preferences of the end users, to a demand-based approach where users get the service they want and are willing to pay for is urgently required. Implementation of a participatory demand-driven approach will ensure that the public obtain the level of service they desire and can afford to pay. Further, full cost recovery of operations and maintenance and replacement costs will ensure the financial viability and sustainability of the schemes. The conditions under which people would be willing to maintain and operate water supply schemes are:

- If they own the assets,
- If they have themselves installed the handpump, or being actively involved throughout,

- If they have been trained to do simple repairs,
- If they know the government will not maintain the asset,
- If they have sufficient funds for maintenance, and
- If they have to pay for O & M.

Hence, it is possible to institutionalise community-based rural drinking water supply programme if the Panchayati Raj Institutions/local communities are empowered to generate resources and are trained and equipped to plan, implement, use, maintain and replace water supply schemes themselves in coordination with the Government agencies/Private Sector/NGOs.

Swajaldhara

The Government of India has been emphasizing the need for taking up community-based rural water supply programmes and with this end in view a beginning was made in 1999 by sanctioning Sector Reform Pilot Projects on experimental basis. With the experience gained, the reforms initiatives in the rural drinking water supply sector has now been opened up throughout the country by launching the Swajaldhara programme on 25.12.2002. The key Principles of the programme are:

Principles of Swajaldhara

- adoption of demand responsive, adaptable approach along with community participation based on empowerment of villages to ensure their full participation in the project through a decision-making role in the choice of the drinking water scheme, planning, design, implementation, control of finances and management arrangements;
- full ownership of drinking water assets with appropriate level of panchayats;
- panchayats/communities to have the powers to plan, implement, operate, maintain and manage all Water Supply and Sanitation schemes;
- partial capital cost sharing either in cash or kind including labour or both, 100% responsibility of operation and maintenance by the users;
- an integrated service delivery mechanism;
- taking up conservation measures through rain water harvesting and ground water recharge systems for sustained drinking water supply; and
- shifting the role of Government from direct service delivery to that of planning, policy formulation, monitoring and evaluation, and partial financial support.

As per the guidelines issued in June 2003, Swajaldhara will have two Dharas. First Dhara (Swajaldhara-I) will be for a Gram Panchayat (GP) or a group of GPs or an intermediate panchayat (at Block/Tehsil level) and the second Dhara (Swajaldhara-II) will have a district as the project area.

Funds under Swajaldhara are now allocated to the States/UTs and the allocated amount is intimated to the States/UTs. The States/UTs make district-wise allocation and furnish the details to the Department of Drinking Water Supply. On receipt of such information, the funds are released directly to SWSM/DP/DWSM by Department of Drinking Water Supply.

Three Programmes of the Prime Minister

The Honourable Prime Minister in his Independence Day Address (15.8.2002) announced three programmes viz. Installation of one lakh hand pumps, providing drinking water facilities to one lakh Primary Schools and revival of one lakh traditional sources of water. Thereafter EFC memo for the programmes was prepared and the case was processed for Cabinet Approval. CCEA gave the approval in June 2003. The guidelines for implementation of the programmes have since been prepared and circulated to all the states. The programme is to be completed in two years, i.e. 2003-2005. The total cost involved is Rs. 800 crore have been made.[15]

Providing Community Water Supplies

To promote community health an easily accessible water supply should be available that provides sufficient safe water to meet community needs. Household water needs can be estimated by questioning community member about their daily water use. If this is not possible, a minimum water need can be circulated by assuming that the average person uses 25 litres per day for drinking, cooking and personal hygiene. More water will be needed for laundry, but this may be available from other sources such as rivers or ponds.

To ensure that the water is potable, either the water supply should be protected the water should be treated before use. Low-risk water supplies for drinking and other domestic uses can be provided to communities in many ways. Often, unprotected water sources, such as springs, traditional wells and ponds, can be improved and this may be preferable to constructing completely supplies. However, unprotected sources are open to contamination and pose a potential health risk. Community hygiene programmes should therefore promote the use of protected drinking-water sources.

Characteristics of Low-risk Water Sources

- The water source is fully enclosed or protected (capped) and no surface water can run directly into it.
- People do not step into the water while collecting it.

- Latrines are located as far away as possible from the water source and preferably not on higher ground. If there are community concerns about this, expert advice should be sought.
- Solid waste pits, animal excreta and other pollution sources are located as far as possible from the water source.
- There is no stagnant water within 5 metres of the water source.
- If wells are used, the collection buckets are kept clean and off the ground or a handpump is used.

When resources are limited, it may be necessary to decide whether greater emphasis should be placed on the quality of the water, or on its availability. Where sufficient safe water for all is not immediately available, intermediate steps should target the provision of larger quantities of lower-quality water. Deciding on an acceptable level of contamination is difficult and depends on the willingness of community members to pay increased costs for better water, as well as on their willingness to treat water within the home. If payment is required for water use, it must be affordable to the whole community. In only case, water with high levels of contamination, particularly with faces, should never be used. Local health officials should be consulted about the quality of water provided and the level of health risk.

Many rural water supply programmes aim to develop water sources that can be fully managed by users, with only limited additional support from local government. While this can make a sense of community ownership more achievable, it also require communities to make long-term commitments, such as maintenance of improved water sources, and even to contribute financial towards their construction This means that it is important to involve communities during all stages of development of the improved water sources, from initial planning and implementation to long-term management. Community members should be actively involved in selecting the type of water supply they receive and have access to information that allows them to make informed decisions. However, discussions must be balanced and should also consider what the supporting agency considers feasible, not simply what the community desires. On the other hand, solutions chosen solely by outside agencies are more likely to fail.

From the outset it is also essential that community members are fully aware of the short and long-term implications of their choices, for while it is relatively easy to build an improved water supply sustaining, it is often a major problem. For example, boreholes with hand pumps are often recommended to communities, but this technology requires relatively expensive maintenance, and access to spare parts and tools is essential. In one country, spares for handpumps were available only in the capital city, a two- or three-day journey for remote communities. As a result, the hand pumps were likely to fail in a very short time and the investment would have been wasted.[16]

K. Pandimurga Chinnan in his article, "No Fresh Water—No Future" in *Yojana*, Vol. 48, Feb. 2004 clearly indicated the essential steps for tackling water crises.

The main constraints that are faced in the water sector are inadequate trained personnel, inability to mobilise internal and external resources, inadequate project preparation, uncoordinated development approach, institutional weakness, technological shortcomings, poor quality of water resources itself, water losses through leakage intermittent services, haphazard garbage collection and disposal systems, inadequate drainage of surface run off, non-involvement of community in project planning development, operation and maintenance activities, etc. The following suggestions for solving the water crisis are given below:

- A large share of water to meet new demands must come by saving water from existing uses through comprehensive reform of water policy.
- New strategies for water development and management are urgently needed to avert severe national, regional and local water scarcities that will depress agricultural production, damage the environment and escalate water-related health problems.
- Major institutional policy and technological initiatives are required to ensure efficient socially equitable and environmentally suitable management of water resources.
- In facing the enormous challenge of meeting the requirements of water supply for domestic irrigation and industrial uses it is natural to expect that the R&D sector should play an important rule.
- Since a major portion of water resources are used in agriculture the farmer's co-operation is a must in the process of water management at all levels. An efficient irrigated cropping system also can sustain India's large and expanding population. During the years of poor monsoon, the farmer can go in for crops demanding less irrigation such as gram, barley and mustard during the rabi system.
- Attention should be paid by researchers and extension personnel in increasing the production per unit area/per unit of water in agriculture.
- Water management programmes should be implemented in a systematic way with integrated coordination of all relevant government departments at State and Central level. There is a need for revision of water legislation/ground water control regulation acts to maintain water table at a reasonable depth for sustainability.
- Clearcut water rights system is indispensable for the sustainability of our agriculture.

- Integrated watershed development actions have to be taken to use rainwater, soil water, ground water and run off water to increase production in rainfed areas.
- A data base should be created among all water boards and corporations for effective transfer of best practices.
- Immediate steps should be taken for drastic reduction of wastage of water in all sectors and protection of water sources from industrial pollution.
- The beneficiaries role should be modified from passive recipients to active participants in water conservation activities. As woman know better all the matters related to water, participation even from the selection of the site for water projects to the maintenance is important.
- Above all, a strong political will of government to frame appropriate water policy and equally important indomitable conscience of water users to utilize water judiciously are absolutely necessary for sustainable utilization of water.

CRITICAL APPRAISAL

I. Need of Sectoral Reforms

Provisions of high quality and sustainable drinking water services for all the citizens, particularly the rural poor, is critical to enhance the economic productivity of any nation. Supply of safe and quality drinking water to the rural community remains a significant issue in the governance in India. The traditional approach for implementing programmes for supply of drinking water in rural areas was top-driven, the result being that the community involvement was minimal and the problems of providing drinking water in all villages could not be addressed fully. What were needed, therefore, were reforms in this sector and a new programme, namely, Sector Reforms Project (SRP), was introduced by the Government of India.

The Rajiv Gandhi National Drinking Water Mission introduced the Sector Reforms Project in selected districts of the country in 1999. The Project envisaged community participation in creating and maintaining drinking water sources and sanitation facilities. It redefined the role of the government from being a "provider" to that of a "facilitation." The Project was to be driven by demand originating from within the community in contrast to the erstwhile practice of thrusting a source on the community without involving them.

Reforms Objectives

The Sector Reforms Project envisaged mission approach and emphasized creation of institutions that are relatively more independent and focused. The basic approach was "decentralized governance." Some of the objectives of Mission were:

(a) Increasing community participation and creating awareness the water is a resource, which has to be paid for.
(b) The operational and maintenance aspects of the source created would be the responsibility of the community.
(c) The community needs to consider imposition of user charges for maintenance of the source.
(d) Full freedom to the villagers in the selection of a water source and its implementation.
(e) Gender sensitive approach towards drinking water problems.
(f) Emphasis on quality of drinking water and reliability of the reforms.[17]

2. Sustainability

The Government has accorded the highest priority to rural drinking water for ensuring universal access as a part of policy framework to achieve the goal of reaching the unreached. Despite installation of more than 3.5 million hand-pumps and over 116 thousand piped water supply schemes, in many parts of the country, the people face water scarcity almost every year thereby meaning that our water supply systems are failing to sustain, despite huge investments. The examination of sustainability issues of drinking water supply as well as systems has, therefore, become imperative.

World Bank, in its Review Report (1998), has made the following findings of much interest on India's Water Resources Management Sector:

(i) Water is becoming an increasingly scarce resource in India, its finite and fragile water resources are depleting, yet it continues to be used inefficiently on a daily basis in all sectors, while various sectoral demands are growing rapidly.
(ii) The Current approach emphasizes development of water resources and construction of new infrastructure under a top-down, supply-oriented and fragmentary framework.
(iii) The present institutional arrangement in India, including central, state and local institutions, and both formal and informal structures, do not enable comprehensive water allocation, planning and management.
(iv) Existing organizations, furthermore, lack capacity in key management areas as well as effective mechanisms for implementation.
(v) Appropriate economic incentives for efficient water use and conservation are lacking on various levels, thereby impacting negatively on water provision and usage in these sub-sectors.
(vi) The absence of appropriate direct water pricing, and lack of adequate application of other economic and financial incentives at the sub-sector level has also served as an obstacle to the smooth transfer of water between sectors and states.

(vii) Supporting technological and informational systems, to enable effective planning and management of water are also weak.

(viii) The current situation in water service delivery in India is, in general, characterized by a vicious circle of inadequate financial allocations to the sector (particularly for O&M) and inefficient and bloated service institutions, which have led to poor quality and unreliable services, user dissatisfaction with their services, and an unwillingness of users to pay for those services. The inadequate resources generated by the sector due to low prices and user unwillingness to pay for services further undermine sector financial resources contributing to a perpetuation of the circle. The end result is a sector that has become unsustainable.

(ix) The vicious cycle of the drinking water sectors (both rural and urban) varies due to the varied and desegregated institutional structures that make up the RWSS and UWSS sub-sectors within the states in India.

Further, GWSS, Assessment Report—2000 identified similar sector constraints viz. (i) financial difficulties, (ii) institutional problems, (iii) inadequate human resources, (iv) lack of sector coordinating, (v) lack of political commitment, (vi) insufficient community involvement, (vii) inadequate O & M, (viii) poor water quality, (ix) insufficient information and communication and lack of hygiene education are equally applicable to India.

Acknowledging the necessity to involve local community or community-based organization for sustainability of the systems, the following necessary elements are identified:

- Community mobilization and capacity building.
- Community share in the capital investment.
- Community ownership and control.
- O & M and management by the community.
- Dependable water source to meet community needs.

Having achieved appreciable physical coverage of habitations with water supply system through the normal "supply-driven" and "cent per cent Government funded" programme, it is now, high time to reorient the programme-approach. The present water resources scenario is critical, especially the status of ground water exploration and availability is causing a lot of concern. Apart from the severe threat to sustainability of the sources due to indiscriminate ground water use, water quality problem has emerged as a major issue adding a new dimension. Taking into account all the constraints relating to proper management and conservation and protection of ground water source *vis-a-vis* the action needed to be taken at different levels, a multi-pronged integrated approach with a well conceived mix of professional, technical, administrative and legal aspects with a focus on "community-based-demand-responsive approach would pave the way for making sustainable rural drinking water supply in the country.

Providing safe and adequate water to the people is one of the several challenges that our country is encountering. The problem is particularly severe in rural areas. Government has been addressing this as a priority issue since the commencement of the first five year plan. An overview of the rural water sector indicates that still a lot needs to be done. The problem is multi-dimensional and area specific in nature. Several factors like increased urbanization, negligence of traditional water sources, poor water management, resource depletion due to over exploitation of existing resources, lack of co-ordination between departments and poor institutional set-up in addressing the problem have led to the severity of the problem over the years. It is important to understand the existing situation and the complexities in order to address the problem in the context of project design and implementation and factors affecting sustainability of Rural Water Supply (RWS) programmes. Sustainability through water conservation and water management is seen as the best option.[18]

3. Poor Availability

The annual per capita availability of freshwater in 1951 was 5,177 cubic meters, that declined to 1,869 cubic meters in 2001. It is likely to fall further to 1,341 cubic meters in 2025, and in 2050, it will be 1,140 cubic meters. It is generally presumed that if per capita level falls to 1,000 cubic meters, it could seriously affect the health and economic activity of the entire country. At this level, water crisis will be seen in 25 percent of India's geographical area, affecting 21 percent of the total population. Already, 5.5 percent of the country's geographical area and 7.6 percent of the population are facing acute water shortage, with availability less than 500 cubic meters.[19]

4. Poor Quality of Water

"Lack of reliable data, however, makes it difficult to appreciate the magnitude and impact of the crippling and incurable diseases like fluorosis and arsenical dermatitis. Fluoride contamination affects districts in 15 states and excess arsenic affects 8 districts of West Bengal. Fluoride levels are high in Andhra Pradesh, Gujarat, Haryana, Karnataka, Punjab, Rajasthan, Tamil Nadu and U.P. and iron levels are high in the north-eastern and eastern part of the country. Similarly, salinity is high in Gujarat, Haryana, Karnataka, Punjab, Rajasthan and Tamil Nadu. The number of quality affected habitations with excess fluoride/arsenic/salinity/iron, etc. is about 1.54 lakh.

Towards following up the quality problems as outlined, a large number of district water testing laboratories have been established in Panchayat Raj Engineering Department in different States under an elaborate action plan of the RGNDWM. In the present socio-economic condition, reaching the vast rural areas of the country with decentralized water quality-monitoring programme is an almost impossible task and the formidable problem is to bring water samples from the remote parts of the districts to the labs. Although samples may be collected and brought to the labs for examination, pooling them at one place for subsequent transportation is extremely difficult. Also, to collect and bring samples regularly for chemical/bacteriological quality assessment has also been not easy because of storage problems.

Therefore, there is need for introducing simple bacteriological quality assessment tests such as the H2S Strip test, which can be done by people themselves. Routine quality assessment (both chemical and bacteriological) can be done in the local field labs that may be established in schools or PHCs.

Research studies in 144 countries by Esrey and Nookes (1992-93) show that interventions like Safe Disposal of Excreta; Household and personal hygiene, Quantity and quality of water can make significant difference in the overall health and quality of life of people, especially that of children.

A Status of Water Quality

Providing safe water has been one the major focuses in the recent years with the increasing levels of contamination observed in the ground water sources. Under the National Drinking Water Mission by the Government of India, a submission on water quality monitoring is integrated as a part of drinking water supply programme. Water quality testing has been conducted in all the rural areas of the state. Major contaminants found are excess fluoride, iron, nitrate and hard water problems. 66 million people in India are estimated to be consuming groundwater with unsafe levels of flouride. Nearly 30 million people in the eastern states are estimated to be at risk of consuming water with higher than acceptable arsenic levels (Kolavalli and K.V. Raju, 2003).

Reasons for Quality Decline

Degradation in water quality has been observed due to various reasons. Contamination of ground water sources due to disposal of untreated sewage, disposal of industrial effluents without treatment, disuse of wells, extensive usage of chemical fertilizers. over exploitation of ground water and poor sanitation and hygiene.[20]

5. PRIs must be made Responsible for Water Supply

Lack of safe drinking water was been identified as major causes of sickness and death, especially of the children. Therefore, rigorous efforts need to be made by all to sustain, safeguard and provide drinking water to the people. Community has to be mobilized and sensitized to save India from a water scarce country to a water resource country. This is possible if we learn from our traditional water resource management and harvest the knowledge and transfer to the modern local self-governments—the Panchayati Raj Institutions (PRIs).

The three-tier Panchayati Raj Institutions (PRIs) are increasingly being recognized as the cornerstones of people-centered and self-reliant village development programmes. Therefore, PRIs can play a major role in managing and maintaining drinking water supply in the villages.

6. Harvesting Rain Water

Rain is the first form of water in the hydrological cycle. Rainwater offers advantages in water quality both for irrigation and domestic use. Rainwater is naturally soft (unlike well water), contains almost to dissolved minerals or salts, is free of chemical treatment and is relatively a reliable source of water for households. Rainwater collected and used on site can supplement or replace other modern sources of household water. Generally, the conservation/harvesting of water refers to collection and storage of rainwater and other allied activities aimed at prevention of losses through drain off, evaporation and seepage, etc. Rainwater conservation makes droughts less severe, rivers will have water throughout the year and soil holds greater level of moisture and consequently, there is increase in agricultural yield and thus economic conditions of rural poor is appreciably improved. All this leads to regeneration of vegetation and forests and thus overall environment of the region is positively impacted.[21]

In a document of Rajiv Gandhi National Drinking Water Mission, Deptt. of Rural Development, Ministry of Rural Areas and Employment, GOI, 1999, "Guidelines for Implementation of Rural Water Supply Programme."

HUMAN RESOURCE DEVELOPMENT

A National Human Resource Development Programme (NHRDP) has been launched by the Mission from 1994 based on the Human Resource Development Policy Document evolved jointly by the central and state governments. The NHRDP, *inter alia,* aims at training at least one grassroots level trainee through district level trainers who in turn may be trained at selected institutions forming the Indian Training Network (ITN). Under the NHRDP the States and UTs should set-up state level HRD cells for planning, designing, implementing, monitoring and evaluating an appropriate and need-based HRD programme. The HRD programme should aim at empowerment of Panchayati Raj Institutions/Local Bodies with the objective of enabling them to take up operation and maintenance activities related to rural water supply systems. It should also aim at capacity building of local communities by giving requisite training to mechanics/ health motivators/masons, etc. especially women to operate and maintain handpumps and the components of other water supply systems as well as to generate demand for adequate sanitation facilities. To train the grass-root trainees, the States/UTs may build be a pool of district level trainers who could be sent for training to the participating and key institutions. The States/UTs should establish state level HRD cells. The suggested staffing pattern, norm for equipment alongwith delineating of major functions already communicated vide D.O. Letter No. W.IIO38/1/94-HRD dated 15.9.94 and D.O. letter No. W-IIO43/1/95(Media) dated 31-12-1997.

INFORMATION EDUCATION AND COMMUNICATION

The emphasis of IEC programme should not be on hardware aspects but should be aimed at front loading software with the objective of generating a felt need which would result in an increased demand for safe drinking water and better sanitation facilities. Awareness on matters related to water borne diseases manifestations and symptoms should be created. The services of the State Publicity/Public Relations Department should be utilised to provide publicity to the rural water supply programme through mass media to disseminate information about the programme, highlighting the achievements, emphasis on use of safe water to overcome water borne diseases, etc. The importance of using safe water, using water as a socio-economic goods and the problems related to water quality in any specific area should be highlighted. This could be done by bringing to the public knowledge through appropriate methods like folk songs, folk drama, documentary films, pamphlets, brochures and other local means suited to the area. Publicity should also be given in the local newspapers about the action plan for coverage of habitations actually covered on year to year basis with other details like the type of schemes provided, the service level, delivery system, agency responsible for operation and maintenance, etc. 100%.

MONITORING AND INVESTIGATION UNITS

The Government of India has been providing assistance to the States to establish and continue special investigation divisions from the Fourth Five Year Plan to carry out investigation, planning and feasibility study of the schemes. The special monitoring cell and investigation unit at the State headquarters should be headed by an officer suitably qualified and of suitable level for monitoring and investigation with necessary supporting staff. Monitoring unit shall be responsible for collecting information from the executing agencies through prescribed reports and returns (Progress Monitoring System), maintenance of the data and timely submission of the prescribed reports and returns to the Central Government by due dates. The unit shall also be responsible for monitoring at field level of aspects of quality of water, adequacy of service and other related qualitative aspects of the programme. The Unit shall also maintain water quality data in coordination with the concerned Department, Central/State Ground Water Board; details of different technologies developed by institutions for tackling different problems and to provide the same to the field level executing agencies. The Monitoring and Investigation Units should also have technical posts of hydrologists, geophysicist, computer specialists with data entry operators, etc. A Quality Control Unit should be an integral part of M&I Units and should work in coordination with the R&D Cell. This unit will be responsible for controlling/regulating the quality of construction works in water supply schemes and will ensure practical application of latest technologies in the field. The expenditure will be borne by the Central Government and the State Governments on a 50:50 basis.

MONITORING AND EVALUATION

Central Government takes up monitoring and evaluation studies through reputed organisations/institutions from time to time. The State Governments may also take up similar monitoring and evaluation studies on the implementation of the rural water supply programme. 100% financial assistance will be provided by the Centre to the States for taking up such evaluation studies with prior approval of the Mission. The reports of these studies should be made available to the Mission and immediate collective action should be initiated as a follow up to improve the quality of programme implementation.

MANAGEMENT INFORMATION SYSTEM

For effective planning, monitoring and implementation of various schemes under different programme, Information Technology (IT) based Management Information System provides for the following:

(i) Maintenance of micro-level status of water supply to ensure planning and monitoring based on micro-level data,

(ii) Assistance for computer facilities up to division level in phases to ensure latest technology for processing and storing data and its communication from one office to another through NICNET,

(iii) Assistance for conducting training programmes; and

(iv) Development of customised software for enabling States/UTs to fully utilise for power of computer systems for planning, monitoring and implementation of various activities in the sector. 100% Central assistance will be provided for all MIS activities including training during the plan period.

RESEARCH AND DEVELOPMENT

To strengthen the R&D facilities in the concerned Departments in various States, State Governments are encouraged to establish R&D cells with adequate manpower and infrastructure. R&D Cells are required to remain in touch with premier technical institutions within the State. The network of technical institutions may follow the guidelines issued by the Mission from time to time for effective implementation of the rural water supply programme. R&D Cells are also required to be in constant touch with the Monitoring and Investigation Divisions and the Monitoring and Evaluation Study Reports for initiating appropriate follow up action. The R&D Cell should keep in constant touch with the documentation and information centre of the Mission and visit at the Mission's web site. The Mission will provide necessary assistance to the States.

PROVISION OF DRINKING WATER IN RURAL SCHOOLS

All the States are required to compile data regarding district-wise rural schools in existence and number of them having drinking water facilities. The remaining rural schools and Anganwadis are to be provided with drinking water facilities. A part of this work will be accomplished through the funds provided by Tenth Finance Commission and the rest would have to be covered under the rural water supply programme, in addition to the work of covering NC and PC habitations. Expenditure for this purpose would also be shared by the Central and State Governments on 50:50 basis from the funds allocated for ARWSP. States would be required to fix target for coverage of rural schools on an yearly basis and intimate its achievement to the Mission on monthly basis along with the progress reports being submitted to intimate coverage of NC and PC habitations. This activity is to be carried out in coordination with NEP, DPEP, DWCRA, Anganwadis, Department of Social Welfare and Department of Education. All the rural schools should be covered with drinking water facilities by the end of the 9th Plan.

CONCLUSION

Organizing IEC Campaign in a Village Panchayat

The Information, Education and Communication (IEC) campaign is aimed at creating awareness in the community about safe drinking water and its relationship with their health, with a view to changing their behaviour to use, maintain, protect and sustain the assets created for safe water supply. Therefore, the PRIs can play a key role in changing the attitude of the users of water supply and sanitation programme being implemented by Village water and sanitation committee/District water and sanitation Mission. The Village Panchayat should be concerned more with the village level activities. Hence, the members should be familiar with the objectives of the campaign with a focus on:

- To put an end to indiscriminate open defecation by creating a felt need among households for construction of individual latrines.
- To create awareness about the need for safe disposal of children's excreta.
- To create awareness about the collection, storage, handling and consumption of safe drinking water.

- To create awareness in the community about sanitary aspects of water supply, including keeping water source pollution free, safe disposal of waste water and solid waste.
- To create a sense of participation in the community so that the people are involved in the water and sanitation programme from the pre-planning stage to execution of and evaluation.
- To create a sense of competitiveness among individuals and families on sanitation through social marketing.
- To create a sense of willingness to pay for the creation of common and household assets and their operation and maintenance.
- To promote low-cost location specific appropriate technologies.
- To facilitate participatory planning and development through PRIs.

After the formation of the VWSC, the Village Panchayat must take initiative to organise campaigns to create awareness about the importance of safe water supply and sanitation. Since a VWSC member is link person between the village community and DWSM/DWSC/CBOs/NGOs it has an important role to play as an initiator and facilitator. The PAI/VWSC can organize following activities to create demand from the people for better water supply and sanitation facilities.

- The PRIs are expected to organise or to help community to organize the following with the active participation of the panchayat members.
- Organize Jathas/prabhat pheris in the village.
- Contact local folk artists to include messages of hygiene practices.
- Contact schoolteachers to promote school sanitation.
- Actively participate in the WATSAN Committee meetings.
- Provide feedback to the Gram Sabha and the Panchayat Samiti.[22]

The strategies of Rural Water Supply Programme hitherto adopted revolve around the basic premise that provision of safe drinking water is the responsibility of the Government. Increased outlay by the Government, particularly in the last one decade and, a change in technology focus to handpumps fitted on the tube wells and bore wells, had resulted in an impressive increase in the total rural water supply coverage. However, the availability of potable drinking water in rural areas, especially during the summer months, is still not satisfactory. Eventhough about 1 lakh habitations are covered every year, the number of problem habitations has not declined proportionately.

To focus in future would be:

- To ensure coverage of all rural habitations especially to reach the unreached with access to safe drinking water.

- To ensure sustainability of the systems and sources.
- To preserve quality of water by institutionalising water quality monitoring and surveillance through a Catchment Area approach.

Notes and References

1. WHO: Abel Wolman's Charter, *World Health*, January 1977, p. 17.
2. WWF, UNICEF: Fresh Water for India's Children and Nature, April 1998, pp. 1-2.
3. WHO: Nikolai P. Napalkov, Editorial, *World Health*, July-August 1992, p. 3.
4. WHO: Richard Helmer, News from the Waterfront, *World Health*, July-August 1992, p. 4.
5. WHO: Dennis B. Warner and Louis Laugeri, The Legacy of Water Decade, *World Health*, July-August 1992, p. 7.
6. WHO: Bruce M.W. Fisher, We must not lose hope, *World Health*, July-August 1992, p. 17.
7. WHO: Willy Brandt, *World Health*, August-September 1982, p. 3.
8. WHO: David Donaldson, Frank A. Butrico and Guillermo Davila, The Americans Attainable Goals, *World Health*, August-Sept. 1980, p. 25.
9. WHO: "Million in Need", *World Health*, December 1986, p. 4.
10. WHO: *World Health*, Water is Development, December 1986, p. 16.
11. IGNOU: "Public Health and Hygiene", Environmental Sanitation and Safety, p. 27.
12. IGNOU: "Public Health and Hygiene", Environmental Sanitation and Safety, p. 30.
13. IGNOU: "Public Health and Hygiene", Environmental Sanitation and Safety, p. 36.
14. India 2004, Ministry of Information and Broadcasting, GOI, New Delhi, p. 673.
15. GOI, Ministry of Rural Development, Annual Report, 2004-05, New Delhi, pp. 121-30.
16. Healthy Village—A Guide for Communities and Community Health Workers, WHO, pp. 19-21.
17. Ashutosh Jindal, "Community Participation in Drinking Water supply", *Kurukshetra*, March 2004, pp. 36-37.
18. Dinesh Chand, Towards Sustainable Rural Water Supply, *Kurukshetra*, March 2004, p. 3.
19. *Kurukshetra*, October 2003, p. 10.
20. K.V. Raju and S. Manasi, "Water For Rural Areas", *Kurukshetra*, October 2003, p. 33.
21. V.P. Rajvedi, "Rainwater Harvesting", *Kurukshetra*, October 2003, p. 63.
22. Dr. S.Ponnuraj, "Role of Panchayati Raj Institutions in Drinking Water Supply", *Kurukeshtra*, Oct. 2003, pp. 21-22.

CHAPTER 3

HEALTH EDUCATION FOR RURAL SANITATION

The concept of sanitation was earlier limited to disposal of human excreta by cess pools, open ditches, pit latrines, bucket system, etc. Today it connotes a comprehensive concept, which includes liquid and solid waste disposal; food hygiene; personal, domestic as well as environment hygiene.

—*Author*

Health Education for Rural Sanitation

It is well known that a direct relationship exists between water, sanitation and health. Consumption of unsafe drinking water, improper disposal of human excreta and lack of personal and food hygiene have been the major causes of many diseases in developing countries, including India. High Infant Mortality Rate (IMR) is also attributed largely to poor sanitation. It was in this context that Centrally Sponsored Rural Sanitation Programme (CSRP) was launched in 1986.

To keep the household and village environment clean and to reduce health risks, solid waste (refuse) should be disposed of properly. Untreated refuse is unsightly and smelly and degrades both the quality of the environment and the quality of life in the community. It also provides a breeding ground for disease vectors, such as mosquitoes, flies and rats. If waste is not properly disposed of, animals can bring it close to the home and children can come into contact with disease vectors and pathogens. To be effective, solid waste disposal programmes require action at both household and community levels—if only a few households dispose of waste properly, the village environment may remain dirty and contaminated. Community members should decide how important solid waste management is and determine the best ways to achieve waste-management goals.[1]

Sanitation has become a yardstick of socio-cultural development of a nation. It is an important health index of any developing country. Since health and sanitation has an important bearing on the productivity, sanitation also has a correlation with economic progress of a country.[2]

In the Johannesburg Earth Summit it has been agreed to halve, by the year 2015 the proportion of people who do not have access to basic sanitation, which would include action at all levels to develop and implement efficient household sanitation systems, improve sanitation in public institutions, especially schools, promote affordable and socially and culturally acceptable technologies and practices, promote safe hygiene practices and integrate sanitation into water resources management strategies.

Sanitation is a broad term that includes disposal of human excreta, wastewater, solid wastes, domestic and personal hygiene, etc. Human excreta is the cause of many enteric diseases such as cholera, diarrhoea, dysentery, typhoid, infectious hepatitis, and those based on worm infestation, etc. Studies reveal that over 50 infections can be transmitted from diseased person to healthy ones by various direct/indirect routes from human excreta that cause nearly 80% of sickness in developing countries.

The health implications of this state of affairs as said are appalling. Improved hygiene and sanitation help reduce sickness from diarrohoea considerably. Intestinal worms infect about 10% of the population of developing countries that can be controlled through better sanitation, hygiene and water supply. As per the WHO report globally 200 million people are infected with schistosomiasis, of whom 20 million suffer seriously. Basic sanitation facilities reduce the disease by up to 77%. Sanitation facilities help check transmission of many faecal oral disease by preventing human excreta contamination of water and soil.[3]

Objectives

The objectives of the RCRSP is to bring about an improvement in the general quality of life in the rural areas. The policy changes envisaged shall help achieve the objective by:

(a) Accrelerating coverage of rural population.
(b) Generating felt need through awareness creation and health education.
(c) Covering schools in rural areas with sanitation facilities.
(d) Encouraging suitable cost effective and appropriate technologies.
(e) Consequently bringing about a reduction in the incidence of water and sanitation-related diseases (as evinced by fall in the infant/child mortality rates and incidence of diarrhoeal diseases.)

Strategy

The programme will be implemented as community led and people centred. A demand driven approach will be adopted with increased stress on awareness building and meeting the demand with alternate delivery mechanisms. Subsidy for individual units will be progressively reduced and phased out. Rural school sanitation will be introduced as a major component and entry point for wider acceptance of sanitation by the rural masses.

Some of the major elements of the Programme include:

CHART 3.1

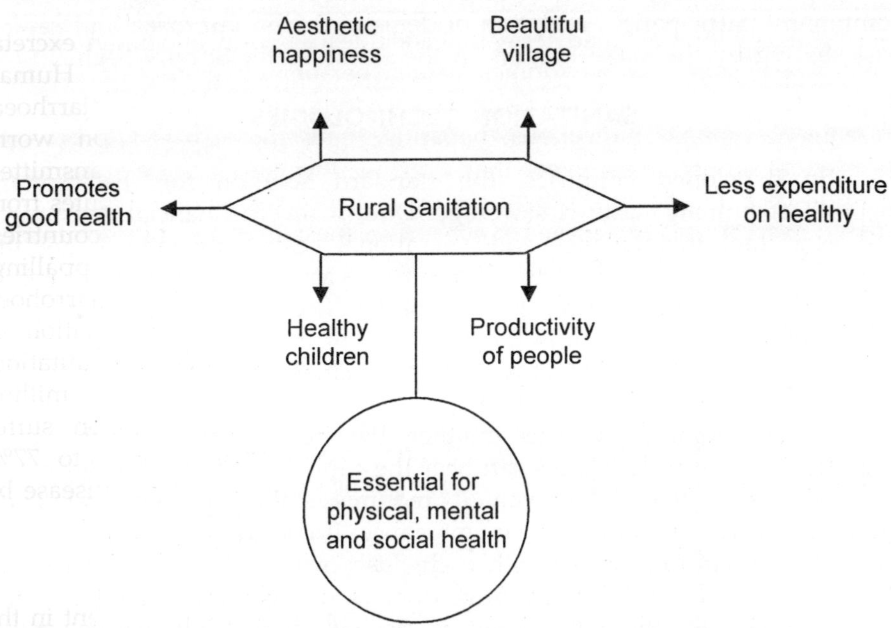

(i) Shift from a high subsidy to a low subsidy regime.
(ii) Greater household involvement (Demand Driven Approach).
(iii) Technology improvisations according to customer preferences and location specific.
(iv) Development of back-up services—Central Sanitaryware, Production Centres (PCs) at District/Block levels, Rural Sanitary Marts (RSMs) as retail outlets, Trained Masons.
(v) Stress on software-intensive IEC Campaign-closer liaison with Prasar Bharti and other media.
(vi) Emphasis on School Sanitation.
(vii) Seek Institutional Finances for latrine units, production centres and rural sanitary marts.
(viii) Dovetail funds from other Government of India (GOI)/State programmes aimed for rural development (IRDP, IAY, JRY, etc.) to supplement the efforts being made under the TSCs.
(ix) Involve Co-operatives, Women Groups (such as DWCRA, RMK, etc.), Self Help Groups, NGOs, etc.

It has been envisaged that during the 9th Plan, the PHEDs shall be transformed into multi-disciplinary organisations. Their professional capabilities shall have to be enhanced so as to handle the IEC, HRD and MIS activities, etc., as well. Water and Sanitation Missions will be constituted at the State and District levels, to institutionalise community-based water and sanitation programmes. These Missions shall be responsible for implementing the Total Sanitation Campaigns (TSC) as well as implementation of the reforms measures—involving increased community participation, adoption of demand driven approach and capital cost sharing by the stake holders in the Rural Water Supply Sector. [4]

SANITATION TECHNOLOGIES

In developed countries, the standard solution for the sanitary disposal of human waste is sewerage. Due to severe financial constraints and exorbitant maintenance and operational costs, sewerage is not the answer to solve the problem of human waste management in India. Sewerage was first introduced in the world in London in 1850, followed by New York in 1860. Calcutta in India was the next city in the world to have this privilege in 1870, yet only 232 town cities of 4,700 in India have sewerage coverage but too partially.

In developing countries neither the government nor the local authorities or the beneficiaries can bear the capital or the maintenance cost of sewerage system. Moreover, it requires skilled person and good management for operation and maintenance. It consumes a lot of water to clean the human excreta, so with each flush over 10 litres of clean water goes down the drain. We build huge dams and irrigation systems to bring waster, which on the other hand is flushed down, into an expensive sewage system, all to end up polluting our rivers and ponds. Most of our rivers get choked up because of the domestic sewage load from the cities. This has lead to heavy pollution of rivers and urban groundwater aquifers.

Sewerage systems are built to protect public health but badly managed sewers can become a serious health hazard. There can be serious outbreaks of waterborne diseases from:

I. River pollution because of sewage outfalls.
II. Ground water contamination because of leaky sewer lines.
III. Contamination of piped water supply systems because of leaky sewer lines leading to infiltration of pathogens into drinking water pipelines.[5]

Water Supply and Sanitation are very important components of urban infrastructure services for improvement of quality of life and health standard of human habitat. While there has been perceptible improvement in access to drinking water, the provision of sanitation facilities has not received adequate attention. The status of sanitation in urban areas is even worse than the water supply scenario. Sewerage systems are not yet accessible to 54 per cent of the urban population and refuse collection and disposal has yet to reach 28 per cent of the population. Out of the more than 3500 urban areas in India only 200 towns have a sewerage system. However, even these 200 sewerage systems cover only parts of the urban areas they serve. Also the systems are in many cases old and need repairs, up-gradation rehabilitation and replacement. Toilets are not available for close to 26 per cent of the urban population. In many areas open defecation is still prevalent and it is one of the main cause for many diseases. The provision of proper sanitation in rural/urban areas will ensure personal hygiene and community health. While sewerage systems are prohibitively expensive, the twin pit latrine system based on UNDP design has become more popular and acceptable low cost on site disposal system.[6]

Low cost sanitation is rightly seen as a most appropriate solution to the dehumanizing practice of carrying night soil. The problem of manual scavenging is not unidimensional but a multi-dimensional one because it involves social, economical, political, financial, humanitarian and cultural aspects. In order to achieve the goal of eradicating manual scavenging during the 10th Five Year Plan a concerted effort is needed at levels. Awareness campaign at National level for the hygiene and human dignity can change the mindset and help in 11 abolition of dry units and open defecation. The acceptability and adaptability of the technology will not only improve the sanitation situation in the country but also put an end to the social stigma on the nation.[7]

Community management of WES services and the adoption of good hygiene practice are critical to achieving sustainable improvements in people's live. Encouraging health-promoting attitudes and behaviours plays a major role in these efforts. At the community level, for example, people's willingness to take on new responsibility and costs will make it more likely that communities will manage their water systems and not depend solely on outside assistance. Within the household, clean water washing and other practices are not routinely followed, the promised health benefits do not materialize. Likewise, access to latrines does not ensure that people will use and maintain them. Behaviours related to sanitation are particularly difficult to both understand and change. The private nature of sanitation undoubtedly accounts for some of this difficulty, as does the fact that sanitary control and disposals of excreta may not be viewed as a problem in villages surrounded by substantial open space.

In recent years, UNICEF and its partners have experimented with new ways to engage people in planning for, using and maintaining WES services, which encompass:

- Community participation,
- Gender considerations,
- Intersectoral convergence, such as linking sanitation with broader health and economic concerns.

These three elements merge in new strategies and approaches. For are to participate productively in programmes, they must first understand how gender considerations affect their roles and responsibilities. Likewise, linking sanitation with everyday concerns, such as diarrhoeal disease control, can increase community involvement.[8]

LESSONS FROM INDIA

The WES programme in India yields lessons that other countries may find useful in adapting aspects of the programme to their own conditions and needs:

1. Long-term commitment and partnerships produce results: UNICEF has supported India's WES programme for several decades, coordinating its activities closely with the Government, NGGs and the private sector. The depth of this support contributes to UNICEF's credibility and access in India.
2. An external agency such as UNICEF has greater freedom than a government does to test new approaches: This relative freedom suggests an important role for UNICEF in WES and in other sectors to develop and test new approaches and build capacity among its partners.
3. Partnerships can maximize results, but they must be closely coordinated and mutually advantageous for each participant. Partners should build on each other's capabilities, strengths and comparative advantages to have greatest impact.
4. Local realities must be taken into consideration in implementing policies made by the central government: To be effective, a national policy framework must be shaped by local realties, including behaviours and values.
5. It is crucial to develop technology (pumps and other hardware) suited to local conditions, especially where water is scarce: To ensure access to clean drinking water for all children, it is especially important to create technical solutions that are feasible and sustainable.
6. A balance must be maintained between technology and the social/and behavioural aspects of WES services: Technological improvements must be accompanied by changes in behaviours and a focus on how communities use and maintain systems if lasting improvements are to be made in people's lives.
7. Gender and poverty need priority attention when programmes are planned, implemented and monitored: These issues are key to community participation, education, training and other aspects of WES.
8. Cost data are needed for comprehensive and effective analyses: These data help programmes improve decision-making, especially in an era of limited resources and need for greater accountability.
9. Convergence among sectors can maximize impact in a community: Efforts to improve people's lives have greatest impact when they combine health, education, nutrition, water and environmental sanitation. For example, improving

sanitation and water facilities in schools will help increase enrolment and retention, especially of girls.

10. Going to scale too quickly has adverse repercussions: It is tempting to expand on pilot projects that seem successful. However, it is better to move slowly to ensure that promising approaches are replicable on a larger scale.[9]

CENTRAL RURAL SANITATION PROGRAMME

Rural Sanitation is a State subject. The efforts of the States are supplemented by the Central Government through technical and financial assistance under the Central Rural Sanitation Programme (CRSP). The programme was launched in 1986 with the objective of improving the quality of life of rural people and provide privacy and dignity of women. The concept of sanitation was expanded in 1993 to include personal hygiene, home sanitation, safe water, garbage and excreta disposal and waste water sanitary toilets for households below the poverty-line (BPL), conversion of dry latrines to water-pour flush toilets, construction of village sanitary complexes for women, setting up of sanitary marts, intensive campaign for awareness creation and health education, etc.

Keeping in view the experiences of the Central Government, State Governments, NGGs and other implementing agencies and the recommendations of the Second National Seminar on Rural Sanitation the strategy for the Ninth Plan was revised and the programme was restructured with effect from 1 April, 1999. The restructured programme moves away from the principle of state-wise allocation of funds primarily based on poverty criteria to a demand-driven approach in a phased manner. Total Sanitation Campaign (TSC) ahs been introduced and the allocation based programme was phased out by 31 March, 2002. The TSC is community-led and people centred. There will be a shift from a high-subsidy to a low-subsidy regime. The TSC approach emphasizes the awareness building component and meets the demand through alternate delivery mechanism. School sanitation has been introduced as a major component and as an entry point encouraging wider acceptance of sanitation among rural masses. The States/UTs are required to formulate project proposals under the TSC in order to claim Central Government assistance.

Under the TSC, so far 179 projects in 27 States/UTs have been sanctioned with the total project outlay of about Rs. 1,952 crore. The Central, State and Beneficiary/Panchayat contribution are about Rs. 1,180 crore, Rs. 408 crore and Rs. 364 crore respectively. The components sanctioned in the 179 projects are (a) construction of 165 lakh individual household latrines; (b) 1.64 lakh toilets for schools; (c) 20,000 sanitary complexes for women; (d) 8,024 toilets for Balwadis/Anganwadis, and (e) 1549 rural sanitary marts/production centres. Besides, funds have been earmarked for start up activities, Information, Education and Communication (IEC) and administrative charges.

The total number of household toilets constructed upto 2001-02 are 98,65,980 (provisional)

The Working Group constituted by the Planning Commission has recommended and outlay of Rs. 3,663 crore for Rural Sanitation in the Tenth Five-Year Plan. During 2002-03, Rs. 165 crore have been provided for the Programme, of which Rs. 16.50 crore is earmarked for North-Eastern States.[10]

RURAL SANITATION

In the rural India, the low levels of household sanitation (only about 22 percent of households are estimated to have toilet facilities as per Census 2001) and the haphazard provision of environmental sanitation infrastructure (e.g. drainage) occasioned by un-coordinated planning and inadequate finances render the settlements in the villages as potential sites for a host of diseases like Schistosomiasis, Dysentry, Japanese Encephalitis, Malaria, Dengue fever and Trachoma. Indirect loss of working days due to repeated episodes of these and other diseases such as asthma, tuberculosis, jaundice, results in huge economic loss. About 1,00,000 usually suffer from morbidity in terms of asthma. tuberculosis, jaundice, and malaria by age and sex in rural India.

The practice of open defecation in India is borne out of a combination of factors—the most prominent of them being the traditional behavioural pattern and lack of awareness of the people about the associated health hazards. In certain cases, lack of access to affordable and appropriate technology is also one of the constraints.

The Central Rural Sanitation Programme (CRSP) was launched in 1986 in the Ministry of Rural Development with the objective of improving the quality of life of rural people and to provide privacy and dignity to the women. The programme provided 100 percent subsidy for construction of sanitary latrines for Scheduled Castes, Scheduled Tribes and landless labourers and subsidy as per the prevailing rdtes in the States for the general public.

The programme was supply driven. Highly subsidized and gave emphasis for a single construction model. Based on the feedback from various agencies, the programme was revised in March 1991 incorporating some changes in the subsidy pattern and also included village sanitation as one component. Based on the recommendation of the National Seminar on Rural Sanitation in September 1992 the programme was again revised. The revised programme aimed at an integrated approach of rural sanitation. Since its inception and up to the end of the 9th Plan, 94.5 lakh latrines were constructed for rural households under the CRSP as well as corresponding State MNP. The total investment made has been Rs. 621 crore under the CRSP and Rs. 1045 crore under the State sector MNP. This has led to only a marginal increase in the rural sanitation coverage. On an average Annual increase in the rural sanitation coverage has been only 1 percent, which was insignificant.

The CRSP was restructured in 1999 with a provision for allocation based component of CRSP to be phased out by the end of the 9th Plan, i.e. 2001-02. The Total Sanitation Campaign (TSC) under restructured CRSP was launched with effect from 1.4.1999 following a community led and people centered approach. TSC moves away from the principle of state-wise allocation, primarily based on poverty criterion to a "demand-driven" approach. The programme gives emphasis on Information, Education and Communication (IEC) for demand generation for sanitation facilities. It also gives emphasis on school sanitation and hygiene education for changing the behaviour of the people from the younger age itself.

The components of TSC include start-up activities, IEC, Individual house hold latrines, community sanitary complex, school sanitation and hygiene education, Anganwadi toilets, Alternate delivery mechanism in the form of Rural Sanitary Marts and Production centers and administrative charges.

VARIOUS COMPONENTS OF TSC

Start-up Activities

The start up activities include the setting up of Water and Sanitation Missions in the States/UTs and the respective districts. Conducting of preliminary surveys (after a phase of IEC, has been carried out) to assess the demand and thereafter preparation of the District TSC project proposals for seeking Government of India assistance. Upto 5% of the total TSC project cost has been earmarked for the above and shall be 100% funded by the GOI.

IEC Activities

With the setting up of the Missions in the Districts, the NGOs/ Alternative Mechanisms and their volunteers shall start the process of information dissemination related to various aspects of the water and sanitation sector, create awareness to the extent that he/she motivates them to construct their own latrines and soakage pits for solid and liquid waste disposal. The willingness of the people to construct latrines is translated/ interpreted as demand generated. The motivator shall be given his/her incentive from the funds earmarked for IEC. The incentive shall be based on his/her performance, i.e. in terms of motivating the people to the extent that they construct the latrine and soakage pits. At least 15% of the total TSC project cost has been earmarked for the above and the funds in a ratio of 80:20 will be provided by the GOI (80%) and the State (20%), respectively.

Alternate Delivery Mechanism [Central Production Centres (PCs)/RSMs]

The IEC activities shall help generate demand. The preliminary survey thereafter shall reveal the quantity of demand based on which the supply of related goods (squatting; slabs/plates with water seal pans, pipes, etc.) shall be selected and ensured, keeping in view the cost factor (predetermined).

The Central Production Centres at the district/block level (depending upon quantity of demand and the spatial concentration of demand) shall be established. The PCs could be opened and operated by NGOs/ Panchayats. Up to 5% (subject to a maximum of Rs. 35.00 lakh) of the total TSC project cost has been earmarked for establishing PCs with a notional earmarking of Rs. 3.5 lakh per PC/RSM envisaged.

Provision of Hardware

As stated earlier, for the purpose of this scheme, a duly completed household sanitary latrine shall comprise of a Basic Low Cost Unit (BLCU) without the super structure (Cost of superstructure shall be borne by the beneficiary). As per the "Technological Options for Implementation of the Rural Sanitation Programme" Handbook, the simplest and least expensive BLCU on an average is estimated to cost between Rs. 625 and Rs. 1000. Maximum subsidy shall be available for the least expensive sanitary latrine, i.e. costing upto Rs. 625. Units with the higher cost (i.e. between Rs. 625 to Rs. 1000) shall be eligible for a lower subsidy.

The financing pattern (subsidy) for the BLCU's is given in Table below:

Sl. No.	*BLCU Cost (Rs.)*	*Contribution (as %age) to the cost*		
		GOI	*State*	*Beneficiary*
1.	Upto Rs. 625	Upto 60%	20%	20%
2.	Between Rs. 625 and Rs. 1000	Up to 30%	30%	40%
3.	>Rs. 1000	Nil	—	—

The BLCUs costing upto Rs. 625 shall be open to 80% subsidy, to be shared between the GOI (60%) and the State Government (20%) and shall not exceed Rs. 500 (i.e. Rs. 375 GOI share and Rs. 125 state share in a BLCU costing Rs. 625. The beneficiary is expected to make a minimum contribution of 20% to the BLCU cost.

The BLCUs costing between Rs: 625 and Rs. 1000 shall attract a subsidy of 60% to be shared equally between the GOI (30%) and the State Government (30%), subject to a maximum of Rs. 500 the beneficiary is expected to make a minimum contribution of 40% to the BLCU cost.

No subsidy will be provided to beneficiaries opting for BLCUs costing more than Rs. 1000. The extent of GOI participation will be fixed. However, states are free to generate greater beneficiary participation with a view to reduce their financial liability and ensure greater sustainability. States/UTs wishing to adopt a single flat rate of subsidy, will be free to do so, subject to a maximum of Rs. 500 inclusive of both GOI and State shares.

SUBSIDY DISBURSEMENT

Subsidy disbursement shall be subject to close supervision and monitoring and linked with the construction activity so as to ensure sincere and full involvement of the community, thereby ensuring the sustainability of campaign. The construction (assuming that the beneficiaries opt between the two models viz. (i) single pit brick lined, and (ii) single offset pit (brick lined) with provision for (2nd pit) linked subsidy disbursement shall be effected in the manner as under:

- Once the institutional framework for implementing the TSC in the State/UT has been set-up, the IEC activities shall be initiated through the NGOs/Alternative Mechanisms networking. The preliminary survey shall follow wherein a demand (for sanitary latrines) estimation shall be made which shall be the basic input of a TSC project proposal. The demand estimation shall be based on the number of sites of 3×3 metre suitably raised/ developed by the beneficiaries as a part of their contribution in kind. It must also be ensured that the site is at least 3 metres away from the Drinking water source. The final beneficiary list shall be drawn by the motivator after physical verification of the sites which will bear countersignatures of the beneficiaries and one villager attesting to each as witness. Based on this list the TSC project proposal shall be prepared. Wherever the beneficiaries are not in a position to provide a 3×3 mtr space, provision for a Community latrine may be considered.
- With the acceptance of the TSC proposal, submitted for the district, the PCs shall be established. Once the PCs are established and production commences (at rates approved by the District Water and Sanitation Committee) the list shall be sent to the PCs in the respective areas for supply of goods and services. The PC shall have its schedule of production, delivery and construction at site (TSC village) by its trained masons. The payment for the goods (bricks, cement, mortar, squatting plate, pit cover, pipe, etc.) and services shall be made to the PC directly from the District Mission. The amount shall exclude that remaining portion of the total contribution of (20% or 40%) which the beneficiary is to make. This amount shall be collected directly from the beneficiary by the skilled mason on behalf of the PC. The motivator shall oversee, assist and supervise all through. The payment to the PC shall be effected after the motivator physically verifies the construction work. The District Water and Sanitation Committee will take the help of field level Government/PRI functionaries for verification. The duly filled and signed schedule of completion shall be sent to the District Mission by the NGOs/Alternative mechanisms concerned.

- Based on the verified schedule (shall include verification of completion of construction work of soakage pits) the District Mission shall release the NGO motivator's incentive.
- A TSC village shall be rewarded if it completes the works/ activities planned in the scheduled manner/time. The reward amount may be fixed by the District Water and Sanitation Mission and may be given to the village panchayat, preferably, in kind.

SCHOOL SANITATION (HARDWARE AND SUPPORT SERVICES)

Children are more receptive to new ideas and therefore the school is the best suitable institution in changing the conditioned habits of people from open defecation to the use of lavatory through motivation and education. The experience gained by children through use of toilets in school and sanitation education imparted by teachers would definitely be carried home and passed on to parents, in most cases who do not have formal education. This has long heen neglected. The Tenth Finance Commission had also drawn attention to this issue and has provided funds for toilet facilities in primary and upper primary schools. This initiative needs to be supported and pushed further.

School sanitation shall form an integral part of every TSC. Accordingly, it is proposed to allow the construction of toilets in schools. The school authorities and Parents Teacher Association (PTA) shall be responsible for mobilising an initial corpus of 5% of the unit cost. The unit cost shall not exceed Rs. 20,000. Once this is in position, the construction of the unit can he taken up. The GOI/State share shall be 60% and 30% respectively with the balance 10% coming from the Panchayats/ beneficiaries.

While drawing up the Action Plan for School Sanitation, it shall be ensured that the total number of schools to be provided with sanitary facilities under TSC have to be estimated taking into account, schools to be taken up under JRY, DPEP, Tenth Finance Commission funds., etc. and ensure that actual break up is clearly mentioned. Construction of the sanitary facilities in the schools shall be done preferably by the construction wing of the DPEP and under close supervision of the Parent Teacher Association. It may also be ensured that approval for the construction of all new schools shall be accorded only if the sanitary and drinking water facilities are integral parts of the plan.[11]

Total sanitation campaign is being implemented in 451 districts of the country. The project outlay for 451 TSC projects sanctioned so far is Rs. 4413.19 crore. The Central, state and beneficiary contribution are Rs. 2620.89 crore, Rs. 979.90 crore and Rs. 812.40 crore respectively. During the current year, 53 projects have been sanctioned. The physical and financial progress of the TSC projects is available on the Departmental web site at www.ddws.nic.in.

PROGRESS

During the current year, the TSC programme has taken off in the right direction and the implementation has been improved tremendously. The monitoring mechanism was strengthened while the hand holding exercises including Capacity development activity has been improved substantially. Some of the key areas of improvement made are as below:

Monitoring Mechanism

Progress is monitored through review meetings taken up by Secretary (DWS). In addition, review Missions are sent to various TSC projects to assess the extent of implementation as well as support the project authorities in implementing the project in an effective manner. In addition to the above, a Mid-term evaluation study of the TSC progrnmmc has been initiated. Over and above, the On-line monitoring of TSC programme has been launched and many States are now feeding their performance On-line on the Departmental web.site at www.ddws.nic.in

Ninnal Gram Puraskar, an award scheme for achieving 100% open defecation free environment has been launched on 2/10/2003 to the Panchayati Raj institutions (PRIs). The individuals and Organizations other than PRIs who play a key role in achieving this feat will also be rewarded. This has generated sufficient enthisiasm amongst the PRIs. Large number of applications were received. The scrutiny process has been completed and the award will be granted in February, 2005.

- HRD training modules for Capacity Development of grass-root level, district and state level officials involved in TSC implementation has been finalized. Training of TSC implementation officials is structured through 4 National Resource Centres at ESI, Ahmedabad, RKNLSM, Kolkata, GRI, Dindigul and SIPRD, Kalyani, WH.
- Booklets on Community participation in water supply and sanitation has been finalized through NIRD, Hyderabad.
- During the current year special thrust was given on School sanitation and hygiene education. Modules on Food hygiene to environmental sanitation has ocean prepared and printed in two technical notes called "School Sanitation and Hygiene Education and Angwanwadi toilet designs." These technical notes have been circulated to all the states. Decision has been taken to cover all Government schools in the country with safe sanitation facilities by 2005-06. Accordingly, an Action Plan for school water and sanitation has been initiated and all the states have been requested to comply for the same.
- Realizing the facts that poor rural men population who do not have adequate land for construction of individual latrines, the

earlier Women complex has been expanded to a Community complex. Further, hygiene education in schools has been highlighted. Featuring these changes which also include provisions for coverage of all Anganwadi toilets and Ninnal Gram Puraskar, the revised TSC guidelines has been made in January 2004. One of the most important features of these revised guidelines is emphasis of coverage of Individual latrines for APL households without subsidy/incentive through proper change of mind set. These are hosted in the web site and the guidelines are being distributed to all the states and district implementing agencies. Further, all the states have been asked to translate the revised TSC guidelines and SSHE technical notes into their regional languages so as facilitate the grass-root level workers also in effective TSC implementation.

- Inter-sectoral Co-ordination meetings with other Ministries/ departments at the Secretary level was held with DWCD, Health and Elementary Education. Co-ordination with external agencies for enhanced facilitation for TSC implementation through UNICEF, WSP-SA has been taken up.
- National Communication strategy has been worked out for the National and District levels utilizing the services of UNICEF and Ogilvey and Mather. The TV spots have been developed.
- As a result of the above initiatives taken up, 24.68 lakh individual household latrines, 32364 school latrines, 1190 women community complex, 6068 Anganwadi toilets have been constructed during the current year along with establishment of 904 Rural sanitary marts and production centers.

GENDER BUDGETING UNDER CRSP

Central Rural Sanitation Programme (CRSP) administered by this Department is meant for providing sanitation facilities in the rural habitation. All the inhabitants of the rural areas irrespective of cast, creed and sex benefit of this programme.

Under Rural sanitation programme there is a special provision for construction of Community Sanitary Complexes for women in order to ensure better hygience conditions and support dignity of women. Separate toilet blocks for girl student in each co-education rural Government schools is being provided under TSC.

However, since the bifurcation cannot be made on gender lines in respect of rural sanitation sector, it is not possible to earmark separate budget provision and fix separate physical targets in respect of this programme.[12]

Physical and Financial Progress

Plan Period	*CRSP (GOI) releases (Rs. Crore)*	*Latrines constructed (units)*
Eigth Plan period, 1992-93 to 1996-97	260.33	4337609
Ninth Plan	—	—
1997-98	96.66	1387080
1998-1999	64.90	1631272
1999-2000	92.00	1087604
2000-01	130.86	698393
2001-02	130.46	734516
Tenth Plan	—	—
2002-03	141.10	2471945
2003-04	205.00	4513884
2004-05 (as on 3.2.2005)	294.10	2841053

OTHER RELATED MATTERS

Maintenance

It is essential to train the community, particularly all the members of the family in the proper upkeep and maintenance of the sanitation facilities. The maintenance expenses of individual household sanitary latrines should be met by the beneficiaries where as that of sanitary complexes for women may be at the cost of the panchayats/voluntary organisations/charitable trusts.

Annual Action Plan

(i) The State shall prepare an Annual Action Plan one month before the commencement of the year on the basis of the shelf of schemes and taking into account the size of the allocation as well as carry over funds. Annual Action Plan should indicate clearly targets under each component for each quarter. A copy of the Action Plan should be sent to Government of India by 30th April.

(ii) While preparing the Action Plan, the completion of the incomplete works should be given priority over new works. It should be ensured that the works taken up are completed as per schedule to avoid cost escalation.

Cost Escalation of the Schemes not Allowed

There is no need or scope for delay in implementation resulting in cost overrun. Hence no additional funds shall be allowed under the TSC as well as the "allocation-based" Sanitation Programme towards cost overrun.

Schedule of Inspections

Monitoring through regular field inspections by officers from State level and district level in essential for the effective implementation of the programme. The inspection should be to check and to ensure that construction work has been done in accordance with the norms, that the community has been involved in construction, that the latrines are not polluting the water sources and also to check whether there has been correct selection of beneficiaries and proper use of latrines after construction. Such inspection should ensure that the sanitary latrines are not used for any other purpose, as has happened some times in the past.

Reports and Returns

The following reports and returns will be sent by the States/UTs:

- An Annual Action Plan for the schemes to be taken up during the year shall be furnished by 30th April of the year to which it relates.
- Monthly progress report will be furnished by the 20th of the succeeding month.
- Quarterly progress report shall be furnished by the 20th of the succeeding month.
- Annual Report of achievements under the programme during the year shall be furnished by 30th April of the succeeding year.

These reports shall enable authorities both at Centre and the State level to monitor the progress of the performance and to take appropriate collective measures.

Evaluation of the Programme

The implementation of the programme, results achieved and its impact will be evaluated at the end of each year by the Government of India through reputed Organisations. The States/UTs may also undertake the Evaluation of the programme through the reputed agencies in the States. Follow-up action taken by the States/UTs should be intimated to GOI from time to time. Any further modifications in the programme could be formulated based on the results of such evaluation.

Audit

The funds released under the Restructured Rural Sanitation Programme will be subject to audit by the Comptroller and Auditor General of India.

ALLOCATION-BASED SANITATION PROGRAMME

Introduction

In order to allow time for proper grounding of the new approach, the existing "allocation-based" programme will also be continued and will be progressively phased out. While the third year of the 9th Plan period will have 50% funds earmarked for the existing scheme, only 30% will be allocated for the fourth year, followed by 10% during the fifth year of the Plan period, mainly to handle spillover costs and small pending commitments.[13]

Programme Components

The components of the programme are as under:

- Construction of individual sanitary latrines for households below poverty line with subsidy (80%) where demand exists.
- Construction of exclusive village sanitary complexes for women, where adequate land/space within the premises of the houses do not exist and where village panchayats are willing to maintain.
- Setting up of sanitary marts and production centres.
- Construction of toilets in schools.
- Total sanitation of village through the construction of drains, soakage pits solid and liquid waste disposal.
- Intensive campaign for awareness generation and health education for creating felt need for personal, household and environmental sanitation facilities.

Brief Details of each of the Components

(a) Construction of Individual Latrines

The pattern of subsidy prescribed under TSCs will be followed.

(b) Conversion of Dry Latrines

As regards conversion of dry latrines, as per records, there are no such latrines in the rural areas. However, the Baseline survey does point to the existence of such latrines. A sum of Rs. 50 lakh shall be earmarked for this purpose for the third and fourth years of the 9th Plan. Unutilized balances shall be merged into the general pool of the resources of the Programme.

(c) Village Sanitation Complexes for Women

Though public latrines have not proved to be very successful in the past in view of the difficulties experienced by rural women in some areas, where individual household latrines are not feasible, village sanitary complexes exclusively for women could be attempted on a pilot basis. Upto 10% of the annual funds can be utilized to provide public latrines in selected villages during the plan period, where the panchayats/charitable trusts/NGOs offer to construct and maintain village complexes exclusively for the use by women.

(d) Rural Sanitary Marts (RSMs)/Production Centres (PCs)

Upto 5% of the allocation, subject to a maximum of Rs. 35 lakh/ district @ Rs. 3.5 lakh per unit can be used to set-up RSM/PCs.

(e) Total Sanitation of Village

Other Sanitation facilities such as drains, soakpits, solid and liquid waste disposals, etc. should be taken up as far as possible under Jawahar Rozgar Yojana (JRY) or any other programme for providing civic amenities in the Panchayat. Where this is not feasible due to other priorities and non-availability of adequate financial resources, the facilities can be taken up under allocation-based sanitation programme. For village that achieve more than 50% sanitation coverage in the below poverty line (BPL) segment, total sanitation packages can be taken up with 50% GOI assistance. No project will be sanctioned by the GOI, duration of which exceeds beyond the 9th Plan period. The facilities may include provision for construction of cattle troughs, sanitation of cattle sheds including provision of drinking water facilities, disposal of solid and liquid waste and Insecticide sprays for mosquitoes/flies.

(f) Campaign for Creation of Felt Need

This is a very important aspect of the programme. While government machinery for publicity may be useful to some extent, a well-orchestrated programme of publicity, health, education and creation of required facilities only can make any change in the attitude of the people. Support of the reputed local voluntary organisations, autonomous institutions, social, political and religious organisations who carry conviction with the people can be enlisted in creating the felt need. These organisations should be selected for their reputation for good and adequate infrastructure already available with them. These details should be collected at the field level. These organizations should be selected for environment creation and generation of felt need-based on clear norms such as number of years of good work, extent of good work, availability of infrastructure, extent of geographical coverage, etc.

These voluntary organizations should be encouraged to prepare projects covering various components of the programme but with focus on generation of felt need and construction of individual sanitary latrines. The incentive scheme provided under TSC for the NGOs/volunateers will be applicable for this also.[14]

CONCLUSION

There is a need of integrated approaches for water, waste disposal and health.

In areas where drainage and sanitation are poor, water runs over the ground during rainstorms, picks up faeces and contaminates water sources. This contributes significantly to the spread of diseases such as typhold and cholera, and may increase the likelihood of contracting worm infections from soil contaminated by faeces. Flooding itself may displace populations and lead to further health problems.

It is often essential that community members participate in maintaining drains. In Indonesia, for example, residents agreed to clean the drains in front of their houses every day and this was inspected twice a week. Community members responded well to friendly inspectors who provided support for clearing the drains. Maintaining the drains soon became part of the daily routine for responsible community members.[15]

Responsibility of Panchayati Raj System

1. Provide health education to people outlining the importance of sanitation to individuals and community.
2. Provide health education through demonstration of the impact of insanitation on the health of the people.
3. Encourage people's participation in making their house and village clean and beautiful.
4. Provide essential items for keeping the village clean.
5. One day a month may be celebrated as cleanliness day.
6. Encourage school children to keep their village clean.
7. Remove the weeds harmful to health.
8. Do plantation to make the environment of the village good.
9. Provide health education as not to throw things any where except in the space provided.
10. Encourage co-operative effort to promote sanitation.

Notes and References

1. Healthy Villages—A guide for communities and community health workers, WHO, p. 52.
2. Building Materials and Technology Promotion Council India, BMTPC, "Water and Sanitation for Cities", World Habitat Day, 6 Oct. 2003, p. 22.
3. *Ibid.*, p. 4.
4. Rajiv Gandhi National Drinking Water Mission, Ministry of Rural Development, GOI, New Delhi, pp. 2-3.
5. Building Materials and Technology Promotion Council India, BMTPC, "Water and Sanitation for Cities", World Habitat Day, 6 Oct., 2003, p. 22.
6. *Ibid.*, p. 4.
7. K.Subramanian: *Shelter*, Vol. 6, No. 3, October 2003, p. 48.
8. *Ibid.*, p. 52.
9. UNICF: Learning from Experience, Water and Environment Sanitation in India, p. 9
10. *Ibid.*, p. 15.
11. India 2004, Ministry of Information and Broadcasting, GOI, New Delhi, pp. 579-80.

12. Rajiv Gandhi National Drinking Water Mission, Ministry of Rural Development, GOI, New Delhi, pp. 10-13.
13. Rural Development Book, pp. 132-35.
14. Rajiv Gandhi National Drinking Water Mission, Ministry of Rural Development, GOI, New Delhi, pp. 18-19.
15. Healthy Villages—A guide for Communities and Community Health Workers—WHO, p. 50.

CHAPTER 4

HEALTH EDUCATION FOR RURAL HOUSING

Good-quality housing is a key element for ensuring a healthy village. Poor housing can lead to many health problems, and is associated with infectious diseases (such as tuberculosis), stress and depression. Everyone should therefore have access to good-quality housing and a pleasant home environment that makes them happy and content. Specific aspects of housing quality are described in the following sections:

- Problems associated with poor housing.
- Cramped and crowded conditions give rise to poor hygiene by providing places for vermin to breed and transmit diseases via fleas, ticks and other vectors.
- Poor household hygiene leads to food and water contamination within the home.
- Poor indoor air quality leads to respiratory problems and inadequate lighting leads to eyesight problems.
- Stress is higher for individuals living in poor housing and poverty.

—*WHO: Healthy Villages*

He

Hou
upon the
inmates le
estimates
areas is al
1991 censu
14-15 lakh
requiremen
addition to
every year
constructed
areas. In
facilities
Hou
economic
The banks
demand fo
by various
G. S
Yojana, Jan
in the form
regulations
budgetary
construction
This is als
Banking in
form of gro

Health Education for Rural Housing

EXISTING SITUATION

Housing is not a luxury but a basic necessity as all activities depend upon the quality of housing because government housing energies the inmates leading to productivity and happiness. As per the provisional estimates made available by 2001 census, the housing shortage in the rural areas is about 149 lakhs as compared to 137 lakh housing shortage per year 1991 census. Under the IAY, for the last three years, on an average, about 14-15 lakh houses are being constructed every year whereas the annual requirement is about 30 lakh houses per annum as per the 2001 census. In addition to this, it is estimated that about 10 lakh shelterlessness are added every year. Thus, the total requirement is about 40 lakh houses are constructed leaving the gap of about 25 lakh houses every year in the rural areas. In addition to the number of houses, the quality of houses and facilities in them are very poor causing many diseases and a dull life.

Housing Constitutes not only a basic necessity but also a crucial economic activity in view of its contribution to the construction industry. The banks, of late have been alive to the potential of this industry since the demand for housing remains insatiable even as the supply is constrained by various structural deficiencies and institutional obstacles.

G. Srinivasan in his article, "The Big Push in the Housing Sector" in *Yojana*, January 2004 clearly states that the Government's thrust on housing in the form of facilitating steps such as the Reserve Bank of India (RBI) regulations pertaining to priority sector lending, fiscal concessions and budgetary support has started yielding handsome returns through construction of dwelling units to lakhs and lakhs of people over the years. This is also corroborated by the latest Report on Trend and Progress of Banking in India 2002-03 of RBI. Assistance to the housing sector in the form of gross bank credit flows had gone up from Rs. 6203 crore (38.4 per

CHART 4.1

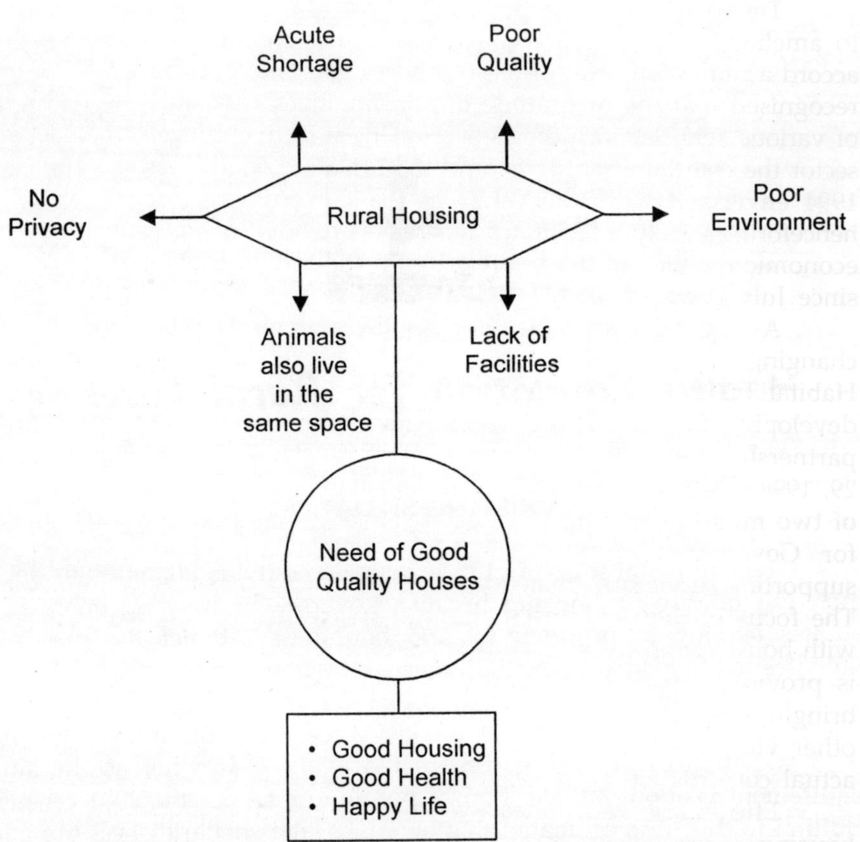

cent of the gross bank credit) in 2001-02 to Rs. 12,308 crore (55.11 per cent) during 2002-03. In order to increase further credit flow to the housing sector, the limit of housing loans for repairing damaged houses was raised from Rs. 50,000 to one lakh in rural and semi-urban areas. Because of the escalating demand for housing in rural and semi-urban areas as also the compulsive need to improve financing to housing sector here, the banks are being directed to extend direct finance to the housing sector upto Rs. 10 lakh per individual as part of priority sector lending with the approval of their Boards.

On its part, the Central government has come out with a series of well-meaning policy ballast to the housing sector in order to augment investment in housing. These include fiscal sops. Lowering of interest rate on housing loans, enhancement of bank finance for housing to the extent of 3 per cent of their annual incremental deposits, support to HUDCO and other housing finance institutions in the public sector.

THE NEW POLICY SHIFT

The long-range objective of the NHP was to stamp out houselessness to ameliorate the housing conditions of the inadequately housed and to accord a minimum level of basic services and amenities to all. It deservedly recognised that the magnitude of housing stock demands the involvement of various agencies including government at different levels, the cooperative sector the community at large and the private corporate sector. The NHP of 1994 envisaged a tectonic shift in the Government's role which would henceforth be only a facilitator than as a provider in tune with the changed economic realities of the reformist path the Indian economy had traversed since July. 1991.

As the NHP provided for review and modification in the light of changing scenario in the housing domain the National Housing and Habitat Policy was unveiled in 1998 to address the issue of sustainable development infrastructure development and for wholesome public-private partnership for delivery of shelter. This policy, laid in Parliament on July 29, 1998 was to foster surpluses in housing stock and facilitate construction of two million dwelling units each year in pursuance of National Agenda for Governance. It also sought to ensure that housing along with supporting services is treated as a priority sector at par with infrastructure. The focus of the policy is robust public-private a partnership for dealing with housing and Infrastructure impediments. Accordingly, the Government is providing fiscal fillips carrying out regulatory and legal reforms and bringing about an enabling milieu. The private and cooperative sector the other vital pillars in the partnership, would come forward to undertake actual construction activities and invest and run infrastructure services.

Efforts are well under way to prop up institutional mechanism for housing finance so that they do not get saddled with non-performing assets. One such proposal is the Mortgage Credit Guarantee Scheme of the National Housing Bank. This would cover housing loans extended by nationalised banks thereby protecting lenders (banks) against potential default. The NHB had begun securitisation of housing loans and has been making operational foreclosure of mortgage (rights of creditors to acquire the property). This would preclude borrowers from willfully defaulting on repayments now. It is also praiseworthy that the prudence of lending bodies has kept the non-performing assets to the barest in this significant segment of the economy. With foreclosure laws in place lending institutions will become freer and flexible in loan disbursals. These measures are salutary in that they minimise the cost of funds to the banks and housing finance companies while simultaneously enhancing the effective yield. This would also help bolster the profitability of the lending banks which are flush with funds but could not find savvy borrowers.

SCHEMES

Indra Awaas Yojana

The Ministry of Rural Development is implementing Indira Awaas Yojana (IAY) with a view to providing financial assistance for shelter to the rural poor living below poverty line. The details of the Scheme alongwith its performance are given below:

(a) The Government of India is implementing Indira Awaas Yojana (IAY) since the year 1985-86 to provide assistance for construction/up gradation of dwelling units to the below poverty line (BPL) rural households belonging to the Scheduled Castes. Scheduled Tribes and freed bonded labourers categories. From the year 1993-94, the scope of the Scheme was extended to cover non-Scheduled Castes and Scheduled Tribes rural BPL poor subject to the condition that the benefits to non-SC/ST would not be more than 40% of tile total IAY allocation. The benefits of the Scheme have also been extended to the families of Ex-servicemen of the armed and paramilitary forces killed in action. 3% of the houses are reserved for the rural Below the Poverty. Line physically and mentally challenged persons. The IAY became an independent Scheme with effect from 1.1.1996.

(b) The funding pattern of the IAY is shared between the Centre and State in the ratio of 75:25. From 1999-2000, the allocation of funds under the Indira Awaas Yojana to the States/UTs is being made on the basis of the poverty ratio, as approved by the Planning Commission, and rural housing shortage, as specified in the Census. Both parameters have been accorded equal weightage. Similarly. allocation to Districts in the States/UTs is made on the basis of proportion of SC/ST population of the District to the total SC/ST population of the State and housing shortage. The ceiling on construction assistance under the IAY currently is Rs. 25,000 per unit for the plain areas and Rs. 27,500 for the hilly/difficult areas. The ceiling on upgradation of unserviceable kutcha house to pucca/semi pucca house is Rs. 12.500 for all areas. This ceiling came into effect from 1.4.2004.

(c) On the basis of allocations made and targets fixed. District Rural Development Agencies (DRDAs)/Zilla Parishads (ZPs) decide Panchayat-wise number of houses to be constructed under IAY and intimate the same to the concerned Gram Panchayat. Thereafter the Gram Sabha selects the beneficiaries, restricting its number to the target allotted from the list of eligible households. No approval of other authorities is required. The Panchayat Samities/Zilla Parishads IDRDAs should, however, be sent a list of selected beneficiaries for their information.

(d) As the need for upgradation of unserviceable kutcha houses in the rural areas is acutely felt, therefore, with effect from 1.4.2004, upto 20% the total funds can be utilized for conversion of unserviceable kutcha houses into pucca/semi- pucca houses and for providing subsidy to the beneficiary availing loan under the credit-cum-subsidy scheme of Rural Housing (RH). Amaximum assistance of Rs. 12,500 per unit is provided for conversion of unserviceable kutcha houses into pucca/semi-pucca houses.

(e) Further, the dwelling units should invariably be allotted in the name of a female member of the beneficiary household. Alternatively, it can be allotted in the name of both husband and wife. The Sanitary latrine and smokeless chullah and proper drainage are required for each IAY house latrine could be constructed separate from the IAY house on the site of beneficiary. The construction of the houses is the sole responsibility of the beneficiary. Engagement of contractors strictly prohibited. No specific type design has been stipulated for an IAY house. Choice of design, technology and materials for construction of an IAY house is the sole discretion of the beneficiaries.

PROVISION OF ADDITIONAL FUNDS FOR NATURAL CALAMITIES

5% of allocation is kept at central share to meet the exigencies arising out of natural calamities and other emergent situations like riot, arson, fire, rehabilitation. The State Government should make necessary recommendation for additional funds in this regard which are to be shared by the Centre and State on 75:25 basis. The maximum limit for such assistance is Rs. 50.00 lakh per district. The relief will be as per the norms of IAY.

During the year 2004-05, the country is affected by various natural calamities. Majority of the victims are from rural areas, their dwelling units get partially or fully damaged apart from other losses. An amount of Rs. 400 crore has been sanctioned for the 20 flood-affected districts of Bihar as Additional Central Assistance under the Indira Awaas Yojana II (IAY). Similarly, on 26.12.2004, a large number of houses were damaged due to Tsunami tidel waves in the region of South-East coast and in some parts of South-West coastal areas of India and for this purpose an amount of Rs. 200. crore are likely to be released under the Indira Awaas Yojana (IAY) in order to provide immediate financial assistance for reconstruction of houses in the rural areas.

PERFORMANCE UNDER IAY

About 121 lakh houses have been constructed under IAY since

inception of the Scheme with an expenditure of Rs. 21419.64 crores (upto 31st December, 2004). During the Tenth Five Year Plan, i.e. last two years, the progress of IAY is as under:

Year	*Funds Utilized Centre + State share) (Rs. in crores)*	*Targets Houses constructed/upgraded (No. in lakhs)*	*(No. in Lakhs)*
2002-03	2795	13.14	15.48
2003-04	2580	14.84	13.61
2004-05*	1377	17.76	5.75

* As reported by the State Governments (upto 31st December, 2004).

During the current financial year 2004-05, the central allocation under IAY is Rs. 2900 crore with a target of 17.76 lakh houses. Out of this allocation, Rs. 2422.86 crore have been released under the scheme (upto 31st December, 2004).

Discontinuation of the Schemes such as Innovative Stream for Rural Housing, Samagra Awaas Yojana and Rural Building Centres

The small schemes under Rural Housing namely Innovative Stream for Rural Housing and Habitat Development, Samagra Awaas Yojana and Rural Building Centres (RBCs) have been discontinued and merged with the main scheme, i.e. Indira Awaas Yojana (IAY) with effect from 1.4.2004.

NEW INITIATIVES

Unit Cost of the Indira Awaas Yojana Houses

The ceiling on construction assistance under the IAY has been enhanced from Rs. 20,000 to Rs. 25,000 per unit for the plain areas and from Rs. 22,000 to Rs. 27,500 for the hilly/difficult areas. The ceiling on upgradation of unserviceable kutcha house to pucca/semi pucca house has also been enhanced from 10,000 to Rs. 12,500 for all areas. This ceiling came into effect from 1.4.2004.

Construction of Sanitary Latrines and Smokeless Chulhas

Sanitary latrine and smokeless chulha will be provided with each IAY house. In case, the beneficiary is unable to construct sanitary latrines due to some reasons, an amount of Rs. 600 would be deducted from the assistance to be provided for construction of the new IAY house or for upgradation of an unserviceable kutcha house. Similarly, where smokeless chulha is not possible, deduction will be Rs. 10.

Loan for IAY Beneficiaries

In addition to the assistance provided under the IAY, loan for construction of IAY houses or for upgradation of unserviceable kutcha houses can be obtained from the banks/other financial institutions if the concerned State Governments/DRDAs take the responsibility in order to coordinate with the financial institutions to make available the credit facilities to those beneficiaries who are interested.

Ownership of IAY House

Under IAY, the houses can be allotted in the name of male member of a deserving BPL family if there is no eligible female member in that family is available.

Equity Support to HUDCO

To meet the housing requirement of economically weaker sections in rural areas and to improve the outreach of housing finance in rural areas, equity support to HUDCO is being provided. During the first two years of the Tenth Five Year Plan, the equity support to HUDCO by the Ministry of Rural Development was as under:

Year	*Equity Support To HUDCO (Rs. in crores)*
2002-03	50.00
2003-04	10.00
2004-05.	5.00

Not yet released.

Provision of Houses for Physically and Mentally Challenged Persons

Under the IAY Guidelines, 3% of the IAY funds are reserved for construction of houses for the rural. Below the Poverty Line (BPL) physically and mentally challenged persons belonging to SCs/STs. As per the information received from the various States/UTs, about 45,083 houses have so far been concerned for the physically and mentally challenged persons under the Scheme.

North-Eastern Region

From the financial year 2000-01, a separate non-lapsable provision working out to 10% of the total budget of Rural Housing was earmarked for North-Eastern States. During the current financial year 2004-05, an amount of Rs. 250 crore has been earmarked for the North-Eastern Region for with a target of 150301 houses. Of this, an amount of Rs. 190.83 crore has already been released and about 69,380 houses have been constructed under the Indira Awaas Yojana (IAY).

Success Stories in Rural Housing and Habitat Development

Smt. Bhagyamma w/o Late Chikkaraju of Alkere village in Mandya Taluk is from BPL family. She is wage labourer and a widow belongs to Scheduled Caste having two female school going children, one is 7th and second one is 5th standard. She is the only wage earner in the family. Before she was staying in a thatched hut. Grama Sabha decided her name for house grant under the Indira Awaas Yojana (IAY) and to construct house herself without involving contractor she came forward and constructed house to her own satisfaction along with smokeless chulha and sanitary latrine as per guidelines. Now she feels much better having own pucca house to live.

Gender Budgeting under IAY

In order to provide social security to women, it is provided in the Indira Awaas Yojana (IAY) guidelines that the houses constructed is to be allotted in the name of female member of the beneficiary household Alternatively, it can be allotted in the name of both husband and wife under the Programme. When there is no eligible female member in the family, available/alive, IAY house can also be allotted to the male member of a deserving BPL family.

However, IAY guidelines do not provide separate earmarking of provisions and physical targets benefiting women. During 2003-04, 5.22 lakh houses were allotted exclusively in the name of women members, while 4.15 lakh houses were allotted in the name of both husband/wife. During 2004-05 (upto 31st January, 2005), 4.49 lakh house were allotted exclusively in the name of women members and 2.26 lakh houses allotted in the name of both husband/wife.

Congested

In small houses there are many things stores—grains, garments, utensils, animals, feet, etc. which allow little space for people living in the house.

Hence there is a need of health education to people to provide them guidance as to how they should live and enjoy a life free from disease.

PROBLEMS

1. Lack of knowledge

People in the villages are ignorant and they are not provided all the benefits under various schemes resulting in low quality housing. There is a lot of corruption in these schemes sponsored by Governments.

2. Lack of Health Education

The villagers do not give much importance to hygiene, hand washing and other facilities resulting into many diseases caused by poor house environment.

3. High Population as Compared to House Capacity

Many people live in a house which has been constructed for 4-5 members. How can they enjoy while sitting, sleeping and existing care should to taken about the size of the house *vis-a-vis* renders.

A visit to villages in Hungary by the authors revealed that villages are heaven possessing all the facilities of the city—good quality housing, lighting, ventilation, decorative as well as pure air of nature with good plantations. While a visit to an Indian village in despressing as the houses are unplanned, insufficient and unclean from where the outsiders want to run away. That is why government officials visit the villages and come back to the city on the same day. Housing is a basic necessity but it must of good quality so that the residents can enjoy the quality of life.

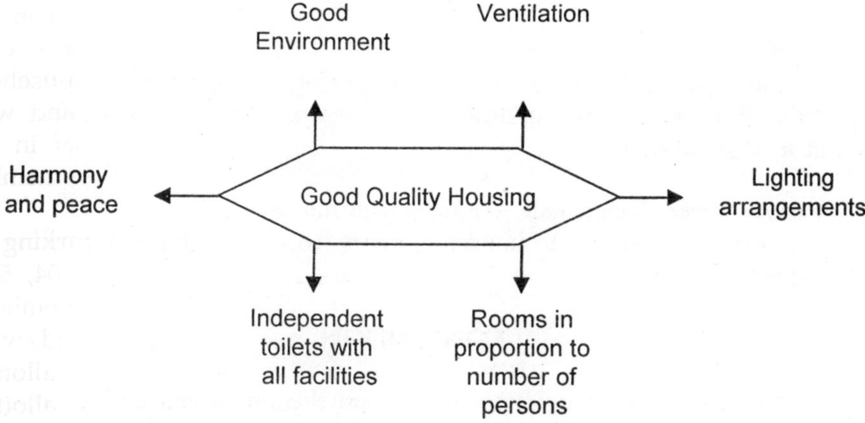

Improvement: Health Education

Panchayati Raj Institutions, i.e. gram Panchayat's must take the initiative to provide health education to the people to help three houses clean. This can avoid them from many diseases and make the villages healthy and beautiful.

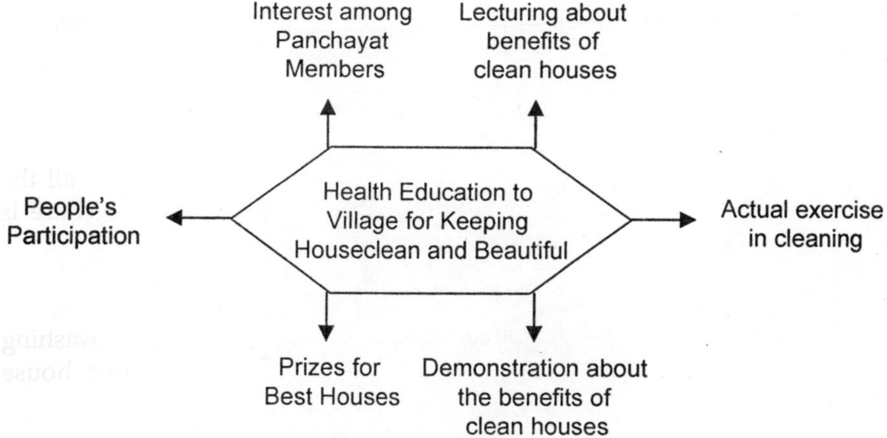

Problems of Housing in Indian Villages

1. Unplanned

Since the villages have expanded without any planning, the houses are congested causing unhealthy environment.

2. Approach Unhealthy

The roads outside the houses is unclean, dirty and insufficient. Children ease in the street resulting into garbage outside the houses.

3. Foul Smell during Rainy Seasons

During rainy seasons, water collect in the locality as there is no drainage resulting into communicable and infectious diseases.

4. Small Houses

Houses are disproportionate to the persons living in the house. If any one falls ill, he cannot be separated to an independent room resulting into the spread of disease.

5. Plastics, Paper, Dung remain Scattered near the Houses

A grim picture of the houses appears from outside area which is full of rubbish material.

CONCLUSION

The emphasis of housing should not be on bricks and mortar but comforts. The houses should be simple with all facilities. There is a need of research to ensure good housing at a minimum cost.

APPENDIX 4.1

Ventilation

Adequate home ventilation is particularly important where wood, charcoal and dung are used for cooking or heating, since these fuels give off smoke that contains harmful chemicals and particulate matter. This can lead to respiratory problems, such as bronchitis and asthma, and make tuberculosis transmission easier. Women and small children are particularly at risk from poor ventilation if they spend long periods within the home or in cooking areas. Where cooking is done indoors, it is essential that smoke and fumes be removed from the house quickly and efficiently. Ventilation may be improved by constructing houses with a sufficient number of windows, particularly in cooking areas. Alternatively, houses can be constructed using bricks with holes drilled through them ("air-bricks"), which allow fresh air to circulate within the house.

Lighting

Poor indoor lighting can have many harmful effects on health and well-being. A poorly lit working environment in the home can lead to eyesight problems, for example. This is a particular concern for women working in indoor cooking areas. Poor lighting within the home can also make people feel more depressed. These problems can be remedied by adding windows to the house to increase the amount of natural light, which is much stronger than light from candles or lamps. In communities where it is important that privacy within the home is maintained, windows can be located where it is difficult for people to see into the house, or constructed with a mesh or lattice work which allows light to enter while guarding privacy. Increasing natural light is also important for home cleanliness: if a house is dark, it is more difficult to see dust and dirt and thus more difficult to clean properly.

Disease Vectors in the Home

Unless homes are kept clean and steps taken to prevent insects from entering, the homes can become infested with disease vectors. In eastern Mediterranean areas, for example, sand flies thrive in the dirt inside houses and transmit leishmaniasis; and in Central and South America, triatomid bugs live in the cracks of walls and in thatched roofs and transmit American trypanosomiasis (Chagas disease). Insect disease vectors can be reduced by keeping food covered and properly disposing of waste. If mosquitoes or flies are a problems windows and doors should be covered with mesh screens and kept shut at night, and mosquito nets placed over beds. Cleanliness within and around home areas significantly reduces the risk of disease transmission.

Overcrowding in Homes

Overcrowding in homes causes ill-health because it makes disease transmission easier and because the lack of private space causes stress. Overcrowding is related to socio-economic level, and the poor often have little choice but to live in cramped conditions. In principle, increasing the number of rooms to live in should improve the health of the people who live there, but increasing house size is often difficult. Careful planning of family size can also help to reduce overcrowding. If community members feel that overcrowding is a problem, they can take the initiative and press landlords to provide more space for tenants at affordable prices. This may necessitate working with local government and pressure groups to ensure that the housing laws and tenancy agreements are revised, and that everyone has access to houses adequate for their family size.

Source: WHO: Healthy Villages, Geneva, 2002, pp. 61-64.

CHAPTER 5

VILLAGE SOCIO-ECONOMIC PROGRAMME: ADMINISTRATION FOR HEALTH PROMOTION AND EDUCATION

"For the realisation of the intended Plan objectives, the quality of design and effectiveness of implementation of the Plan programmes are as important as the availability of resources. Past experience has shown that many development projects and programmes having laudable objectives, have failed to deliver the result/because of the inadequacies in design and implementation."

—*Author*

Village Socio-economic Programme: Administration for Health Promotion and Education

This chapter deals with a critical appraisal of the rural development programmes in view of economic, social and infrastructural betterment of the rural people and areas. The underlying theme of all programmes is sustainable growth that could be achieved through empowerment of local communities, awareness building and popular participation. The ultimate purpose of democratic decentralisation is to ensure a fair standard of living to the rural masses living in abject poverty, squalor, disease, illiteracy, environmental pollution, etc. through well designed developmental programmes. The newly elected local authorities provide the institutionalised means for consolidating many of the gains brought about through community development activities, serving as channels of information for community education purposes, as catalysts to bring together people with common interest and as a stimulus to self-help effort at the village level. Without social and economic welfare development, the health services would become in effective. Hence, poverty removal in *sine qua non* for promoting good health.

CONSTITUTIONAL PROVISIONS RELATING TO WELFARE STATE

The Directive Principles of State Policy enshrined in our Constitution, though not enforceable by any court, IAY down principles fundamental to the governance of the country. Article 37 clearly states that it will be the duty of the State to apply these principles n making laws. Article 38 relates to promoting the welfare of the people, Article 39 IAYs down the broad policy which the State should follow for ensuring adequate means of livelihood for its citizens, protection of interests of children and women, etc.

Article 40 relates to organising village Panchayats while Article 41 deals with the right to work, to education and to public assistance in some cases. Article 43 relates to securing a living wage and Article 46 to the educational and economic interest of the weaker sections of society. Article 47 relates to standard of living, Article 48 to organisation of agriculture and animal husbandry and Article 48A to protection and improvement of the environment and safeguarding of forests and wild life. Thus, the Constitution contains provisions relating to the broad directions to be followed by the State in relation to the welfare and development of people of the country.

The rural development programmes, designed for the socio-economic transformation of the lives of millions in India, have passed through an interesting evolutionary process. Different types of experiments and a series of strategies have been tried to uplift the rural masses from poverty, morass and depression in the past with different degrees of success and failure. Through trial and error, serious efforts have been made to enrich the contents of the rural development programmes from time to time; but the goal of emancipating the masses from the shackles of poverty, hunger, frustration and disease does not yet appear to be within our reach. New strategies, therefore, need to be tried to attain the desired objectives. The United Nations study entitled, "Public Administration—Aspects of Community Development Programmes" classifies programmes broadly into three types for purposes of administrative analysis, as follows.

(a) Adaptive-Type Programmes

Those that are nation-wide in scope but limited for the most part to the catalytic function of stimulating the self-help effort of the people and to liaison with the technical services for support of such efforts. They are termed adaptive-type programmes because they can be attached to almost any department and adapted to the prevailing organisation of government.

(b) Integrative-Type Programmes

Those comprehending not only the general catalytic function at the community level but also the co-ordination of technical services at all levels in ways that will be coherent at the level at which they reach the people to elicit their understanding and active participation.

(c) Project-Type Programmes

Those that are multi-functional but are confined to certain areas. Project-type programmes have also been organised to foster development of special ethnic groups or regions.

According to M.G. Shah, the gamut of rural development programmes involves four aspects, i.e. Economic, Science and Technology, Socio-cultural and Politico-administrative. From economic point of view, development would mean moving away from low income to high income, from unemployment/underemployment to full employment, from subsistence living to higher standard of living, etc. From science and technology point of view, development would mean moving away from traditional methods of production to scientific methods with the sole objective of increasing production. From socio-cultural point of view, development would mean improving literacy, health, removing tradition-bound behaviour, etc. From political point of view, especially under "Panchayat Raj" system, it means decentralisation of decision-making, redistribution of economic power structure, efficient implementation of public policies, etc. To achieve these goals, the Government has created different departments with required skill and expertise.

PRIs are running a large number of programmes of Union Government, State Government and own programmes. We mention here the list of important Union Government programmes and explain some of them.

PROGRAMME FORMULATION

Programme formulation becomes a large and complex task after a positive decision has been taken on a project idea. We have to spell out here all the inputs in a comprehensive form. The manual of health project management lists nine steps required for the project formulation (See Chart 5.1).

CHART 5.1

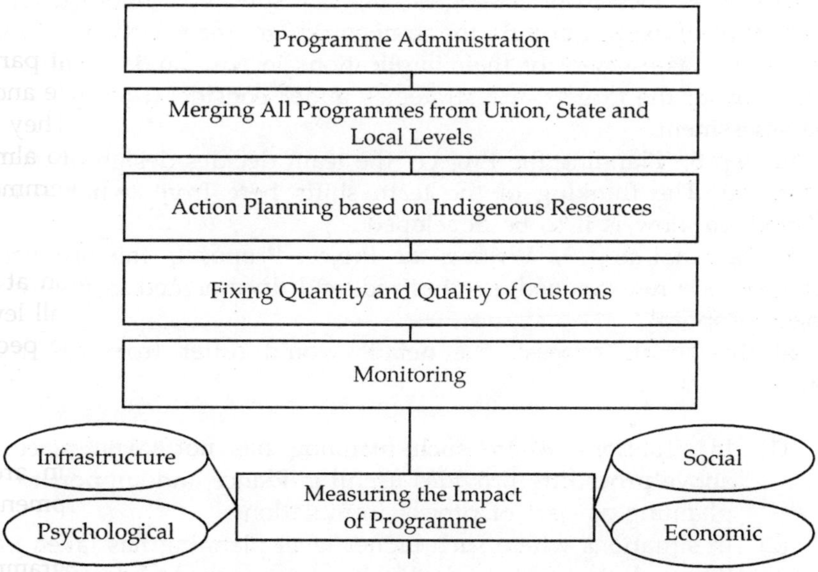

"In step 1, 'Preparation for Programme Formulation', the organization appoints a team to formulate project. A term of reference including time dimension, expected results, resource and problems is decided. The team obtains the necessary data required for the concerned project. Steps 2 and 3 relating to Situation Analysis may be done simultaneously or one after the other.

In step 2, 'Analysis of Organizational Situation', a clear picture of the organizational environment is carried out, i.e. description of the relevant organization and agencies, their decision-making process, past experiences relating to the success or failure of the project, need of current or future levels of the resources for the project, etc. The team should concentrate on producing reasonable and information-based summaries.

In step 3, 'Analysing the Socio-economic and Demographic Situation', the present, and future analysis is done of the socio-economic situation and the demographic situation.

In step 4, 'Analysis and Projection of the Problem', we define the problems and projection of the future situation which is worked out on the assumption that existing trends continue without change in the relevant systems and their policies.

Step 5, 'Getting the Objectives and Targets', entails a statement of the problem-reduction to be achieved through the project and translating them into the kind and magnitude of services (operational targets that would have to be provided at various future times in order to reach the objectives).

In step 6, 'Identification of Potential Obstacles', an attempt is made to predict the potential obstacles that might stand in the way of reaching the operational targets established in step 5.

In step 7, 'Design of Strategies', the key sub-steps involved are the establishment of explicit criteria for strategy design, the selection of flexible strategies, the assessment of their implications in costs and requirements, and revision of the targets and strategies under consideration in the light of the assessment.

In step 8, 'Planning the Project,' the team decides design of efficient performance. The thinking of the team shifts here from 'what is to be developed' to 'how is if to be developed'.

In the final step 9, 'Writing the Project Proposal,' the products of earlier steps are re-examined, synthesized, and documented in the form of a project proposal.

In this whole process, the details would differ from country to country.

(1) In situations where such planning has not taken place, the above procedure provides useful guidance and support to such planning as part of project formulation.

(2) In situations where such higher level planning has taken place, the analytical and general design steps would be considerably shortened and made more specific in content than the procedures now indicated.

After the project has been formulated, there is a need to examine its soundness. J.P. Gupta says that in the appraisal of a project, following questions need to be answered (See Chart 5.2).

CHART 5.2

1. Technical	1. Is the project sound from the technical and engineering point of view?
2. Economics	1. Is the project in a sector of high priority? 2. Is the project likely to contribute to the development of that sector? 3. Will that contribution justify the investment of scarce resources in the project?
3. Financial	1. Is the enterprise to instruct and operate the project financially sound? 2. What financing will be needed to bring facility into operation and from what sources? 3. What will be the probable operating costs and revenues, prospective liquidity and rate of return?
4. Commercial	1. Have adequate arrangements been made for supply of goods and services needed for construction? 2. Have adequate arrangements been made for the supply of inputs needed in the operation?
5. Organisational	1. Is the organization proposed to carry out and operate the project likely to be successful? 2. Would outside help be needed? 3. Are prospective controls adequate?
6. Managerial	1. What is the quality of the proposed management? It is likely to be adequate to ensure performance not inferior to that to be expected from the appraisal?
7. Social	1. What are the changes caused by the project in the behavioural pattern and the attitude in the population? 2. What are the attitudes of the population towards the projects? 3. Does the project require specific element of social change?
8. Environmental	1. Does the project cause pollution? 2. Does the project disturb the equilibrium of ecology? 3. Does the project fit into the environment?

Project planning has to be more scientific and approval procedure more realistic to ensure that avoidable time and cost overruns are much less frequent. The approval procedure should be linked with early completion of incomplete projects and sustainability of project output. Because of the unrealistic approval procedure, many of the projects are delayed. At the other extreme, less stringent approval procedures encourage a tendency to get too many projects cleared without the requisite financial resources in sight. There is, thus, a need for striking a balance between these extremes. It is important to ensure that rigour in appraisal and planning does not itself become a cause of delay because of repetitive and multi-level examination of technical and economic data. Strict time-tables need to be laid down for completion of the approval processes and preliminary work. Similarly, strict financial procedures should be formulated for the lessons learnt from the experience of executing thousands of development schemes during the last forty years can be briefly summarised as follows:

- There is inadequate analysis of available information during programme formulations. This happens primarily, because there is no established mechanism through which the programme agencies can have ready access to the relevant information regarding the target groups/areas or the findings of evaluation studies. As a result, avoidable errors at the planning stage creep in. For example, in a programme designed for the empowerment of rural women, the basic and well-known fact that most rural women, in India, an illiterate was not explicitly considered while formulating the operational rules and designing the delivery system.
- The operational cost of some programmes tends to be abnormally high, partly because of redundant and ineffective administration and partly due to other inadequacies in planning and implementation
- The general approach in implementation is "top-down" and "large-oriented." Some physical and financial targets are sought to achieved in most programmes. However, evaluation studies by the Planning Commission reveal that the fulfilment of these targets do not necessarily ensure that the programme objectives are being met in many anti-poverty programmes though the targeted number families/beneficiaries/districts/villages have been covered and allotted money has been spent, such programmes have failed in making desired impact on the well-being of the beneficiaries. The implementing agencies are often more concerned with the fulfilment of targets assigned to them than with the actual flow benefits to the target groups.
- Formulation of a multiplicity of programmes in an area of the concern without any specific thrusts can lead to several problems. Available resources are spread too thinly across a large number of projects leading to sub-optimal project outcome.
- For some programmes, separate implementing agencies are created whereas these are actually implemented by the existing departments, who work independently for different components of a programme. This results in lack of focus on target groups, wastage of resources and lack of coordination among the line departments. The creation of such agencies without the necessary institutional changes makes them redundant and affects the implementation quality of programmes.
- Lack of accountability of the implementing agencies either to Government or to the people has been the single major cause of diversion of funds in development programmes.
- Several social sector programmes are formulated without

addreressing the question of sustainability of benefits. The most distressing part of financing of the development projects and programmes under the Five Year Plan regime has been the failure to ensure timely and adequate flow of funds to the implementing agencies.

The essential ingredients of people's participation for self-development, as revealed in the success stories, are assessment of local resources and collective planning, sensitising people and building local resources for collective actions and an umbrella support mechanism to facilitate people's development actions. If these processes and mechanisms are to be multiplied on a wider scale, these will have to be institutionalized. The multiplication process requires a major political commitment by the State to provide the necessary political space and a policy framework for a sensitive support mechanism. This will call for, among other things, simplification of ground rules that would facilitate participation of grass-roots level organisations in the development process, bringing about flexibility and dynamism among the providers of public services and orienting the judicial system for speedy disposal of disputes and sensitivity to the needs of the disadvantaged people.

PROGRAMME IMPLEMENTATION

Proper implementation of the programme is vital and great attention and energy is required to ensure this. In this context, India's Planning Commission said: "The success of the Plan will rest very largely on the efficiency with which it is implemented." The purpose of implementation is to ensure that the project activities are completed as per schedule and within budgetary allocations, and that there are favourable conditions to maintain the desired changes generated by the project, after the project as such is terminated. Project implementation steps are repetitive ones and each project manager will have to adopt the procedures to suit his own situation depending upon the nature of the project and the organizational structures. The stages of implementation have been described in Chart 5.3.

1. Initiating the Project

Obtaining approval for the project proposal, appointing the project manager, preparing the interim budget and beginning the recruitment of other project staff.

2. Specifying and Scheduling the Work

Projecting the details of work and deciding what tasks are to be done by whom and when.

3. Clarifying Authority, Responsibility and Relationships

Obtaining agreement as to who is responsible for ensuring that the

CHART 5.3

Steps in Project Formulation

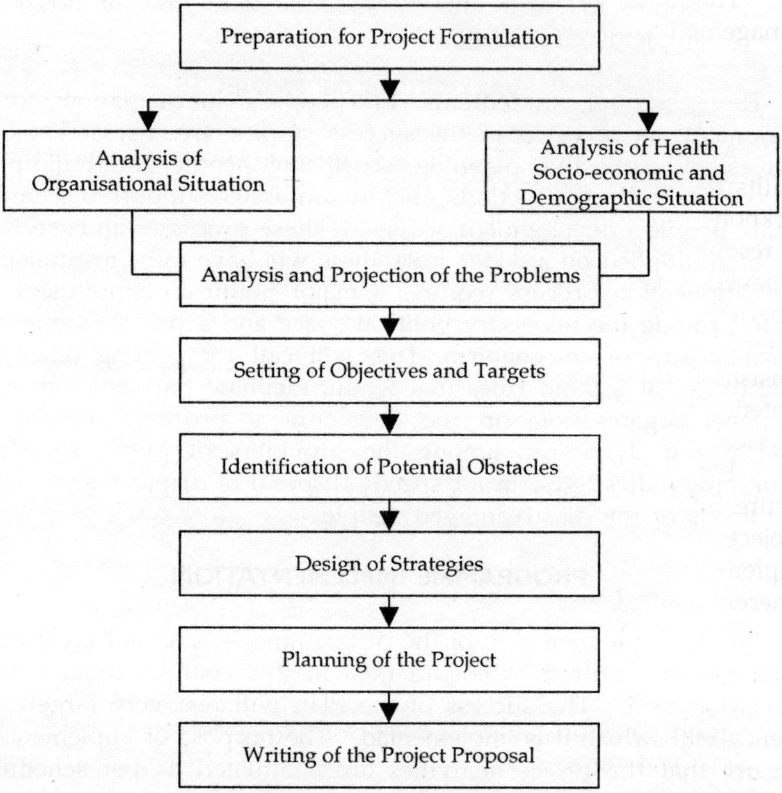

work gets done, distributing decision-making authority among the project team and the existing organizational units, and establishing formal lines of communication.

4. Obtaining Resources

Obtaining the funds, manpower, supplies and equipment necessary for doing the project activities.

5. Establishing the Control System

Determining what information is necessary for project control, identifying sources of such information and setting up reporting systems for the project.

6. Directing and Controlling

Motivating project staff, activities, obtaining information for control and taking corrective action as necessary.

7. Terminating the Project

Handing over responsibilities to existing staff and preparing the final report.

The implementation machinery can resort to modern methods of management to achieve desired results.

EVALUATION OF PROJECTS

All development projects undertaken need to be evaluated for the results they have achieved or failed to achieve. Careful evaluation is the backbone of all projects. It is indispensable as a guarantee of effective use of resources and of accountability for their use. Evaluation of results achieved in a project is required in order to benefit fully from the experience. Evaluation would be futile unless it is carried out in a systematic and co-ordinated fashion with clearly defined objectives and consistent procedures applied by the competent evaluators. Barnabas contends that "to be most effective, evaluation must not be made merely of physical achievements but also of the cost of such achievements."

Evaluation can be effective only if we have well designed format to secure timely, regular and dependable information on the performance of projects. Typically, evaluation must take place at the conclusion of implementation stage of any activity. Such a step ensures the following inherent advantages:

- It would aid in Project Management and control throughout the duration of the Project.
- It would help to ensure compliance with user community objectives before implementation.
- Process of systems design would be evaluated at all stages to aid in improving effectiveness of the Design Teams.
- Cost savings would be realized by modifying systems through evaluation before, rather than after implementation.
- Evaluation would help to ensure that proper design procedures and policies were being carried out.

The need for an effective monitoring and evaluation (M & E) system was felt as early as in the First Plan itself. The First Plan document stated that "with increased investment on development, more attention to systematic assessment and evaluation of the results from public expenditure was necessary."

With every important programme, provision should always be made for the assessment of results. Inspite of considerable development in economic and social sciences, our knowledge of human motivation and social processes is still limited. We cannot always say for certain that a given set of causes will produce a particular, clearly definable, set of results and none other. The Second Plan document emphasized the need for a strong M & E system, for building up a strong development administration, training personnel, informing and educating the public and organizing a sound system of planning based as much on the participation of the people at each level as on the best technical, economic and statistical information available. As a review of the past Plan performance revealed gaps in achievement in various areas of development, the need for a strong M & E system, got reinforced in subsequent Plan documents.

Over the passage of time, elaborate monitoring and evaluation mechanism has been built for efficient development administration and a large number of institutions for training in public administration at the Centre and State level have been created. While the M & E system has proved its utility in development administration, it is not as effective as it should be. The scope and nature of development programmes have been undergoing changes and the interaction between a programme and its environment is becoming increasingly complex. The government now operates under increasing financial and competitive pressures. The M & E system has not shown the necessary dynamism to cope with these changes and complexities. The Working Group on Monitoring and Information System of the Seventh Five Year Plan identified the following programmes:

- Ineffectiveness in identifying/reducing likely delays and problems;
- Large data gaps, delays in data generation and transmission, inadequate data;
- Analysis, feedback not reaching proper users;
- Inadequate information on interlinked projects;
- Information difficult to retrieve in the absence of data bank;
- Information not reflecting the true picture;
- More emphasis on reporting than on action; and
- Inadequate use of monitored information in decision-making.

As stated in the Annual Report of the Ministry of Rural Development, 2004-05, The Sampoorna Grameen Rozgar Yojana (SGRY) was launched on 25th September 2001 by merging the on-going schemes of Jawahar Gram Samridhi Yojana (JGSY) and Employment Assurance Scheme (EAS).

Objectives

The objectives of the Programme are to provide additional wage employment in the rural areas as also food security, alongside the creation of durable community, social and economic infrastructure in the rural areas. The programme is self-targetting in nature with special emphasis to provide Wage Employment to women, scheduled castes, scheduled tribes and parents of children withdrawn from hazardous occupations.

Strategy

The Scheme is exclusively implemented by the Panchayti Raj

Institutions (PRIs). Programme was implemented in two streams till 2003-04. The First Stream was implemented at the District and Intermediate Panchayat levels. 50% of the funds and foodgrains were available under the First Stream, which were further distributed between the Zilla Parishad and the Intermediate Panchayats in the ratio of 40:60 respectively. The Second Stream was implemented at the Village Panchayat level, and 50% of the funds and foodgrains were earmarked for the Village Panchayats and distributed among them through DRDAs/Zilla Parishads. Now, from 2004-05 the programme is implemented as one integrated Scheme. The programme resources are shared by all the three tiers viz. District Panchayat, Panchayat Samiti and the Gram Panchayat in the proportion of 20:30:50. Each level of Panchayat is an independent unit for formulation of Action Plan and executing the scheme. The details of activities/works taken up by the PRIs are as under:

(i) District Panchayats

20% of the resources are reserved at the District level and are to be utilized by the District Panchayats/DRDAs preferably in the areas suffering from endemic labour exodus/areas of distress as per the Annual Action Plan approved by the District Panchayats/DRDAs.

(ii) Intermediate Level Panchayats

30% of the resources are allocated among the Intermediate Level Panchayats. While allocating the resources, equal weightage is to be given to the proportion of SC/ST population and of rural population of the respective Intermediate Level Panchayat areas to those of the Districts. The workers will be taken as per their own Annual Action Plan approved by the Intermediate Level Panchayats. However, while selecting the works, to be taken up, preference will be given to the Areas, which are backward. Calamity Prone or face migration of labour.

(iii) Gram Panchayats

50% of the resources are allocated among the Gram Panchayat (Village Panchayat) for generation of supplementary wage employment and creation of demand driven community village infrastructure, includes also durable assets to enable the rural poor to increase opportunities for sustained employment.

SPECIAL SAFEGUARDS FOR THE WEAKER SECTIONS AND WOMEN OF THE COMMUNITY

(i) 22.5% of the annual allocation (inclusive of foodgrains) allocated both at the level of District and Intermediate Panchayats shall he earmarked for Individual/group beneficiary Schemes of SC/ST families living below the Poverty Line (BPL).
(ii) Minimum 50% of the Village Panchayat allocation (inclusive of

foodgrains) shall be earmarked for the creation of need based village infrastructure in SC/ST habitations/wards.

(iii) Effort would be made to provide 30% of employment opportunities for women.

SALIENT FEATURES OF THE SGRY

- The Sampoorna Grameen Rozgar Yojana (SGRY) is Centrally Sponsored Scheme (CSS) being implemented with an annual allocation of about Rs. 6000 crore (Centre + State) and 50 lakh tonnes of foodgrains.
- Under the Scheme, 50 lakh tonnes of foodgrains amounting to about Rs. 5700 crore (at economic cost) is being provided every year, free of cost, to the State Governments and Union Territory Administrations.
- The cost of the cash component of the Programme is shared by the Centre and State in the ratio of 75: 25.
- The payment of foodgrains is made by the Ministry of Rural Development to the Food Corporation of India (FCL) directly.
- About 100 crore mandays of employment are envisaged to be generated every year in the rural areas.
- Every worker seeking employment under the SGRY will be provided minimum 5 kgs. of foodgrains (in kind) per manday as part of wages.
- The balance of wages will be paid in cash so that they are assured of the notified minimum wages.
- The State Governments and UT Administrations will be free to calculate the cost of foodgrains (paid as part of wages) at either BPL rates or APL rates or anywhere between the two.
- Panchayati Raj Institutions (PIUs) can take up works as per the felt need of the areas.

SGRY is a noble programme with unique features. The first ever programme of such magnitude that is fully planned and implemented by the Panchayati Raj Institutions (PRIs) in tune with 73 Constitution Amendment Act. It has to be seen as a huge investment in the capacity building of the vast human resource in the rural areas that has the potential of transforming the face of the economy as a whole. While launching the SGRY, lessons learnt from the past mistakes have been kept in mind and all possible measures to prevent the repetition of earlier mistakes have been ensured. The success of any programme of4his magnitude fairly depends upon the quality of delivery mechanism, which finally rests with the implementing agencies, i.e. The PRIs. Besides, there is an urgent need to change the attitude and the opinion of all concerned towards wage employment programmes. Uptill now these programmes are taken and assessed as social sector programmes or the social safety network programmes. This mindset must be changed. These programmes should not be considered as social sector programmes or merely an intervention to provide social safety net to the target group. The SGRY has an economic aspect as well. Our goals are not merely generation of additional mandays and provide food security to the rural poor but at the same time channelising its vast potential in nation building exercise through the development of human resource and economic infrastructure which may transform the rural face and give boost to the nation's economy. The SGRY therefore, must be taken as an economic programme based on welfare economics. The attainment of objectives of poverty alleviation Programmes will get accelerated if we address the core issue with this mindset and implement programmes accordingly.

NATIONAL FOOD FOR WORK PROGRAMME

A new programme, National Food for Work Programme (NFFWP) has been launched from the month of November 2004, in 150 most backward districts of the country, identified by the Planning Commission in consultation with the Ministry of Rural Development and the State Governments.

Need for Programme

A need for the new programme was felt because the existing resources in the SGRY were not sufficient to meet the requirement of additional wage employment in most backward districts. Moreover, it was felt that the additional resources should be channelised into some focus areas like water conservation and drought proofing which is the principal problem in some States and a major cause of backwardness of certain regions. Some areas are flood-prone and measures for flood control require special attention in these areas in a planned manner. The States were finding difficult to provide State share of funds and therefore, a 100% Centrally Sponsored Scheme was proposed so that the investment in backward areas does not suffer because of lack of resources available with the States.

Objective

The objective of the programme is to provide additional resources apart from the resources available under the Sampoorna Grameen Rozgar Yojana (SCRY) to 150 most backward districts of the country so that generation of supplementary wage employment and providing of food-security through creation of need based economic, social and community assets in these districts is further intensified.

Criteria for Selection of 150 Most Backward Districts

For States (other than special category States and States in the North Eastern (N.E.) region except Assam) most backward Districts have been chosen on the basis of an exercise undertaken by the Planning Commission using three parameters, namely, (i) agricultural productivity per worker, (ii) agricultural wage rate, and (iii) SC/ST population. Same criteria was followed for Assam.

For the special category States and States in N.E. region (except Assam), districts were identified from out of the list selected under Rashtriya Sam Vikas Yojana (RSVY). At last one district has been selected in each State other than Goa. While selecting these districts suggestion received from the State Governments were also considered.

Funding

The programme is being implemented as a 100% Centrally Sponsored Scheme. Foodgrains are also provided to the States free of cost. The transportation cost, handling charges, and taxes on foodgrains are, however, be the responsibility of the States.

For the current year, Rs. 2020 crores have been allocated for the Scheme. In addition, 20 lakh tonnes of foodgrains are also provided to the States. If the present level of SGRY allocation is maintained the annual requirement for the next year under NFFWP is estimated to be about Rs. 5400 crores and 37 lakh tonnes of foodgrains. It is expected that with this level of investment it will be possible to provide 100 days of supplementary wage employment to one member of each BPL family in the rural areas of the identified 150 districts.

Focus of the Programme

the programme will focus on water conservation, drought-proofing and land development as a first priority. Flood control measures, rural connectivity in terms of all-weather roads and other productive works for ensuring economic sustainability may also be included depending upon local needs.

Perspective Plan and Implementation

A five years perspective plan will be got prepared by the collector of the district with the assistance of the experts and in consultation with the appropriate level of panchayats. A gram panchayat and block-wise shelf of projects will be prepared based on priorities. The works for execution will be selected out of the shelf of projects so prepared under the perspective plan. The works will be got executed through line Departments/Panchayati Raj Institutions (PRIs)/reputed NGOs/Self-Help Groups as desired by the collector.

Special Monitoring

besides, furnishing of periodic reports in the prescribed format on monthly basis, strict monitoring and vigilance would be ensured by adopting special mechanism as under:

(a) The Panchayat concerned will have the right to inspect and review the progress of any work under the scheme in its jurisdiction.
(b) For each work sanctioned, there will be a supervisory committee of local people to ensure it that the work has been properly done. Its report has to be kept with the completion report.
(c) District level monitoring will do 100% verification of the works done under the programme.

PRADHAN MANTRI GRAM SADAK YOJANA

Introduction

Pradhan Mantri Gram Sadak Yojana (PMGSY) was launched on 25th December, 2000. It is a 100% Centrally Sponsored Scheme, with the target of connecting through good All-weather roads every habitation that has a population of more than 1000 within 3 years and every habitation with a population of more than 500 by the end of the Tenth Plan. In respect of the Hill States (North - East, Sikkim, Himachal Pradesh, Jammu and Kashmir, Uttaranchal) Desert Areas and Tribal (Schedule-V) areas, the objective is to connect habitations with a population of 250 persons and above.

According to figures made available by the State Governments as a result of a survey to identify the Core network, about 1.70 lakhs Unconnected Habitations need to be connected under the PMGSY. This includes 59,890 Unconnected Habitations with population of over 1000 persons, 81,510 habitations having population between 500-999 and 29,710 habitations having population of 250-499 persons.

National Rural Roads Development Agency (NRRDA)

The National Rural Roads Development Agency (NRRDA) registered under the Societies Registration Act, 1860 on 14th January 2002, extends technical support to the Programme at the Central level through advice on technical specifications, project appraisal, appointment of part time Quality Control Monitors, management of monitoring systems and submission of periodic reports to Ministry of Rural Development. During 2004-05, meeting of the General Body of NRRDA was held on 16th November, 2004. Three meetings of the Executive Committee of NRRDA were held on 17th June, 2004, 31st August, 2004 and 11th October, 2004.

State Level Agencies

'Rural Roads' being a State subject, PMGSY works are executed by State Agencies. The State Governments have identified the Nodal Department as well as the Executing Agencies for execution of the Programme in the States. Most States have set-up State Rural Road Development Agencies (SRRDA) for the purpose, which also serve to coordinate the execution of the Programme in the field.

Technical Agencies

In order to provide a firm technical base for the programme, Principal Technical Agencies (IIT level institutions) and State Technical Agencies (REC level institutions) have been selected to provide technical advice to State Governments and assist NRRDA in technical scrutiny, training, R&D project activities and the like. During 2004-05, three more State Technical Agencies were appointed.

Quality of Works

Pradhan Mantri Gram Sadak Yojana (PMGSY) IAYs special emphasis on Quality of Road Works. Accordingly, Rural Roads Manual (JRC SP 20:2002) has been prescribed as the Technical Manual for the programme. The Quality of Works under programme is determined in relation to the specifications prescribed under Book of Specifications (BoS) published by the Indian Roads Congress (IRC) for Ministry of Rural Development MoRD).

Since rural roads is a State subject and State agencies are executing the programme, ensuring the quality of road work is primarily the responsibility of the State Governments. A three-tier Quality Management Mechanism is envisaged in order to ensure the requisite quality assurance. The First Tier of Quality Mechanism is the in-house Quality Control to ensure the implementation of quality standards through carrying out mandatory tests by Contractor under the supervision of the District Level Programme Implementing Unit (PIU). The supervision by department officers, also forms part of this tier itself and the PIU is required to record the test results in Quality Control Registers

The Second Tier of Quality Mechanism is independent Quality Monitoring System at the State Level to see that the first tier of Quality Control System is achieving its intended objectives. The States are also required to appoint a senior professional as State Quality Coordinator (SQC) who is empowered to coordinate and supervise both the tiers of quality mechanism, through the SRRDA.

The Third Tier of Quality Control Mechanism functions as independent Quality Audit at National Level. Selected retired professionals from State and Central Agencies termed as National Quality Monitors (NQMs), perform independent inspection of the works on systemic randomized basis. The basic objective of this tier of the Quality Mechanism is to see that the First and Second Tier of Quality Control is achieving its intended objectives, the contracts are being managed professionally and systemic issues in Quality and Execution are addressed.

Upto the end of March 2004, 22,000 works were inspected by NQMs out of which 86% are rated "Satisfactory" and 14% rated "Unsatisfactory." Based on experience of inspections carried out by NQMs in last few years the reporting format of NQM has been modified and oriented more towards Institutional Quality Assessment, Contract Management and Quality Assessment rather than only the assessment of Quality of works. During the current financial year, 3230 works were inspected up to December 2004 out of which 73% works have been rated"Satisfactory" and 27% works rated "Unsatisfactory."

I. Swarnjayanti Gram Swarozgar Yojana

A new holistic self-employment programme, namely, Swarnjayanti Gram Swarozgar Yojana (SGSY) was launched on April 1999. With this, the erstwhile programmes, viz. Integrated Rural Development Programme (IRDP), Development of Women and Children in Rural Areas (DWCRA), Training of Rural Youth for Self Employment (TRYSEM), Supply of Improved Toolkits to Rural Artisans (SITRA), Ganga Kalyan Yojana (GKY) and Million Wells Scheme (MWS) ceased to be in operation. SGSY has been devised keeping in view the positive aspects as well as deficiencies of the earlier programmes.

Main Features

(i) Emphasis on mobilization of rural poor to enable them to organize into Self Help Group.
(ii) SGSY—a credit-*cum*-subsidy scheme where credit is critical component and subsidy is only an enabling element.
(iii) Participatory approach in Selection of key activities.
(iv) Project approach for each key activity.
(v) Emphasis on development of activity clusters to ensure proper forward and backward Linkages.
(vi) Strengthening of groups through Revolving fund Assistance (RFA).
(vii) Training of beneficiaries in Group processes and skill development-integral part of the project.
(viii) Marketing support with emphasis on market research, upgradation/diversification of products, packaging, creation of market facilities, etc.
(ix) Provision for development of infrastructure to provide missing critical link. 20% fund (in case of NE State 25%) is earmarked for infrastructure development.
(x) Active role of NGOs in formation and capacity building of SHGs.
(xi) Focus on Vulnerable Groups, i.e. SC, ST, Women and Disabled
(xii) 15% fund earmarked for Special Projects to ensure a time bound programme for bringing specific number of BPL families above poverty line.

- SGSY would provide opportunities for self-employment to the rural poor. The programme would shift to a process-oriented approach in five stages.
    - Social mobilisation for formation of self-help groups;

- Savings among the group and internal lending among its members;
- Provision of a revolving fund;
- Micro-finance; and
- Micro-enterprise development.

- ❑ Network of institutions that promote the self-help movement would be created during the Plan period. Partnership would be forged between NGOs and other community-based organizations, government agencies and other financial institutions. There would be a system of identifying and training local facilitators.
- ❑ Key activities would be planned to respond to the needs of the area. Training Programmes for beneficial linkages with training institutions would be forged.
- ❑ Greater attention would be paid to marketing. Rural haats/ markets at the taluka/district level would be set-up for display of products. Linkages will be developed with private channels, industrial enterprises and export houses for higher value realization for SGSY groups.
- ❑ Special attention would be paid to provide technical support for upgrading technology and standardization of products. Use of information and communication technology would be promoted during the plan period in this regard.
- ❑ The SGRY would be the single wage-employment programme. The programme would have three streams which would seek to address the need of rural infrastructure at the village level, ensure guaranteed employment of at least 100 days in areas facing chronic unemployment/migration and provide relief in natural calamities such as floods, droughts, earthquakes and other contingencies. The projects under SGRY would be chosen with a view to taking up schemes that enlarge the scope for increased economic activity.

Land Reforms

Access to land will be an important element in the poverty alleviation strategy. Tenancy reforms, record of rights of land owners and tenants, computerization of land records, prevention of alienation of tribal lands, and issue of land rights for women will be the major tenets of the land reform agenda.

2. Jawahar Gram Samridhi Yojana

Jawahar Gram Samridhi Yojna (JGSY) is the restructured and comprehensive version of the erstwhile Jawahar Rozgar Yojana. Launched on 1 April, 1999, it has been designed to improve the quality of life of the rural poor.

3. National Social Assistance Programme

The National Social Assistance Programme (NSAP) which came into effect from 15 August 1995, is a Centrally- Sponsored Programme. A provision of Rs. 635 crore has been made for the programme in the budget for 2001-02.

4. Annapurna Scheme

The Annapurna Scheme has been launched with effect from 1 April 2000 to provide food security to those senior citizens (65 years) or above who though eligible have remained uncovered under the National Old Age Pension Scheme.

5. Training

The implementation of various rural development programmes which calls for an efficient and motivated stream of Government as well as non-government functionaries is a very challenging task.

THE PATH AHEAD

Rural poverty alleviation programmes were revamped and re-focused during the Ninth Plan to increase their effectiveness. Programmes that provide self-employment and wage employment to the poor would be implemented with greater vigour during the Tenth Plan.

- The promotion of a movement which enhances social capital and forges linkages with other formal and informal stakeholders engaged in developmental activities would be a major thrust during the Plan. PRIs have created a space for the involvement of the community in governance. There is a need to provide greater attention to effective empowerment of PRIs. The Government recognizes the necessity of building, implementation and monitoring of development programmes. These would be undertaken on a large scale during the Plan Period.

Delivery Mechanism

Poverty alleviation programmes have been designed to address different facets of rural poverty. Micro-credit-linked programmes provide a package of services including credit and subsidy to set-up micro-enterprises. Wage employment programmes address the issue of transient poverty. Besides, schemes for infrastructure development and provision of basic services contribute to the well-being of the rural people. Successful implementation of these programmes requires an appropriate policy framework, adequate funds, and an effective delivery mechanism. Past experience shows that the mere availability of funds is not likely to eradicate rural poverty. Nor is the design of the rural development programmes, no matter how refined, a sufficient condition. The success of these programmes ultimately depends on the capability of the delivery system to absort and utilize the funds in a cost-effective manner. An effective and responsive district-level field machinery with a high degree of commitment, motivation. Professional competence and, above all, integrity has been recognized as one of the prerequisites for successful implementation of anti-poverty programmes.

An effective delivery system has to ensure prople's participation at various stages of the formulation and implementation of the programmes, transparency in the operation of the schemes and adequate monitoring. International experience shows that greater functional and financial devolution to local governments results in higher allocation of resources for social sectors and more efficient use of resources. Such trends in social spending have been witnessed in many Indian states as well.

CONCLUSION

The following suggestions are made to improve the qualitative impact of government programmes:

1. Organising the Poor for Greater Participation

Local institutions like farmers' co-operatives and Mahila Mandals should perform intermediary functions like awareness generation, credit extension, etc. The members of these organisations should also be nominated to the respective standing committees of the Panchayat on rotation basis.

2. Unity of Plan and Policy

A national plan of action supported by national, regional and block level policies should be evolved and adhered to uniformly, all over the country, e.g., *provision of 7 basic minimum services* unanimously adopted at the conference of CMs held in 1996. The method adopted to achieve this goal should be left to the ingenuity of PRIs. Multiplicity of schemes should be avoided.

3. Emphasis on Co-ordination Rather than Control

The Central/State Government Departments should co- ordinate the sectoral activities operating at regional and local levels through an effective computerised *Rural Information System.* The flow of information should be two-ways, i.e. while the PRIs report their progress, central/state level co-ordinators should use this feedback to analyse the problems/shortcomings to suggest necessary policy-changes.

4. Schemes to Originate from PRIs and not State/Centre

The PRIs should not be treated as mere implementing agencies of the schemes and funds devolved to them. They should be sufficiently equipped to collect their own database, analyse their problems and priorities and formulate their own schemes and programmes to develop their area and people. Consolidation of schemes and programme funds at GP level would help provide autonomy to frame need-based projects and shelve schemes having high delivery costs.

5. Simplification of Procedures/Norms

Project planning has to be made more scientific and simplified, to be properly understood and implemented at GP level. The elected members have to increase the rigour of awareness building exercises. There is need for discontinuation of excessive paper work in the name of monitoring, which alienates the elected representatives and gives way to bureaucratisation of programme implementation. Emphasis should be laid on field inspections and result-oriented feedback in terms of number and percentage of village population crossing poverty line. There is a need for standardisation of norms pertaining to financial expenditure at each level, according to the functions entrusted. All sanctioning authority should be delegated to ZP/TP/Gram Sabha.

6. Adoption of Package Approach

The projects should be completed within 2 years and should preferably be undertaken in a cluster approach. The assistance should be given as a package to ensure achievement of tangible results as seen in Sri Kshetra Dharmasthala Model. Sufficient attention should be given to maintenance of existing assets rather than creation of additional assets. Thus, the emphasis should be on cumulative contribution of PRIs rather than annual achievements.

7. PRIs as Corporate Bodies

The PRIs should be trained to develop a business-like approach, i.e., spending government money should not be an end in itself but it should be yielding returns in the form of revenue generation. The vast reservoir of human resources needs to be productively channeled so as to enrich rural economy. The cost-benefit ratio and internal rate of return needs to be worked out and monitored for all schemes.

8. Focus on HRD

A study of economic growth in the post-Independence period clearly indicates that human development through better education, health nutrition and family planning at local levels promotes economic growth as effectively as capital investment in factories. The highest social returns as well as the closest links with both subsequent and simultaneous growth are in primary education, including adult literacy. Educated farmers tend to produce upto 15 per cent more than the uneducated. In this connection, Theodore Schultz says: "It is not possible to have the fruits of modern agriculture and an abundance of modern industry without making large investments in human resources. Social returns on such investments are very high in the long-run." The gains arising out of mass education outweigh its negative aspects, such as educated unemployed or social tensions. The strains and tensions produced by a widening of the base of education in a way are signs of vitality and of the process of change. In such a situation, demand will call forth its own supply, and economic progress will be more rapid.

9. Creation of Satisfactory Monitoring System to Measure and Regulate Performance during Implementation

Most of the programmes included in grass-root planning are never completed within the budgeted resources and fixed time schedules. Programme control is a managerial function that helps the heads of the Departments at the district level to keep the programme functioning as scheduled. It is possible only if realistic advance targets of output are fixed before implementation.

A participatory and result-oriented bureaucracy interacting with an aware and educated populace would interact fruitfully to produce a self-reliant village entity in the right spirit of democratic decentralisation for rural development.

Cluster Approach

SGSY stresses on cluster approach for taking up economic activities. The key activities are to be taken up in clusters. The cluster may not merely be geographic agglomerations but limits where backward and forward linkages can effectively be established. Separate clusters are to be taken up for each activity. More and more Swarozgaris can be added to cluster each year. The cluster approach in the programmes is adopted to facilitate infrastructure and marketing support to the activity.

Project Approach

The SGSY adopts a Project approach for each Key Activity. Project Reports are to be prepared in respect of each identified Key Activity. The Banks and other financial institutions have to be closely associated and involved in preparing these Project Reports, so as to avoid delay in sanctioning of loans and to ensure adequacy of financing. Project report should include all aspects like level of investment required at Swarozgaris level economies of group lending, return from the activity, repayment schedule, technical input required by Swarozgaris, training requirement and mode of training, credit, infrastructure and marketing requirement and identification of resources to develop them, net accruable income from activity.

Training and Skill Development

SGSY is process oriented Scheme which involves organizing the rural poor into Self Help Groups (SHGs), their training and capacity building to enable them to evolve into a self-managed organization. Therefore, the role of Facilitators/SHPIs, field level functionaries of Banks and development functionaries is critical in successful implementation of the Scheme. It has been noticed that wherever functionaries have been trained in the concept and functioning of SHGs, group dynamics, guidelines of the scheme, marketing and entrepreneurship development, etc., the quality of groups as well as overall implementation of the programme has been qualitatively better. It has also been observed that large number of development functionaries do not have access to well organized training Programme.

SGSY IAYs much emphasis on skill development and other training programmes. Since it was observed that a large number of development functionaries/bankers do not have access to well-organised training programmnes, the Ministry had earmarked a separate budget during 2003-04 for organising training programmes for Training of Trainers, Facilitators, Bank officials and development functionaries at various levels. An amount of Rs. 7.39 crores was released to the State Governments/Training Institutes for conducting training programmes under SGSY during 2003-04.

During the current financial year, an amount of Rs. 1.81 crores has been released to the State Governments/Training Institutes for conducting training programmes under SGSY upto December 2004.

As stated in the Annual Report of the Ministry of Rural Development, 2004-05.

PROVISION OF URBAN AMENITIES IN RURAL AREAS

The scheme of Provision of Urban Amenities in Rural Areas (PURA) was announced by the Honourable Prime Minister in his speech on 15th August, 2003 on the concept promoted by the Honourable President of India to bridge the rural-urban divide and achieving balanced socio-economic development. The initial implementation strategy of PURA was to launch the scheme in around 5000 rural clusters across the country in the next five year.

- The scheme aims to meet the gap in physical and social infrastructure in the identified rural clusters consisting of 10-15 villages around towns with population of one lakh or less to further their growth potential. The identified areas of intervention and support are:
  - (i) Road and transportation,
  - (ii) Power connectivity,
  - (iii) Electronic connectivity in the form of reliable telecom, internet and IT Services,
  - (iv) Knowledge connectivity in the form of good educational and training institutions,
  - (v) Market connectivity to enable farmers to get the best price for their produce,
  - (vi) Drinking water supply, and
  - (vii) Health facilities of basic quality and standards.

- These facilities are expected to be created by the Implementing Agencies by converging resources of the on-going Central and State Government programmes. If there is any gap which cannot be funded under any scheme or the available funds under the existing schemes are insufficient for the purpose, such gaps will be funded through PURA. The PURA builds on the existing schemes while providing funds for critical gaps.
- The Ministry of Rural Development is the nodal Ministry for formulation, implementation and monitoring of the scheme. During the current year (2004-05) there is a budget provision of Rs. 10 crore under PURA. The Ministry with the approval of the Planning Commission decided to launch a pilot phase for implementation of the Scheme so that based on the experience of the pilot phase, the design of the Scheme and its detailed guidelines can be worked out.
- It has been decided to launch the pilot phase in seven States selecting one cluster of 10 to 15 villages in each State. The seven States selected for the pilot phase are Andhra Pradesh, Assam, Bihar, Maharashtra, Orissa, Rajasthan and Uttar Pradesh. The detailed project reports have been prepared for each of the selected cluster and have been received in the Ministry.
- A Steering Committee on PURA has been constituted to examine, sanction and monitor the implementation of projects under PURA. The Steering Committee is chaired by the Secretary (Rural Development). The first meeting of the Steering Committee was held on 11th January, 2005. It has been decided that each cluster will be financed to the extent of Rs. 4 crore to Rs. 5 crore. The projects will be of 3 years duration and in the initial phase the schemes to provide physical connectivity in the selected clusters.

DISTRICT RURAL DEVELOPMENT AGENCY ADMINISTRATION

The DRDA has traditionally been a principal organ at the District level to oversee the implementation of different anti-poverty programmes of the Ministry of Rural Development. Since inception, the administrative cost of the DRDAs was met by setting apart a certain percentage of the allocation for each programme. However, keeping in view the need for an effective agency at the District level to co-ordinate the anti-poverty programmes, a new Centrally Sponsored Scheme for strengthening the DRDAs was introduced w.e.f. 1st April, 1999. Under this scheme, the staff costs of DRDA establishments are met by the Central and State Government in the ratio of 75:25.

Objectives

The primary objective of the Scheme of DRDA Administration is to professionalise the DRDA so that they are able to effectively manage the anti-poverty programmes of the Ministry of Rural Development and interact effectively with other agencies. The DRDAs are expected to coordinate effectively with the line departments, the Panchayati Raj Institutions, the banks and other financial institutions, the NGOs as well as technical institutions with a view to gathering support and resources required for poverty reduction effort in the district.

SALIENT FEATURES

Organisational Structure

- Each district will have its own DRDA. The DRDA would be headed by a Project Director, who should be of the rank of an Additional District Magistrate. In respect of such States where DRDA does not have a separate identity, a cell will be created in the Zilla Parishad to maintain a separate account so that these are capable of being audited separately.
- The DRDA is visualised as a specialised agency capable of managing the anti-poverty programmes of the Ministry on the one hand and to effectively relate these to the overall efforts of poverty eradication in the District.
- The DRDA's role will be to facilitate the implementation of the programmes, to supervise/oversee and monitor the progress, to receive and send progress reports and maintaining accounts of funds received for various rural development programmes.
- DRDAs also need to develop synergies among different agencies for the most effective results.
- The DRDAs are expected to deal only with the programmes of the Ministry of Rural Development. If DRDAs are entrusted with programmes of other Ministries or those of the State governments, it should be ensured that these have a definite anti-poverty focus.
- The Chairman Zilla Parishad would be the chairman of the Governing Body of the DRDA. The DRDA shall also have an Executive Committee.

Staffing Pattern

- The staffing structure of the DRDAs include positions for planning for poverty alleviation, project formulation, social organisation and capacity building, gender concerns, engineering supervision and quality control, project monitoring, accounting and audit functions as well as evaluation and impact studies.

Each DRDA should have the following wings:

- Self-employment Wing;
- Women's Wing;
- Wage employment wing;
- Engineering wing;
- Accounts wing;
- Monitoring and Evaluation wing; and
- General Administration wing.

Administrative Cost

The administrative cost per district has been fixed as follows:

Category 'A' district (<6 blocks)—Rs. 46 lakhs
Category 'B' district (6-10 blocks)—Rs. 57 lakhs
Category 'C' district (11-15 blocks)—Rs. 65 lakhs
Category 'D' district (>15 blocks)—Rs. 67 lakhs

The above limits are applicable from the year 1999-2000. The ceilings are raised every year, on a compounding basis, upto 5% to set- off increases due to inflation, etc.

Personnel Policy

The DRDA should not have any permanent staff and should not resort to direct recruitment.

- Employees should be taken on deputation for specific periods to ensure better choice of staff and flexibility in staffing pattern.
- The posts of Project Directors, Project Officers, APO and all technical posts should be manned by officer with proven capability and motivation selected in an objective manner by Selection Committees.
- In the selection of Project Directors and APOs, emphasis should be on selecting officers of young age. Indicatively, the PDs and APCs should not be more than 40-45 years of age. and in any case not more than 50 years of age.

System of Monitoring and Control over the Performance of Scheme

The Central Government has a system of effective monitoring and evaluation through inspections both by Central Government and State Government officials and through Audit Reports. Besides, Vigilance and Monitoring Committees exercise vigilance and monitor implementation of programmes by the DRDAs. The Governing Body of the DRDA also reviews and monitors the implementation of the Annual Plans of the DRDAs.

Council for Advancement of People's Action and Rural Technology

The Council for Advancement of People's Action and Rural Technology (CAPART) is an autonomous Organisation under the Ministry of Rural Development established in 1986 to promote voluntary action towards implementation of projects for the enhancement of rural prosperity and to act as catalyst for development of technologies appropriate for the rural areas.

CAPART as a promoter of different models of development has undertaken the following activity during the year 2004-05.

In the year 2004-05, several steps for initiating re-engineering and repositioning of CAPART in the context of changed national and international scenario had been started by holding of interactive Regional meetings with NGOs at twelve places, e.g. Jaipur, Patna, Hyderabad, Chennai, Kolkata, Bhubaneswar, Guwahati, Ahemadabad, Mumbai, Banglore, Trivandrum and Lucknow. The suggestions of these nearly 2000 NGOs which participated in these interactive sessions were taken into account while preparing the agenda for the final National Brainstorming Session held at New Delhi on 28.12.2004 under the Chairmanship of Dr. Raghuvansh Prasad Singh, Minister for Rural Development and President of CAPART. The meeting was attended by a wide cross section of NGOs from all over the Country, members of the GB, the EC of CAPART, members of its various Committees etc Based on the outcome of this session, further initiatives were taken up by CAPART in the context of its re-engineering and repositioning.

Monitoring and Evaluation

The Ministry of Rural Development places special emphasis on monitoring and evaluation of its programmes being implemented in rural all over the country. Effective monitoring of the programmes is considered very important for efficient delivery at the grass-root level particularly in view of the substantial step up in the allocation of funds for rural development programmes since the Eighth Five Year Plan onwards. In order to ensure this, the Ministry has evolved a comprehensive multi-level and multi-tool system of Monitoring and Evaluation for the implementation of its programmes. Appropriate objectively verifiable performance indicators have been developed for each of the specific programme, both by the Ministry of Rural Development and the State authorities for effective programme monitoring at the District, Block, Gram Panchayat and Village levels so that alarm signals can be captured well in advance for in mid-course corrections.

The Ministry of Rural Development implements a number of programmes through the State Governments/Union Territory Administrations for poverty alleviations, employment generation, development of infrastructure and area development in the rural areas of the country. Substantial Budget Allocations are provided annually to achieve the stated goals. While the programmes are useful in ameliorating rural poverty, there is scope for improving the delivery system in terms of both effectiveness and efficiency which is the primary challenge we are facing today. There is an immediate need to ensure that the programmes are executed as per the Guidelines so that the benefits reach the rural poor and under developed areas in full measure. The system of monitoring is designed to meet this objective and to check any possible leakages.

The important instruments of the monitoring mechanisms are briefly outlined below:

Review by Union Ministers

The Minister of Rural Development and the Ministers of State for Rural Development visit States/UTs and review the performance of programmes with the Chief Ministers, Ministers and officials of the State Government concerned with the implementation of the programmes. Such review meetings provide the much needed impetus in the implementation of the programmes by energizing and motivating the Implementing Agencies. The need for ensuring better utilization of funds and effective delivery of benefits to the targeted groups is emphasized in these review meetings. During the year under report such reviews have taken place in Patna (for Bihar), Guwahati (for North-Eastern Regions), Mumbai, Pune, Bangalore and several other States. These review meetings were very useful in resolving policy issues and problems of programme implementation.

Periodical Progress Reports/Returns

All the programmes of the Ministry are continuously monitored through periodical progress reports received from the State Governments depicting both the financial and physical progress of the programmes. The Monitoring Division has streamlined the data processing system and the Monthly Progress Report is issued by the 10th of every month. These reports give the State-wise and Programme-wise performance of the schemes. District-Level information on the performance of various schemes are also being generated and disseminated to all concerned.

The Monitoring Division has developed a District-wise Data Management System of the Programmes of the Ministry of Rural Development. The system is a web based application and is used for data management of both State and District level data regarding physical and financial progress of the schemes of the Ministry.

CHAPTER 6

HEALTH EDUCATION THROUGH COMMUNITY PARTICIPATION: INFORMATION, EDUCATION AND COMMUNICATION

Information, Education and Communication (IEC) activities are crucial for mobilizing people's participation in the development process. It is now increasingly realized that the willing participation of the people in the development process is a pie-requisite for attaining the objectives of various development programmes. Lack of awareness has been one of the major obstacles in securing people's participation in the development process, in view of which, the IEC activities assume particular significance since they make systematic, coordinated and effective use of information for the education of the people and communicate such information in a manner that makes it 'empowering knowledge'.

—*Author*

Go in Search of People
Begin with what they know
Build on what they have

—*From a Chinese proverb*

Health Education through Community Participation: Information, Education and Communication

According to Dennis E. Poplin (Communities—A survey of Theories and Methods of Research, McMillan, NY, 1972), A community is "a unit of social and territorial organization in which people live, work, attend school, and carry on many other activities, which are a part of daily living. Indeed, communities are unique in that all of a person's needs can potentially be met within them."

Murray G. Ross defines community organization as (Murray G. Ross and B.W. Lappin, Community Organisation, Theory, Principles and Practice, Harpa and Row, NY, Second Ed.) "a process by which a community identifies its needs or objectives, gives priority to them, develops the confidence and will to work at them, finds resources (internal and external) to deal with them, and in doing so, extends and develops cooperative and collaborative attitudes and practices within the community."

Kausar S. Khan, *et al.* in their paper, "A Healthcare Paradox" stress upon people's participation. To quote them "Alma-Ata's challenge to view health as a human rights issue has not been adequately met by most Third World countries. Barring a few examples, health services continue to be either sub-standard; inaccessible, unaffordable and underutilised, or to suffer from varying combinations of these factors.

While governments of many countries, have spent millions on building physical infrastructures at district levels, the overall health status, especially of the urban and rural poor, remains deplorable. It is not more than evident that constructing a hierarchy of health centres, and even staffing them with doctors and paramedics, does not resolve the deeper issue of developing a health system that can achieve the goal of equity in health: universal coverage and care according to need.

This challenge is faced not only by governments but also by the non-governmental sector concerned with the health of the people. There is a pressing need to develop primary healthcare (PHC) systems which are technically sound and predicated on these principles of universal coverage and care according to need, but which at the same time involve communities so as to ensure that their own perceptions of their needs are fully recognised and that they are fully involved in the effort to address those needs."

Even the document "Action Plan for an Effective and Responsive Government" stressed that time has come for a strong message to be conveyed that administration is for the people and not the public servants themselves. There has to be a change of attitude, and public servants purport to offer, but in terms of public satisfaction. Simultaneously, there has also to be a cleansing of the services and codification of the ethics, value systems and the interface with the politicians.

MEANING OF COMMUNITY PARTICIPATION

What exactly we mean by community participation becomes rather enigmatic because every one interprets this term in his own way. The interpretation ranges from taking passive interest in local affairs as by reading newspapers, listening to radio, viewing TV and discussing matters with others, taking part in political activities like attending meetings, conferences, etc. and participating in processions and demonstrations. It may even include protest actions like strikes. It is through participation that citizens at large are associated with the decisions taken by government. Participation can be at various levels and by different sets of people on different issues, in each case drawing different segments of community. It may be manifest in different degrees of intensity.

Broadly speaking, the word participation is used to refer to the role of members of general public, as distinguished from that of appointed officials including civil servants, in influencing the activities of Government or in providing directly for community needs. It may occur at any level from the village to the country as a whole. It may involve decision-making, as in the case of governing bodies of local authorities and it may extend to actual implementation, as occurs when villagers/town-dwellers decide to carry out a community self-help project. The participation may be direct, as in community projects and in the work of private welfare organisations or it may be indirect, through elected officials or representative bodies responsive to public opinion. Individuals may participate through non-governmental or statutory bodies.

The extent of participation—whether direct or indirect—will ultimately depend upon citizens' access to information and opportunity of presenting their views to elected representatives.

Community participation is the process of socio-economic development in which individuals and families assume responsibility and develop their capacity to contribute to development. This enables them to become agents for their own development instead of being passive beneficiaries of development aid. They are not obliged to accept conventional solutions that are unsuitable. They can improvise and innovate to find solutions that are suitable and sustainable. They have to acquire the capacity to appraise a situation, weigh the various possibilities and estimate what their own contribution can be. They are supposed to take active interest while the community must be willing to learn, the health system is responsible for explaining and advising, and for providing clear information about the favourable and adverse consequences of the interventions being proposed, as well as their relative costs.

Health personnel form an integral part of the community in which they live and work. A continuing dialogue between them and the rest of the community is necessary to harmonize views and activities relating to primary healthcare. Such a dialogue enables health personnel to acquire a better understanding of the community's feelings, the reasons for its views, the level of its aspirations and the pattern of its organization and communication. For their part, the people will learn to identify real health needs, to understand the national strategy of primary healthcare and to become involved in and promote community action for health. Thus, society will come to realize that health is not only the right of all but also the responsibility of all, and the members of the health professions, too, will find their proper role.

In the report on Primary Healthcare presented at Alma-Ata by WHO and UNICEF, community participation has been mentioned as the essence of primary healthcare approach. It has been rightly pointed out that "self-reliance and social awareness are the key factors in human development."

Development is a multi-dimensional phenomenon which cannot be achieved unless the community itself is involved. Resources available with any Government are limited especially in the developing countries like India. Communities, according to their capacity, need to mobilise human, financial and material resources to supplement the resources provided by the national Government and other extra-community sources in order to effectively carry out local health improvement efforts. A community input for healthcare into the overall strategies, policies and work plan of the programme, which may range from unsystematic efforts by well intentioned health administrators to understanding varying community situations, to a systematic arrangement for the participation of people in health policy-making and for regular feedback of primary healthcare programme information from communities into the decision-making processes at different levels. Substantial financial and human resources can be mobilised from the community for health some of which may otherwise remain unused, such as the enthusiasm and energy of youth and women for community action. Communities with institutional structures such as local Government, a cooperative society, or a commune, which have a degree of control over the community productive assets, can mobilise resources for community health development programmes more easily than those relying on voluntary and individual contribution. Thus, the community participation is most widely seen as a way to mobilize resources for health that would otherwise not be available. A Government promoting health to meet the diverse needs of the people may be faced with expenditure it could not meet if the entire effort had to be financed out of the public purse. So, in order to cut costs, the intended beneficiaries themselves contribute to the extension of Primary Healthcare coverage.

Community participation involves members of communities in planning, implementing and monitoring of health activities. Thus, community is wholly involved in the programme rather than being asked to either contribute or to take advantage of the services offered under it. Community participation is the process in which individual families assume responsibility for their own health. They come to know their own situation better and are motivated to solve their common problems. This enables them to become agents of their own development instead of passive beneficiaries of development aid. They, therefore need to realize that they are not obliged to accept conventional solutions that are not suitable. They have to acquire the capacity to appraise a situation, weigh the various possibilities and estimate what their own contribution can be.

Community participation is an educational and empowering process in which the people, in partnership with those who are able to assist them, seek to instil a sense of belongingness, self-reliance, confidence and competence to diagnose the problems, prioritise the needs and assume critical responsibilities to manage, control and assess activities that affect them most and take collective actions that are proved necessary. It is a democracy in action. Community participation is of intrinsic value to the population group and ensures the involvement of local population in the decision-making process concerning development planning and implementation through their own efforts with the available local resources. The primary healthcare strategy is based upon effective community participation.

In Community participation, we have to safeguard the interests of the poor and the disadvantaged section of the society. Participation has objectives which the community commonly share. This common sharing makes the members of the community come together to take collective action to achieve the common goal. The goal gets the parameters and defines, in different situations, who the participants are. The roles different participants perform depend upon their capacity and capability like skills, technical knowledge, formal position, education, control over funds, connection with those in power, etc. The hierarchy makes the powerful participants active and others passive. This affects participation in favour of those who have the power to make decisions for and over others.

The poorer groups, who are generally the most affected by the development process, are the least endowed and least powerful. The poor are automatically excluded from the participation process. Decision-making is the first step in the development process. Therefore, a key objective of participation is to find out ways to include the hitherto neglected groups, who are directly affected by the negative impacts of development in the decision-making process.

Participation is a process of giving weightages to the poorer groups in the development process so that they may have a say and control over decisions which affect their lives; participation is a process of empowering the poorest. The indicator of genuine participation is the extent the poorer groups have power over decision-making and over resource management. Achieving sustainable development depends upon the extent of the participation.

Let us now discuss the essentials of participation:

- Full involvement at all levels, i.e. policy-making and planning.
- Framing/Developing programme.
- Implementation of programme.
- Evaluation of programme.
- Empowerment of powerless through giving weightage to them.
- Control over process and monitoring to ensure benefits.
- Keeping people well informed at all stages.
- According due recognition to people's contribution.
- Sincerity of government functionaries in enlisting people's support.
- Harnessing physical/economic/social resources of individual.
- Designing innovative plans for people's involvement in community.
- Empowered relationships.
- Voluntary contribution to programmes.
- Inculcating responsibility among the people for all development activities in the community.
- Ensuring that the people benefit from all development activities of the community.
- Selfless desire to work for the community.
- Respect faith in people's capacity and value the opinions and experience of the people.
- Develop on the basis of equal partnership.

P.K. Bajpai in his article, "People's Participation in Government" in *IJPA*, Oct.-Dec. 1998, rightly mentions that meaningful participation is concerned with achieving power, i.e., the power to influence the decision that affects one's livelihood. So power is the key variable to influence decision-making and lack of it not only causes but also perpetuates the ill-being of the poor. Thus, participation, power and well-being are interlinked. Indian experience has been altogether different as policies and programmes meant for development of poor have rendered only intoxicating impact and have genuinely not been concerned with sharing power.

Government must understand that consciensation of the people and their active participation in the development process, on one hand, and asserting their rights, on the other, does not weaken the authority of the State but is the symptom of true and mature democracy.

PURPOSES

Based upon our earlier observations, let us mention the important purposes that can be served by encouraging people's participation (Refer Chart 6.1).

(i) Creating will and determination among the members of the community for improvement in their present and future life.
(ii) Identification and development of the local resources, thereby generating self-reliance among the community.
(iii) Achieving integrated area coordination among various agencies interested in primary healthcare.
(iv) Mobilising the available manpower for productive and useful activities.
(v) Keeping the members of the community constantly informed about the developments in the area.
(vi) Arranging functional-literacy programmes which can help them in understanding new technology.
(vii) Organising various clubs of youth, women, to serve as centres of discussion and development.
(viii) Providing an open forum for the community to discuss its problems and find indigenous solutions which may be efficient and economical.
(ix) To develop local leaders who can further educate and mobilise the people in the area.
(x) Encouraging the people to adopt modern changes which can accelerate their socio-economic development.
(xi) Arranging extra curricular activities to generate social awareness through well designed publicity.
(xii) Encouraging the people to develop themselves rather than depend upon the Government for all activities and thus become self-reliant which is the key to development.
(xiii) Resource mobilisations from within the community to supplement organised healthcare services and keeping social control in the way resources are utilised.
(xiv) Encouraging non-governmental and voluntary organisations to become active partners in healthcare delivery.
(xv) Encouraging village health committees, panchayats, mahila mandals and youth clubs involvement in healthcare.
(xvi) The healthcare service providers and voluntary agencies should not behave as providers rather they should consciously make

CHART 6.1

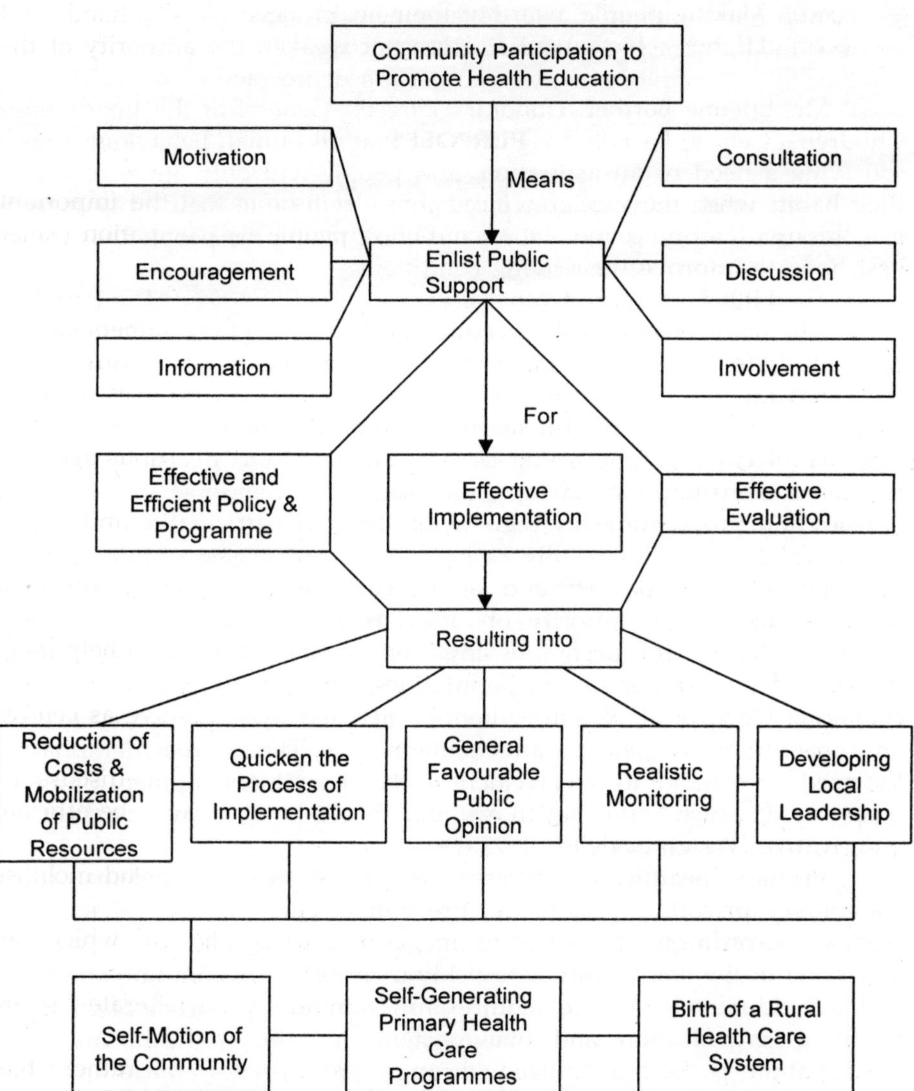

efforts to be viewed as agents of change enabling the community to use its own resources, improve skills to improve its own health.

(xvii) Recognizing the need to develop inter-sectoral coordination and multiple support linkage with health and health-related sectors of development to provide for the interest of varied sections of the community to avoid segmentation.

(xviii) Motivate and strengthen the skill of grass-root level workers to improve their credibility in the community.

(xix) Catalyst for further development.

(xx) Generate kinetic energy for health development.
(xxi) Making people aware of their health needs.
(xxii) Higher achievement at a lower cost.

Mr. Etienne Berthet, Honorary Director-General of the International Children's Centre, Paris has rightly said that all human behaviour aims at satisfying a need or an aspiration, and people will only agree to change their habits when they are convinced that it will be to their advantage. So it is through informing, motivating and encouraging the people that we can best hope to improve their living conditions.

The Fifth Five Year Plan has also recognised this need. The Fifth Plan says, "The involvement, of the people and their elected representatives is a prerequisite for effective planning. A plan which does not take into account their aspirations and preferences can have no operational validity, especially since its successful implementation can be ensured only if the majority of citizens functioning as entrepreneurs and decision-makers in relation to consumption, savings, investment, etc., endorse the envisaged policies and programmes by their whole hearted participation."

WHO and UNICEF, fully aware that the vast masses of humanity live in a state of abject poverty and, as a result, carry a great burden of ill-health, place a high priority on alleviating this burden. The strategy recently adopted for accomplishing this is that of providing primary healthcare to all under served populations, through the integration at the community level of all resources, both human and material, needed to make an impact upon the health status of the people. The approach emphasizes the need for community involvement in the general development process—a process of which better health can and should be both an ingredient and a derivative (WHO/UNICEF, 1977a:3).

Primary healthcare addresses the main health problems in the community providing promotive, preventive, curative and rehabilitative services accordingly. In order to make primary healthcare universally accessible in the community as quickly as possible, maximum community and individual self-reliance requires full community participation in the planning, organisation and management of primary healthcare. Such participation is best mobilized through appropriate education which enables communities to deal with their real health problems in the most suitable ways.

Dr. Hiroshi Nakajima, Director-General of World Health Organisation stresses the need of exploiting people's potentialities. To quote him:

> "People are the true measure of the success of policies and programmes. At the same time, people are the determinants of success. Experience teaches us that, whether in the most sophisticated cities or in the most remote villages, when people act with determination and understanding in pursuit of goals they deem essential, they achieve success. Previously insoluble problems are

solved and resources are mobilized. Miracles happen, "We must learn to harness the energy, wisdom and will of the people we serve."

Health functionaries should have firm conviction in the ability of the people to participate. Judith long-staff Mackay in his Article, "Profile of a Health Advocate" rightly says: Health advocates are crusaders for health-people with a strong sense of mission.

Dr. H. Mahler, Director-General of World Health Organization in his Article, "Health for All—Everyone's Concern", stresses the need of people's participation. To quote him:

> "Its primary responsibility is to promote individual and social awareness leading to people's involvement and self-reliance. If the individual, the family, the community do not fully realise the value of health, nor the potential consequences of the health hazards to which they are exposed or to which they voluntarily expose themselves, our goal of health for all will not be achieved. Nor will it be achieved if the people do not fully become involved in efforts to control disease and promote health."

The focus placed by the PHC approach on community involvement means that decision-makers, in developing new policies for health education, must understand and accept the need to make provision for communities to define and pursue their own goals, to mobilise their own resources, and to control and evaluate their own efforts.

It also means that mechanisms must be developed or strengthened to ensure that individuals and communities can express their views on their country health policy and take an active part in the planning and delivery of health programmes, including health education. We have to find ways of building up this process of community involvement to a point of providing continuous guidance from the grass-root to national policy-makers. Eventually, national priorities should evolve from the synthesis of local priorities.

PROCESS OF COMMUNITY PARTICIPATION IN HEALTH PROGRAMMES

I. Analysis of the Needs and Requirements of the People in the Community

The understanding of the community is the first ingredient of the process of participative management, since the community consists of many heterogeneous groups. Such understanding would help us in assessing the positive as well as negative factors that will influence the success of the participation process. This analysis must be done on scientific lines and efforts should be made to locate the informal leaders through the process of sociometry, who can be helpful in changing heterogeneity into homogeneity to avoid the wastage that would result from the friction among the different groups.

2. Designing the Health Programmes to Meet the Needs of the People with the Involvement of the People

The Health workers in the areas must design the PHC programmes which meet the priority needs of the community. It would be desirable to involve the opinion leaders—both formal and informal, so that they can give information which one has not come across during the survey already made. This will also kindle interest in them.

3. Educating the People through Formal and Informal Channels to make them Aware of the Programme and Utilising the Resources Available with them

After designing the programme and getting it approved from their headquarters, it becomes the duty of Health workers to educate the people through formal and informal channels so that they become aware of the potentialities of the programmes. Here the health workers can also assess the resources which can be tapped locally with no cost or very little cost so that the people can manage the health programmes later on themselves.

CHAPTER 7

INTER-SECTORAL CO-ORDINATION: VITAL FOR HEALTH PROMOTION AND EDUCATION

"Closely allied to the concept of community participation is the fact that these programmes cannot be planned and implemented by the health sector alone. Only a multi-sectoral approach can set in motion the processes that lead to self-sustaining development. The benefits of visiting a health centre will be short-lived indeed if the person returns to the same environment that caused his ill-health in the first place. All conditions must improve—educational, economic, social, and of course health—if there is to be any real, lasting improvement."

—*Author*

Inter-Sectoral Co-ordination: Vital for Health Promotion and Education

Alma-Ata-Declaration has desired multi-sectoral approach as one of the basic principles underlying Primary Healthcare approach so as to enable the health organisations to attain 'Health For All'.

The health status of the community is influenced by the various sectors such as Agriculture, Broadcasting and Information, Public Health Engineering, Education, Social Welfare and Rural Development. The programmes and schemes like Nutrition, Adult Education, Water and Sanitation, Integrated Child Development and Social Marketing need to be coordinated into an overall development effort.

National Institute of Health and Family Welfare in its document "Management Training Modules For District Health Officers" (New Delhi, 1990) states that the health and family welfare programme cannot function in isolation. The activities of other sectors directly as well as indirectly influence health development. Therefore, primary healthcare has to become a part of overall socio-economic development, including agriculture, irrigation, animal husbandry, education, social and women's welfare, housing and public works, communication, rural development, cooperatives, industries, panchayats and voluntary organizations. At present, extension workers and functionaries of these sectors/departments are operating in the field with few linkages of coordination. Mechanisms for coordination at the Central, state and district levels need to be developed so that the activities of the workers of all these sectors could be coordinated at the grass-root level. Arrangement should be made for working as a team, each member knowing who is doing what and for what purpose, so that programmes could be implemented in a more complimentary manner avoiding unnecessary duplication of efforts.

Coordinated planning at the community level will make it possible to link Primary Healthcare closely with other sectors and with other agencies. The District Health Officer, therefore, needs to develop sound coordinating mechanisms at Community, Sector, Block and District levels. At present, extension workers of these sectors are operating in the field with few linkages. Mechanism for coordination at the Central, State and District levels also need to be developed so that the activities of the workers of all these sectors could be coordinated at the grass-root level.[1]

Arrangements should be made for working as a team, each member knowing who is doing what and for what purpose so that programmes could be implemented in a more complimentary manner, avoiding unnecessary duplication of efforts.

Coördination means bringing about consistent and harmonious action of persons and programmes with each other towards a common goal. The coordination is lacking in the field of healthcare administration resulting in poor delivery of health services. Professor Mofide (Iran) has rightly indicated the prevailing atmosphere when he states: "In the majority of countries with some or all of these problems (environmental) pollution, uncontrolled population growth; nutritional deficiencies; the high risk of disease: shortages and maldistribution of trained staff; and insufficient financial, material and physical resources, there exists also a fragmentation of responsibilities for the delivery of healthcare, with overlapping, conflicting, and competing organisations within the health system and widely scattered funding mechanisms with the little control over costs. Health services authorities give only token recognition to those segments of the services that are not under their direct executive or financial control, and often plan only for that part of the national budget that is said to be their responsibility. The state of affairs is unjustified and harmful.[2]

Resources for the healthcare delivery are limited in the developing world. An effective health approach and strategy requires the coordinated efforts of sectors and agencies that can contribute directly or indirectly to the promotion of healthcare. Such coordinated efforts would promote health services that will be more efficient and effective from both the standpoint of the providers and that of the beneficiaries. The need of coordination is so great that according to Findlay, "It expresses the principles of organisation in toto; nothing less."[3]

The essential requisite to achieve coordination is to develop meaningful linkages with sectors of social and economic development, which can influence the promotion of healthcare, e.g., agriculture, public works, housing, communication, education, etc.

The second step is to pool the efforts of all health agencies at all levels in a system to achieve maximum output—public and private; national and international; curative and promotive; peripheral, intermediate and central; western medicine and traditional medicine. This would avoid the dangers of dysfunctional attitudes.

Third, there is the need of welding different aspects of health services into a total health package, e.g., integration of maternal and child care, family planning, prevention of communicable diseases, health education, environmental sanitation.

Coordination and linkages on a systematic, rather than on *ad-hoc*, basis will definitely reduce costly duplications of effort and lead to increased health coverage of the needy population and neglected areas, while making the optimum use of the resources. Most of the countries in their reply to the WHO admitted that the lack of coordination in healthcare delivery system is a serious challenge. To quote WHO:

"The consensus of opinion is that the most important managerial problems are foreseen in the continued reduction of the imbalance of the system and the lack of integration in the distribution of care with the existence of parallel systems with different objectives. Fragmentation and division of responsibility between the different levels of care have led to a lack of effective communication between the health and social welfare agencies. . . As there are several agencies providing medical care there is overlapping and duplication of activities . . . . The major managerial problems . . . is to recognise the various components of this system in a way that reflects complementarity eliminates duplication and minimizes waste of resources."[4]

This problem becomes more acute in a federal country like India, where health is a State subject. It becomes important to coordinate the health programmes at the national level. The dilution of health standards in the State may affect adversely the whole country. There is a need, therefore, to give more powers to the central authority by making health a Concurrent subject. One of the health experts went on to say: "The present health situation in developing countries, especially India, is in a chaotic condition as non-scientific and realistic attempt is visible to coordinate the available inputs to produce maximum output. We can locate a large area without any healthcare facilities while in some areas, every third shop or house is providing medical care."[5]

How can we achieve effective coordination? According to Dr. White, its achievement may require.

"The most delicate insights, the most mature wisdom, and perception of a truly artistic quality."[6]

It has to be achieved through formal as well as informal. methods.

The effective coordination and linkages would automatically result from effective planning, policy-making, and manpower planning.[7] After planning and policy-making, the effective instrument to achieve coordination is to design a sound organisation. Dr. White says:

"An organisation characterised by clear lines of authority, adequate powers, well-understood allocation of functions, absence of overlapping and duplication of effort and proper delegation of work in itself reduce the necessities of coordination."[8]

Besides, if the organisational boundaries are properly demarcated, there would be little scope of confusion and misunderstanding and coordination would naturally flow from this inherent structure.

The coordination among different agencies, however, can be obtained through mutual consultation or information. This mutual consultation should be encouraged through setting up of inter-departmental agency/ committees for joint planning, joint decision-making and joint action in areas concerning more than one agency. While achieving coordination, we may keep the cost factor in mind. Such inter or Intra-agencies can serve a useful purpose when the members come duly prepared with a sense of urgency and commitment. According to Key, "a session of an inter-departmental committee tends to be a place where departmental representatives come well prepared to defend their positions and level more convinced than before of the correctness of their attitudes."[9]

We are to take care that the benefits achieved through coordination should surpass the expenditure incurred to obtain coordination.

Besides formal methods, we should adopt informal methods which are as effective as the formal ones, e.g., the Central Council of Health and the Central Council of Family Welfare (India) used the informal methods to achieve coordination among the different States and between the Union Government and the State Governments. "It is the most powerful cement in the whole executive structure."[10]

We must encourage such informal methods at all levels of Government.

We must try to achieve coordination to obtain coherency in all the agencies dealing directly or indirectly with healthcare, all the systems of medicines, all the persons responsible for healthcare (team work) and at all the levels through well designed formal and informal channels with minimum costs to fulfil the goal—the betterment of the health of mankind irrespective of the status and location and to obtain optimum benefits from available and potential resources.

According to Dr. Halfdan Mahler, "there is one more illustration that health can only be attained through a combination of diverse measures in the health and other related sectors. These measures have to be applied within communities to deal with the full range of problems whose combined effects ravage the health of people. With the possible exception of smallpox eradication (which had unique features—the exception that proved the rule), attempts to deal with single cowman cable diseases in ways that were at best parallel and at worst divergent have proved to be ineffective. There is no escape from the need to deal in a concerted manner with those factors that in the final analysis are common to most of these diseases, This is the rationale for primary healthcare accessible to all in a spirit of social equity, and for health systems based on primary healthcare."[11]

The health and family welfare programmes cannot function in isolation. The activities of other sectors directly as well as indirectly influence health development. Therefore, primary healthcare has to become a part of overall socio-economic development, including agriculture, irrigation, animal husbandry, education, social and women's welfare, housing and public works, communication, rural development, cooperatives, industries, panchayats and voluntary organizations. At present, extension workers and functionaries of these sectors/departments are operating in the field with few linkages or coordination. Mechanisms for coordination at the Central, state and district levels need to be developed so that the activities of the workers/functionaries of all these sectors could be coordinated at the grass-root level. Arrangements should be made for working as a team, each member knowing who is doing what and for what purpose, so that programmes could be implemented in a more complimentary manner avoiding unnecessary duplication of efforts.

Ale ya El Bindari Hammad[12] (*World Health*, March 1986, p. 3) in the Article, "Inter-sectoral Cooperation in Primary Healthcare" rightly mentions the need of forging alliances with other sectors of development to ensure good health. To quote him:

> Improvements in the health status of a population cannot be achieved simply by expanding and developing the health services. The prevention and control of disease and the promotion of health require a concerted effort for the improvement of human well-being as a whole. In this task, what has been defined as "healthcare" has to be supported by improvements in the social and economic infrastructure, and contributions from various sectors other than health.

In the initiatives embodied in WHO's Health for all strategy, inter-sectoral action has been emphasised and articulated as part of the health strategy, mainly because of the basic re-ordering of health priorities. Today the major emphasis is on the prevention and control of disease and the promotion of health through primary healthcare. This shift in priorities has immediately highlighted the inter-sectoral character of healthcare. Agriculture and nutrition, housing, sanitation, water supply, literacy, health education and greater self-reliance in healthcare are all integrated in the current primary healthcare strategies.

Achievement of the Health for all goals will depend vitally on sound inter-sectoral action directed at specific health goals. On the one hand, eliminating the major causes of prevalent sickness and preventing any specific cluster of diseases will require action in all those areas outside the health sector which currently contribute to the incidence of those diseases. And on the other, the broader aim of increasing well-being and resistance to disease as a whole while promoting and maintaining good health will require the combined efforts of many sectors not immediately related to health.

Neither the individual nor the household perceives well-being as fragmented into sectors even if that well-being stems from a specific economic sector, or from education, or from health, or from employment. Well-being is a single unified condition. The same is equally true of the well-being of a community. It is with this perception in mind that health planners and health workers need to act when drawing up strategies or putting primary healthcare into practice. This will ensure that the health component is placed in the context of social development as a whole, and that other sectors are mobilised and motivated to lend their support towards achieving health goals. World Health Organization is also committed to this ideal.

More than ever before, the experts responsible for planning national economies are recognising that a country's health forms part of an integrated process of development.

The experience of the world's industrialised countries showed that diseases associated with poor sanitation, illiteracy and poverty were eventually controlled, not by spectacular medical breakthrough, but by improvements in urban services, housing and the environment, higher levels of education and better diets.

The moral for all the world today is that the health sector cannot do it alone! Many other ministries, services, institutions, official and unofficial bodies, and all levels of administration down to the community and the family must become involved in health.

So the drive towards the goal of Health for all by the year 2000 can only be inspired and fuelled by concerted inter-sectoral action. Our graphic model suggests only the eight elements included in WHOs definition of Primary Healthcare education about health, proper nutrition, safe water and basic sanitation, maternal and child care including family planning, immunization, prevention and control of locally endemic diseases, appropriate treatment of common diseases and injuries, and provision of essential drugs. (See Chart 7.1)

But these symbolise a huge range of factors to which other sectors besides health must contribute if all people are indeed to attain a level of health that will permit them to lead a socially and economically productive life.

No sector engaged in socio-economic development can function properly in isolation. In the context of primary healthcare it is necessary to involve all the developmental departments in a coordinated effort. The inputs of one department have got to be synchronised with those of other departments—a total effort at the grass-root level. Success in the field of health and family welfare will largely depend on successful implementation of various programmes of social and economic development simultaneously. Particular mention may be made of education, social

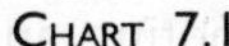

CHART 7.I

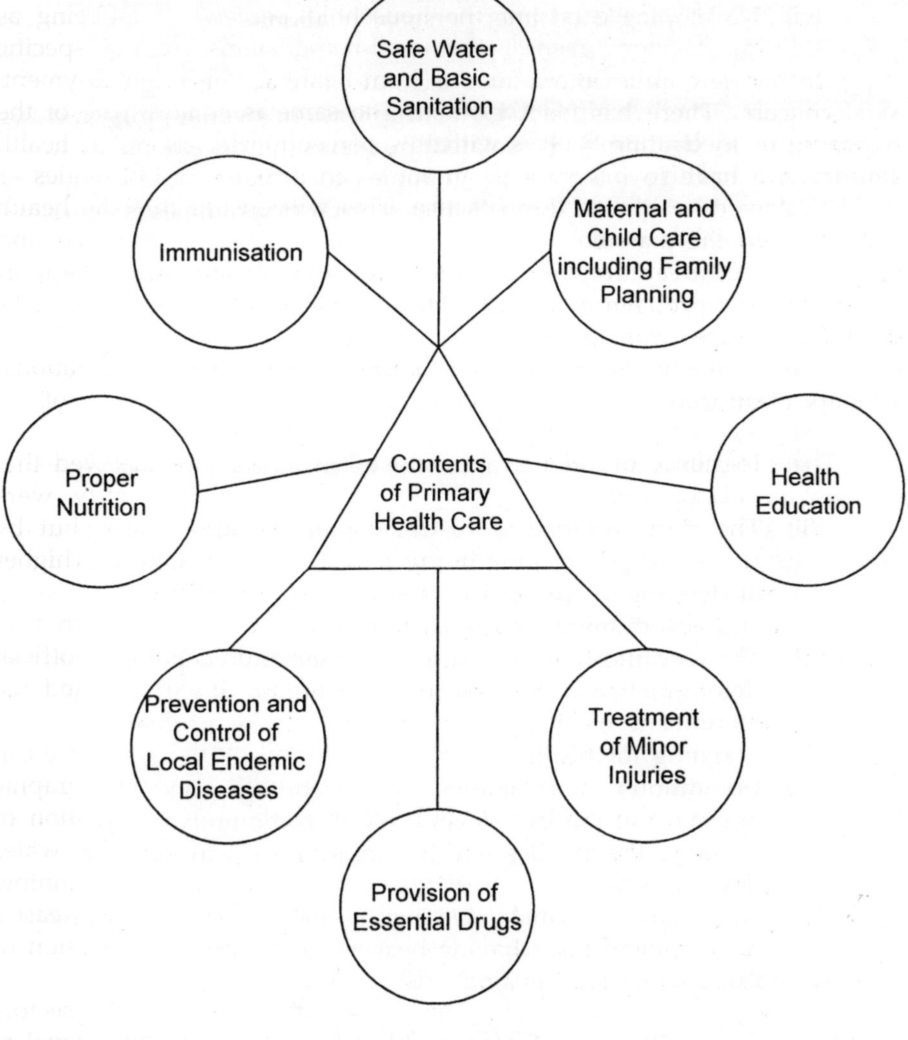

welfare, agriculture, animal husbandry, food, industry, works and housing and communication with which health development programmes should be linked for the success of health and family welfare programmes.

ESSENTIALS OF INTER-SECTORAL CO-ORDINATION

(i) Clear-cut demarcation of the role of different sectors of development in the promotion of health.

(ii) Arranging meetings among collaborative organisations to sort out duties and responsibilities.

(iii) Developing informal relationships.
(iv) Creating interest in other organisations.
(v) Joint monitoring of the programmes.
(vi) Developing good inter-personal relations.

In the new millennium, inter-sectoral coordination is going to be of vital concern. There has been lot of duplication, overlapping, and high expenditure in dealing with isolated problems of development. In 21st century, we have to integrate programmes to achieve multi-dimensional benefits. Area development through Inter-sectoral programmes is going to be the tool with the planners.

In the 21st century, resources for health may not be unlimited. The solution to the problem of Primary Healthcare in new millennium lies in pooling resources from the sectors having impact on Primary Healthcare directly or indirectly. Following are recommended to be pursued to ensure Primary Healthcare:

(i) Health is an input into, as well as an outcome of socio-economic development.
(ii) The clear formulation of development policies, plans, actions and strategies keeping in view the focus on health. It also aims at defining of role and responsibilities of participating agencies and determining functional linkages.
(iii) The identification of area for inter-sectoral cooperation and the determination of the specific contribution of each sector to the attainment of the goals proposed in the normal process of planning for health.
(iv) Community participation to encourage an inter-sectoral approach at the local level through community empowerment.
(v) Locating the hurdles which stands in the way of inter-sectoral development.
(vi) Arranging informal meetings among agencies engaged in development tasks having bearing on health.
(vii) Conducting joint evaluations.

Experience with inter-sectoral support for primary healthcare is still in infancy and there is considerable doubt as to how such support can be harnessed. While the health sector must take a lead in promoting cooperation, effective action may require direction from outside the health sector, by a body with executive as well as coordinating powers. There is a need to set-up co-ordinating machinery at all levels.

CASE STUDIES

1. Urban Basic Services Scheme

Government of India, State Governments and UNICEF initiated urban basic services to make the life of slum-dwellers in the cities better and check degradation of cities.

J.S. Saksena and P.N. Govindarajuler in their Article, "Healthcare for Urban Slums with special reference to Bangalore City" have rightly sensed the problem. To quote them:

> "Slum-dwellers have the worst of both the worlds-urban and rural. On one side they suffer from economic hardships, lack of education and absence of health infrastructure like the rural population. On the other hand, they also suffer the ill-effects of overcrowding, pollution and rootlessness characteristics of large metropolitan cities."[13]

They further add that "Most comforts and conveniences of the cities are sustained by the work done by slum-dwellers. As such, the affluent and the privileged have the moral responsibility to try to mitigate and alleviate their suffering. Rural population may be ignorant of the "goodies" they are missing but a slum-dweller is painfully aware of the privations suffered by him due to his constantly rubbing shoulders with urban affluence and conspicuous consumption with resultant frustration and resentment."

The author conducted a research study in Una district of Himachal Pradesh to study the impact of the scheme. The Urban Basic services programmes in Una district was started in 1987-88, but it actually came up in May, 1988 when the first instalment of money was received. The programme is being implemented in all the five towns of the District, i.e. Una, Mehatpur, Santokhgarh, Gagret and Daulatpur. The Analysis of table indicates that out of a total slum population of 27,186 in all the five towns, 14,000 population is being covered under UBS. The interesting feature of the population is that the Bastis are scattered being partly Hilly areas and these Bastis are not typical of Bastis in metropolitan cities in plains like Faridabad, Ludhiana, Delhi, etc. These Bastis do not pose problems to environmental sanitafion—except that the inhabitants, mostly belonging to scheduled castes, are poor and thus the women and children of these Bastis need special care to ensure their development and ultimately the total Development of the area.

There has been an effort to provide coverage of the basic services in all the Bastis. For improving the health services especially for women and children, there has been immunization (cent per cent) both for children and women, training of Dais, supplementary nutrition of children, medical checkup of children in Balwadis and primary schools. To ensure the education among children and women, the Balwadis and Adult Centres for Women have been set-up and to ensure economic independence for women, tailoring and knitting classes were started. There were also classes in food processing and soap-making. To maintain environmental sanitation, hand pumps have been installed, individual community and institutional latrines have been provided. Thus, women and children, especially of weaker sections of the society, have benefitted from the programme. For this, the

Programme Officer has developed a liaison with District Information Officer to maintain Data Bank and information service.

The study found lack of inter-sectoral coordination to make sustained impact. Most of the components in these UBS programmes aim at providing fragments of services, while people need a total package. Most of the people narrated the same stories as given by Sister Agnestia in her article, "Towards Healthcare Directed for Social Transformation" (A Real Life Experience). To quote:

> "Can vitamin tablets satisfy their hunger and care their malnutrition? Can ORS eradicate the repeated attacks of diarrhoea? What was I doing through my health education campaign? I was trying to conceal the real cause of the illness. The fact is that the poor are forced to lead unhealthy lives because of their poverty, which itself is a result of the exploitative and unjust practices of Society. Uncritical acceptance of health messages conveniently removes the responsibility for ill-health from those who exploit and instead place the blame on the very people who are victims of the exploitation."

It is evident that most of the functions carried out by UBS personnel relate to other sectors like Health, Education, Social Welfare, etc. In order to converge the benefits, we suggest the following to ensure effective linkages:

(a) Where services are already provided by other sectors the need is to make these services functional through the intervention of UBS staff rather than venturing their own services like Immunization, Training of Dais, etc.

(b) District Coordinator must see as to what can be provided by other departments without any consumption of resources. For example, all the places for conducting classes for women and children are hired while many such rooms are lying idle and thus can be provided free of cost. Similarly, this exercise need to be done at Municipal level. One is surprised to find that the Municipal Committee/Notified Area committees are charging rents of their unoccupied rooms from this project which is a sad reflection.

(c) Most of the Project staff is vied with the idea that whatever has been budgeted must be spent whether it is relevant or not, e.g. a community latrine was built in an area where most of the houses have household latrines.

(d) Linkage with the Community has not been developed, e.g. for the construction of community services, no community labour was used and thus the expenditure became high with the defeat of basic purpose.[14]

2. Women's Health

Government of India, Department of Women and Child Development Ministry of Human Resources Development presented country report to the Fourth World Conference on Women (Beijing 1995).[15] The report clearly mentions the need of inter-sectoral coordination to promote health of women.

Women's health covers mortality, morbidity, nutritional status and reproductive health. Linked to these are environmental degradation, violence and occupational harzards, all of which have implications for women's health.

The health status of a population is one of the crucial elements in the assessment of the quality of life. More precisely, indicators, namely, maternal mortality (MMR) and morbidity rates, infant mortality rates (IMR), life expectancy, fertility rates, studied along with statistics on female literacy rates, work participation rates, age at marriage, cases of recorded violence, malnutrition, etc., provide pointers to the physical status and well-being of women.

The health of Indian women is intimately related to the socio-economic status of the households to which they belong and their age and kinship/marital status within the households. Given the predominantly patriarchal set-up, women and girls get a lesser share in the intrahousehold distribution of healthy goods and services, compared to men and boys. However, in the intra-household distribution of labour, women get the major share of economic, procreative and family responsibilities. Due to the competing demands on their time and energy, as well as their socialization, women tend to neglect their health. The lesser access to food coupled with neglect invariably leads to a poor nutritional status and a state of ill-health for most women.

Women's health plays an important role in determining the health of the future population, because women's health has an inter-generational effect. The cumulative impact of the low health situation of women is reflected in the high MMRs, the incidence of low-birth weight babies, high prenatal mortality and foetal wastage and consequent high fertility rates.

Asha Das in her article "Child Development and Empowering Women in India,"[16] in *IJPA*, July to Sept. 1997 rightly observes that the major approach for the future will be to bring in holistic approach for women's development. This underscores harmonisation of various efforts in different fronts—social, economic, legal, political and cultural. This calls for consolidation of various programmes and efforts in different sectors of the Government, and their integration in a logical fashion to converge various services and facilities required by women. A sub-plan approach to package all relevant resources and benefits for women's development will be laid down to ensure their systematic focus on women.

3. Community Development Programme (CDP)

The programme of Community Development started after

independence in India was a programme cutting across sectoral boundaries. It embraced education, health, drinking water, roads, agricultural production and cottage industries.

4. Integrated Child Development Services (ICDS)

ICDS, started in 1975-76, is an excellent example of Inter-sectoral coordination. The ICDS Scheme aims to improve the nutritional and health status of pre-school children, pregnant women and nursing mothers through providing a package of services, including supplementary nutrition, pre-school education, immunization, health checkup, referral services and nutrition and health education. In addition, the scheme focusses on effective convergence of inter-sectoral services in the Anganwadi Centres (AWC) which is the place for providing services to women and the children.

5. Integrated Rural Development Programme

In 1976, the Lok Sabha approved the new strategy of rural development, which is commonly known as Integrated Rural Development Programme. World Bank sector paper defines rural development as "Rural development is a strategy designed to improve the economic and social life of a group of people—the rural poor. It involves extending the benefits to the poorest among those who seek a livelihood in the rural areas. The group includes small farmers, tenants and the landless."

R.N. Azad defines it as "integrated development of the areas and the people through optimum development and utilization of local resources, physical, biological and human by bringing about necessary institutional, structural and attitudinal changes by delivering a package of services to encompass not only the economic field, that is, agriculture and rural industries but also the establishment of social infrastructure, and services in the area of health and nutrition, sanitation, housing, drinking water, with the ultimate objective of improving the quality of life of the rural poor and rural weak. Integrated rural development implies functional, spatial, and temporal integration of all these parameters. Thus, Integral rural development is a multifacet framework involving a multi-disciplinary approach. In this process, self-help and community participation have a paramount role."[17]

The IRDP, launched in 1980, is a credit linked self-employment programme of assistance of the already identified rural poor families to augment their income and help them cross over the poverty line. The IRDP is implemented through the District Rural Development Agency (DRDA), which is a broad-based representative body that provides guidance and direction for programme implementation. At the grass-roots level, Block Development Office is responsible for implementing IRDP. At the state and the Central Government levels, the Department of Rural Development and the Ministry of Rural Areas and Employment respectively oversee the programmes implementation.

The ultimate thrust of IRDP need be on enhancing the quality of life of the rural people. The Public Accounts Committee (PAC) of parliament has recently given some suggestion about reshaping the Integrated Rural Development Programme (IRDP).[18]

It lacks a comprehensive approach. A large number of poverty alleviation programmes pertaining to income, employment, quality of life, etc. of the poor are implemented simultaneously aiming at more or less the same group of people. This creates overlapping which results in confusion and weak planning. Secondly, these programmes are implemented by a large number of ministries and departments of the central and state governments. This multiplicity of agencies, without any satisfactory level of co-ordination among them, adds to the confusion. And, thirdly, the IRDP approach aims at providing self-employment to the poor without giving due consideration to the desirability and feasibility of self-employment for the poorest sections of the society. It has been observed that many times the poor, and specially the poorest sections of the population, prefer wage employment. The committee therefore feels that the poor, who are not willing or are incapable of taking up self-employment should be given an option of wage employment. There is a need to integrate wage employment programmes with self-employment programmes.

The committee has recommended that a more comprehensive approach to rural development should be adopted which would aim at redesigning the whole rural economy and society, at elimination of the exploitation of the poor and at providing them with gainful employment, whether under the auspices of the public or private sector or under self-employment. IRDP can be effective only if there is integrated planning and coordinated implementation. The committee therefore suggests that as a first step in this direction, all allied programmes and activities, and the economic infrastructure required for effective implementation of these programmes are integrated and brought under one ministry to avoid overlapping and to enable the government to have an effective control over these programmes. All the programmes must be an integral part of a single development plan formulated by a single development authority and for whose effective implementation one single authority is responsible and accountable.

Notes and References

1. Dr. Hector R. Acuna, Community Participation, in *World Health*, Aug.-Sept. 1977, p. 6.
2. WHO, *World Health* Paper, 55, p. 83.
3. R.M. Findlay, Art of Administration, Edinburgh, Oliver, 1952, p. 48.
4. WHO, Public Health Paper, 55, p. 61.
5. Based on Personal discussion.
6. L.D. White, Introduction to the Study of Public Administration, Macmillan, pp. 213-14.

7. For details refer to the respective Chapters.
8. L.D. White, *op. cit.*, p. 214.
9. V.K. Key, Politics and Administration in White (Ed.), The Future of Government in the United States, p. 155.
10. S.E. Finer, Primer of Public Administration, London. 1950, p. 68.
11. Dr. Halfdan Mahler, "Defeat TB and Forever", in *World Health*, January 1982, p. 3.
12. Ale ya El Bindari Hammad, "Inter-sectoral Cooperation in Primary Healthcare", in *World Health*, March 1986, p. 3.
13. WHO, *World Health*, March 9, 1986, p. 16.
14. S.L. Goel,"Planning and Administration of Urban Basic Services", in S. Bhatnagar and S.L. Goel,"Development Planning and Administrative" ed., New Delhi, Deep & Deep, 1992, pp. 167-206.
15. GOI, Department of Women and Child Development, Ministry of Human Resources Development, Fourth World Conference on Women, Beijing, 1995, (Country Report), p. 84.
16. Asha Das, "Child Development and Empowering Women in India", in *IJPA*, July-Sept., 1997, pp. 392-93.
17. R.N. Azad, Integrated Rural Development Dynamics of Development An International Perspective, New Delhi, Concept, 1977, pp. 419-39.
18. A.K. Debey, "IRDP: The South Asian Experience" in *IJPA*, April-June, 1997, pp. 149-50.

CHAPTER 8

APPROPRIATE TECHNOLOGY AND RESEARCH FOR RURAL (PRIMARY) HEALTHCARE AND EDUCATION

> Technology stimulates science and science acts as a spur to new technology. Social progress depends on both technology and science, but both of these again depends on man's basic desire to live a life that is both physically and intellectually richer and fruitful. A piece of technology may be regarded as appropriate for a community if its design is related to the real needs of that community and its use fulfils these needs. Its use and promotion are based on that community's economic viability and technical competence to support, service, maintain and even improve upon it to suit local conditions. Appropriate technology is thus an approach in which technical innovation and adoption go hand in hand with social and cultural integration.
>
> —*Author*

Appropriate Technology and Research for Rural (Primary) Healthcare and Education

In this chapter, we are discussing two interconnected issues, i.e., (a) Appropriate Technology for Health, and (b) Research for Primary Healthcare.

A. APPROPRIATE TECHNOLOGY

As stated in a WHO document, appropriate means: besides being scientifically sound, the technology is acceptable to those who apply it as well as those for whom it is used. This implies that the technology should be in keeping with the local culture. It must be capable of being adapted and further developed if necessary. As stated in a WHO document, health technology has been defined association of methods, techniques and equipment, together with the people using them." The use of appropriate technology is an important factor that will contribute to the success of primary healthcare. The following are some examples of these technologies

1. Biogas generation for cooking, lighting and refrigeration.
2. Use of plastic moulds for water-sealed latrines.
3. Indigenous cooling system using running water to help maintain the cold chain.
4. Use of bamboo to fortify' concrete-based hand pumps and community maintenance of these hand pumps.
5. Organisation of community maintenance of hand pumps.
6. Rain water storage tanks.

It is not defined in terms of the high level of technology used, but by the attention given to the local conditions and environment. Thus,

CHART 8.1

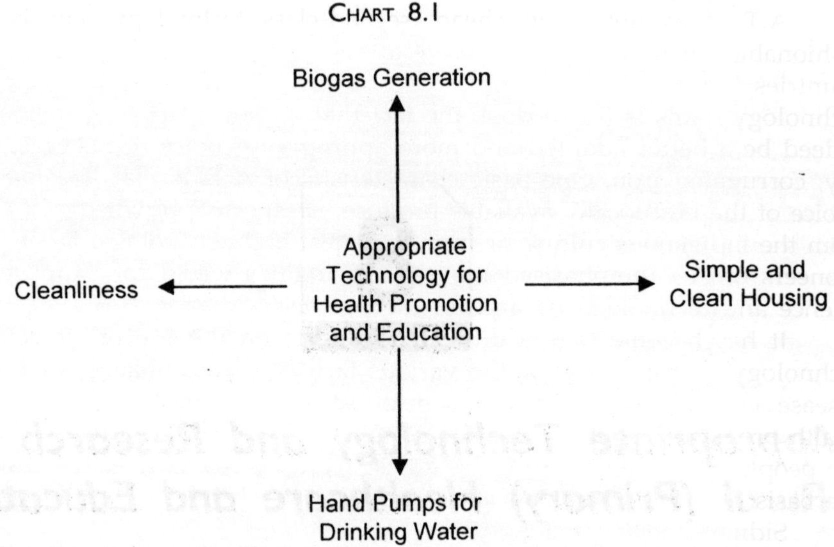

appropriate technology, depends on the local skill, resources and talent. Appropriate technology is the only answer to promote primary healthcare. These were also reiterated by Alma Ata Declaration.

Ashok Khosla in his article, "Technology and Development" in *IJPA*, July to Sept. 1989, pp. 531-32 rightly defines appropriate Technology as: "Technology which serves the goals of development is defined as appropriate technology. Appropriate technology springs from creative, in response to local needs and possibilities. It is relevant and ready for use by the common people, and aims directly to improve the quality of their lives. It derives maximum leverage from the local cultural environment, by drawing upon the existing managerial and technical skills and providing the basis for extending them. It uses the physical potential of an area and maintains man's harmony with nature."

Claudine Brelet in his article, "Appropriate Technology for Health" in *World Health*, June 1985, defines it as:

> Appropriate Technology for health is a concept that has launched thousands of projects and programmes all over our planet, initiated by governments, non-governmental organizations, small local voluntary groups and private individuals.

Generally abbreviated as ATH or A.T. it has been defined by WHO as "technology that is scientifically sound, adaptable to local needs, and acceptable to those who apply it and those for whom it is used, and that can be maintained by the people themselves in keeping with the principle of self-reliance with the resources the community and the country can afford." So from the start, the accent has been put on people's participation, and on their appropriation of the appropriate means to provide and use healthcare.

A.T. does not mean cheap, second-class technology, nor is it a fashionable label that can be used to sell cheap devices to developing countries. Although sometimes scornfully dismissed as "bamboo-technology", this is to overlook the fact that, in some places, bamboo can indeed be a better adapted and more appropriate choice of material then, say, corrugated iron. One basic characteristic of A.T. is that it entails the choice of the best locally available produce, irrespective of whether it stems from the indigenous culture or from the latest high-technology. Indeed, the pioneers of A.T. emphasised the need in today's world for "appropriate science and technology by and for the people."

It has become highly difficult to decide on the use of appropriate technology keeping in view the various factors—need, finances, nature of disease, etc. It has become a fashion to use complex technology for simple health problems thereby increasing costs and non-availability to majority of the people. Hukan Hellberg in his article, "Technology for Health" suggests the basis of decision-making about the use of appropriate technology.

Sidney Nickhe in his article, "Money for Health" in *World Health*, May 1989, writes based on his experience in Kieto district hospital. The costs incurred in running a district hospital are often high because the technology used in providing health services is neither sustainable nor effective. An affordable technology could be helpful to district health managers especially in the areas of support services and energy use.

To cook for the 50 or so patients admitted each month to the Kieto district hospital requires seven truckloads of firewood, each weighing seven tons. This does not only mean deforestation and destruction of the environment, but is also an expensive and inefficient use of resources.

Cooking is done on an open fire where three stones serve as a stove. Money could be saved by using an improved energy-saving stove, which also burns firewood. Such stoves are produced at an appropriate technology centre in Arusha (CAMARTEC) and are sold to institutions which use firewood for cooking purposes. The stoves reduce fuel wood consumption by more than 50 percent compared to the three-stone fireplace. Where energy problems prevail, health services are inevitably adversely affected. For example, refrigerators for preserving vaccines use kerosene but practice shows that the unreliability of fuel supplies may result in spoiled vaccines. The use of kerosene for refrigerators, lighting and sterilising purposes is too expensive for most district hospitals. Alternative sources of energy are available but capital investments are forbidding. A biogas plant could be more efficiently and effectively used at a district hospital than wood-burning systems.

Biogas is produced when bacteria break down organic material under airless conditions. It is a simple technology and when carefully used in rural hospitals where human and livestock dung is easily available, it would come cheaper than using kerosene, firewood or charcoal, with their added labour and transportation costs. Although capital costs are relatively higher—about US 1,000 dollars for material, labour and accessories—biogas is cheaper in the long-run.

Other technological innovations which could be used to reduce running costs in healthcare delivery include:

- use of solar energy for refrigeration, lighting and heating;
- water "harvesting" during the rainy season for hospitals and dispensaries in areas where water is scarce; underground storage of water has been found to be relatively cheap;
- use of Ventilated Improved Pit (VIP) latrines in areas where water supply is unreliable and where resources are inadequate for installing and maintaining flush water toilets; and
- avoiding recently introduced brand name drugs and relying instead on cheap generic products.

Dr. Nashara's five year experiences at the district hospital underline the importance of preventive rather than curative measures. He has seen a steady drain of the resources needed to treat patients suffering from preventable diseases.

"If the environment is kept clean, swamps are sprayed and water is treated, the incidence of diarrhoea can be kept low", he says confidently, since experience has shown him that diseases prevalent in the area have a devastating impact on the community and on available resources.

Primary Healthcare is gaining acceptance as a strategy for bringing basic health services to all the people. Such programmes can have a significant impact on health by focussing on a carefully selected number of health problems that are preventable by means of simple, and relatively low cost, interventions.

Decisions concerning the health technology that is necessary and affordable should be made after evaluating the basic procedures to be carried out in the fields of medicine, surgery, paediatrics, obstetrics and so forth. There is no point in training "Cadillac mechanics" if they are to work on "motor scooters and bicycles."

But man is not a machine and technology does not only mean "nuts and bolts." We need improved technologies and abilities to undertake health advocacy, to inform and communicate about health. We have to create social awareness about appropriate technologies, and to stimulate political will for appropriate decisions about the use of resources that will result in relevant technical solutions. But for all of this, we need to build a sound scientific and technological base in order to give credibility to our persuasion.

Eero Lehtinen and Daphne Fresle in their article, "Medical diagnostic ultrasound" rightly warn against the use of too much modern technology. To quote them:

> New technologies in the field of radiology have sprung up like mushrooms after rain in the last decade.

Indeed, within the last ten to fifteen years medical technology has evolved with a sometimes bewildering rapidity, improving and creating new diagnostic tools which complement, or even compete with, each other. The difficult task for the doctor, health administrator and policy-maker is that of informed choice. Even the richest countries cannot possibly provide the total range of available technology, so high is the cost to patient and society.

The key surely lies in the cost benefit risk equation in its broadest sense. And until we truly view healthcare and the medical technologies, not in isolation but as part of a total pattern of social and economic development, we shall be unable to use to real advantage the extraordinary advances in knowledge which make the present age so challenging and stimulating.

Professor H. Abrams, one of the most prominent radiologists in the United State, concluded his presentation at a symposium on the impact of the new imaging technologies on healthcare by stating:

> "In summary, we simply cannot afford the new technologies. They will cost a great deal and be overused. They will take resource from the poor and have little impact on the health of the sickest segment of the population. A paradox thus unfolds. On the one hand, a nation with high unemployment may well have better things to spend its resources on the computer topography scanning, nuclear magnetic resonance and digital radiography. On the other hand, the individuals who constitute the nation and are subject to illness want nothing less than the best and the newest, if there is the faintest possibility that it may affect their health."

Let us explain with an example. WHO has developed a kit for Dais for ensuring safe delivery. There is no more crucial passage in life than birth. Yet 60 per cent of the world's women do not have access to pregnancy care and safe delivery care, which would dramatically reduce the risk of maternal and newborn mortality. Making available this appropriate technology would be a decisive step towards Health for All.

The basic kit is simple, inexpensive and can be made from locally available materials. It supports three essential factors that will dramatically reduce the risk of infection in mother and child; a clean delivery surface, clean hand (soap and a nail stick), clean cutting of the umbilical cord (a razor blade and cotton for tying-off the cord). A tape measure enables the health worker to monitor the growth of the uterus regularly, in order to detect conditions that require special care. Newborn babies and infants can lose as much as 25 per cent of their body heat unless they are well wrapped up; a simple cap made from several layers of cloth can conserve a large part of their body heat and thus make them less vulnerable to diseases. This is another example of appropriate technology for birth.

There has been a great revolution in technology in medical sciences.

Complicated machines to be handled by experts are available. 21st century is going to be more explosive as far as the innovations in new technology are concerned. However, there is a need to simplify this highly complicated technology, which only a few can afford. We must develop simple technology, which people can afford and sustain, e.g. Oral Dehydration Therapy.

Denise Ayres rightly says, "Few health technologies have as great a potential as oral dehydration therapy (ORT) to make an impact on childhood mortality in developing countries. Simple, inexpensive and effective, ORT can be used not only throughout the health system but at home as well."

Robert J. Gerety in his article, "A New Use for Yeast" said, Plasma-derived vaccines against hepatitis B cannot satisfy the needs of less affluent areas of the world where the disease is endemic. But vaccines produced in yeast by recombinant DNA technology seem likely to fulfil all the needs on a global scale.

Kirsten Staehr Johansen in his article, "International Insulin Pump Study" rightly said, "One of the best examples of medical technology intended for home care of the patient is the miniature insulin pump. No larger than a pack of playing cards, it is usually secured by a belt to the chest or thigh of a diabetes sufferer. An imparted "shunt" (valve) releases insulin into the patient's vein in quantities that he or she can regulate according to need. Insulin is essential for diabetes victims to maintain their blood-sugar level, and without it they risk falling into a coma. The pump can be recharged manually from an external source, or by inserting a cartridge containing fresh insulin."

According to Jan Stjernsward and Peter Ozorio, there is the knowledge to prevent cancer pain, derived from several decades of clinical experience and research, and there are simple and inexpensive methods to ease pain. There are, as well, drugs to provide relief for patients, and to allow the incurably ill to die with dignity.

Yet despite the best intentions, what is known is not applied, and even though pain relief is the only human therapeutic alternative, it is not offered adequately to millions. There is a need of global commitment.

Appropriate technology in health is going to be the greatest challenge of new millennium because of the following reasons:

1. Technology is becoming highly sophisticated with the passing of time.
2. It is highly costly to afford by developing countries on a large scale.
3. Manpower to make use of new technology is not available as it costs in their retention and training.
4. There are many inherent dangers in the new technology to have negative effects on health of the people.
5. Very less attention is being paid to develop appropriate

technology to suit the needs of millions of people suffering from abject poverty and illness.

6. Complicated machines go out of order and we need highly trained specialists to maintain them.

Therefore, in the new millennium, we should focus attention on providing appropriate technology to suit majority of the population.

B. APPROPRIATE RESEARCH FOR PRIMARY HEALTHCARE

W.A. Hassouna in his article, "Solving Peoples' Problems" has rightly said that services research is a relatively new field of scientific endeavour which achieved recognition in the 1960s. It seeks to identify ways and means of taking medical knowledge, expertise and technology out of laboratories, academic institutions and pilot projects, and applying it in order to solve the health problems of the people. It is an interdisciplinary approach which is mainly concerned with action involving all the factors that affect health status through the use of health resources. It assists decision-makers at various levels in making accurate assessments of the health services delivery system and in identifying and testing the changes that can be made so as to lead towards more effective and efficient methods of meeting people's real health needs."

George C. Salmond discusses the need, meaning and scope of research for Primary Healthcare.

CHAPTER 9

HEALTH EDUCATION OF REFERRAL SYSTEM FOR HEALTH PROMOTION

"Referral system coordinates the health system to promote health promotion and education."

—*Author*

Health Education of Referral System for Health Promotion

Referral system is an indispensable element of healthcare to ensure adequate and quality healthcare to the people. Without scientific planning for referral services, we are witnessing huge crowds at secondary and tertiary healthcare institutions. The cost of treatment at secondary and tertiary levels is very high. If there is a proper referral system, it would result into:

(a) adequate facilities at each level of healthcare,
(b) quality services based on standard norms,
(c) less rush at secondary and tertiary level,
(d) increased competence of personnel at lower levels,
(e) less cost,
(f) develop permanent linkages among primary, secondary and tertiary healthcare,
(g) create interest among health professionals in identifying rural health problems and their solution,
(h) optimum use of resources,
(i) encourage research in local problems,
(j) keep the health systems effective, efficient, responsive, and
(k) result in the satisfaction of the ailing humanity.

Karnataka Health System Development Project in its report, defines ideal referral health system as:

> Conceptually a multi-tier system which combines preventive, curative and specialised care is efficient when it provides patients access to levels of care that are appropriate to their health needs with a

minimum of inconveniences and delay. It works best when the lowest tier is easily accessible to the community and provides the bulk of the preventive care as well as curative care services for common illnesses. Patients with more complex problems are identified in a timely and systematic manner and referred to the appropriate high level. Each successive level provides services that are more complex and therefore more expensive. In such a system, the higher tier provides technical leadership and support for the lower tiers, and the community has confidence in the quality of care provided at each tier and the patients understand they will be in accordance with patient needs.[1]

CHART 9.1

Patient Referral System

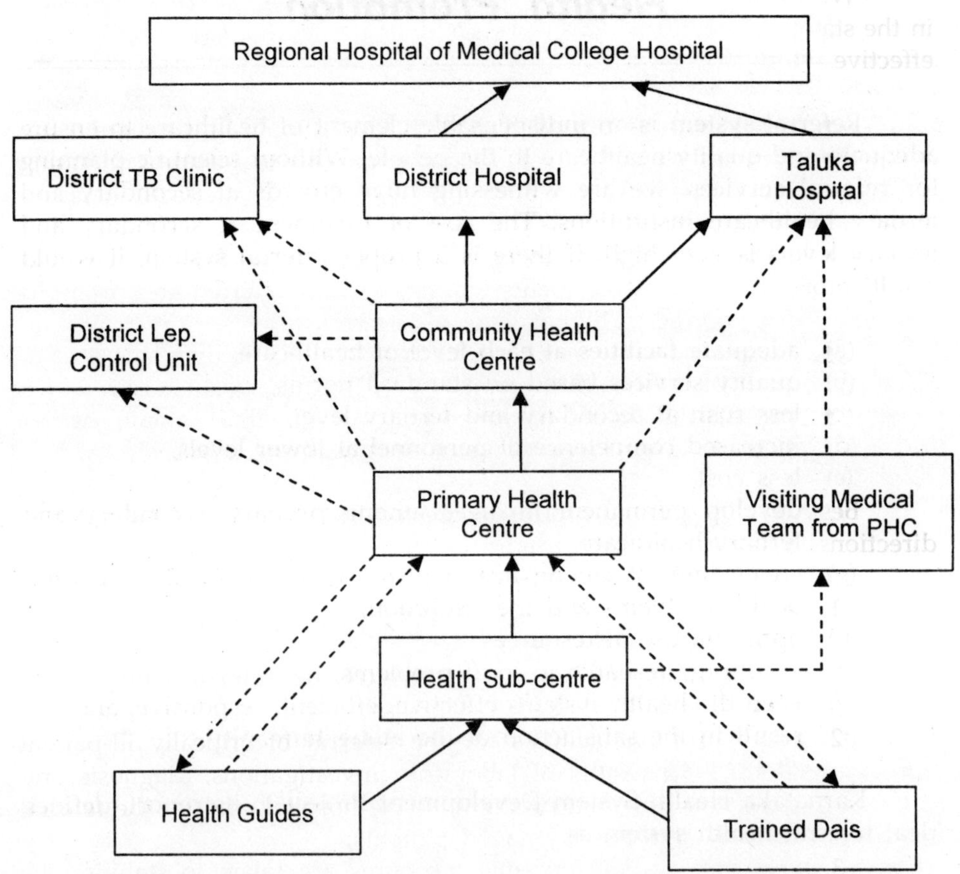

Source: NIHFW, Management Training Module for Health Assistants (Male and Famle), New Delhi, 1987, p. 129.

As health services are extended to rural areas, and as more and more responsibility for healthcare is placed on paramedical staff, a patient referral system becomes the means for ensuring quality healthcare to all patients. A good patient referral system is an essential component of primary healthcare. In India, health assistants are the supervisors responsible for maintaining a functioning patient referral system between sub-centres, the primary health centre and community health centre,

A simple patient referral system is shown in Chart 9.1. Patients enter the system at the sub-centre level; if adequate treatment is not available at the sub-centre, they are referred to PHC and CHC, where appropriate treatment is available. In certain unusual situations, one or more of the referral levels may be skipped; for example, a patient with a serious head injury may be referred from a PHC directly to a Regional Hospital. But normally, a patient will move up the referral system, step by step, as shown in the Chart 9.1.[2]

World Bank appointed a working group to establish referral system in the states assisted by it. The work group suggested the following to make effective referral systems:

- services to be provided at each level should be defined;
- services should be of adequate quality to inspire confidence among patients that they will be treated in an effective manner at that level;
- patients and the community must have the confidence that if the need arises, the patients will be properly referred and promptly transported to higher level of healthcare;
- the public is aware about the type of services available at each level of the health system; and
- procedures should be followed to ensure that patients do not skip the lower levels at which they could be effectively treated.[3]

Besides, the working groups suggested the following administrative directions to streamline the procedure of referral system:

1. ensuring that referrals are made to the nearest properly equipped referral centre to provide treatment at the earliest, rather than the hospital to which the referring hospital is administratively linked;
2. transportation facilities for the referral of critically ill-patient along with results of laboratory investigations, diagnosis and treatment provided by the referring hospital, and for the referral of poor and disadvantaged patients;
3. ensuring that all possible measures are taken to stabilise the patient before referral;
4. avoiding unnecessary delays in the receiving hospitals by, for example, publicising information on clinic hours, laboratory

hours, X-Ray hours, giving priority to referred cases, simplifying admission procedures, etc.;
5. maintaining registers or records at both the referring hospitals and the receiving hospitals. This information will facilitate the monitoring and evaluation of the referral system in terms of the number of cases, purpose of referral, destination or source of referral, etc;
6. issuing guidelines in respect of referrals from private sector;
7. the District Surgeon will review once a month, the working of referral system and also visit the institutions each quarter for inspection; and
8. the referral hospital will attend to the referred patients on top priority.[4]

Mrs. Indira Gandhi, Prime Minister of India, while presiding over a function at Lady Hardinge Medical College at Delhi, rightly mentioned (quoted by Dr. P.N. Chhuttani, Ex-Director, PGI, in his article, "Decentralisation Needed" published in Medical View Point column of *The Tribune*, dated 4-5-1980) that "The referral system has entirely failed in almost all our larger towns and cities. Consequently, there is growing overcrowding at our major hospitals whose services stand diluted. In the larger cities there is the multiplicity of the controlling authorities, i.e. the Government, the Municipal Corporation, the Municipal Committee, Voluntary Organisations, private Hospitals, etc." She further stated that "there is no common meeting ground and hospital services have become almost totally unregulated. Consequently, the conditions in our capital city are chaotic. The poor and the needy flock towards the larger, better known hospitals in the hope of better treatment and care only to find that they have to wait for days to be examined, much less to find a place to stay. Patients wander from hospital to hospital. Besides facing considerable inconvenience, their efforts to seek relief cause duplication of work and expenditure. It is thus necessary that every big city must have an apex body, perhaps called the hospital board, to establish referral hospitals for every zone."

How can we get out of this chaos to design a system of patient care? The answer is introduction of Regionalisation. Regionalisation connotes the development of graded patient care within a defined geographical or functional area from lower to higher levels, adapting the health services to the characteristics and needs of the area and thus, ensure the optimum utilisation of resources. The essential characteristics of regionalisation are:

(a) Two-way flow of patients,
(b) Two-way flow of records,
(c) Two-way flow of services,
(d) Two-way flow of personnel,
(e) Mobile units,

(f) Centralised administration and decentralised execution,
(g) Coordinating education programme for the region,
(h) Communication and transport between components, and
(i) Coordination with other community health services.

Thus, regionalisation would ensure the best utilisation of time of the specialists and provision of comprehensive healthcare to the patients nearer their homes, with all the benefits of specialities. The regional area should neither be too large nor too small, but should be such as to ensure adequate span of attention. It would also automatically develop referral system scientifically.

The referral system presents the following five aspects:

(a) It has to be built into the organisational structure of the medical services of a country. The rule should be that only when one unit cannot provide what a patient needs should the patient be referred to the next higher unit in the chain.
(b) The problem has to be organised both internally and externally. 'Internally' means that patients in the hospital have to be referred from the in-patients to the out-patients department just as soon as their health situation permits. The 'externally' referred system exists among the several Institutions on different levels of the hierarchy.
(c) The referral system, must be established for the purpose of diagnosis and treatment and used for both in-patients and out-patients.
(d) It is a two-way system. Patients should be referred to higher level institutions for diagnosis and treatment when necessary, but they should also be referred back to the referring institution as soon as possible.
(e) The referral system concerns not only patients and diagnostic facilities but also the personnel of the medical services. This is also a two-way system, so that human knowledge and skills are utilised fully and are continually developed through consultations and the interchange of ideas and experience.

The specialists from the regional hospital must come to the District hospital and the specialists from the District hospital to the health centre on a regular basis as consultants, to hold specialist clinics and give guidance; the medical and paramedical personnel should go to the higher level institution regularly for in-service training.

REFERRAL SYSTEM IN PUNJAB

Punjab Health Systems Corporation, established with the assistance of World Bank, has initiated Referral System in the State under the World

Bank protect. The Punjah Health Systems Corporation has taken up 151 health institutions, including District Hospitals, Sub-Divisional Hospitals, Area hospitals and 86 Community Health Centres to improve secondary healthcare.[5]

The Referral Manual for health systems in the State of Punjab has been compiled to issue administrative guidelines and referral protocols. The contents have been taken from Staff Appraisal Report, State Health Systems Development Project II, document of the World Bank, Feb. 20, 1996. The norms of services at Community Health Centre, Sub-Divisional Hospitals and District Hospitals, Equipment Norms, Norms of Staff has been collected from Project Proposals for the development of Secondary Level Healthcare Systems in Punjab, September 1995. Referral Registers have been designed with the help of APVVP, Hyderabad. The Referral-*cum*-Feedback cards in different "colours" have been printed. For Primary Health Centres, Pink colour, Blue colour for Community Health Centre, Green colour for Sub-Divisional Hospitals, White colour for District Hospital. Reporting formats for CHC/SDH/DH have been designed.[6]

Two registers, both by referring institutions and referred institutions, are to be maintained to keep proper records. Besides, there are large number of details, which have been drawn to make the system functional. However, the systems has not taken roots and is still in infancy. (For columns in the Register, See Dummy Tables 9.1 and 9.2).

Let us take up a case study of referral systems introduced in two of the blocks in Punjab (Ropar District). There are 17 districts in Punjab. Punjab has a vast network of Public Healthcare facilities comprising of 217 hospitals, excluding three tertiary level hospitals, 104 community health centres, 484 primary health centres and 1462 subsidiary health centres, dispensaries. The tertiary care facilities in Punjab consist of three Government Medical Colleges, two private medical colleges, i.e. Dayanand Medical College and Christian Medical Colleges, Ludhiana and a prestigious Post-Graduate Institute of Medical Education and Research (PUIMER), Chandigarh.

The Punjab Health Systems Corporation proposes to strengthen the functioning of the referral system in hospitals through the following measures:

- Renovating and upgrading hospital buildings to provide appropriate space for services.
- Upgrading and updating clinical skills of medical officers and staff nurses through an effective training programme.
- Providing ambulances for transporting critical patients.
- Installing phone, fax and paging systems in hospitals.
- Financial power to Senior Medical Officers in charge of the hospitals to purchase one item up to Rs. 2,000 (Rupees two thousand only) and Deputy Medical Commissioners upto Rs. 5,000 (Rupees five thousand only) and Civil Surgeons/

TABLE 9.1

Referral Register to be Maintained by the Hospital which is Referring the Patients

Sl. No.	*Registration No.*	*Name of Patient*	*Age*	*Sex*	*Date and Time of receiving the patient for the first time*	*Name of Institue where referred*	*Diagnosis*	*Condition at the time of sending referral, date/time*	*Sent by whom*	*Action taken*	*Feed-back received*

TABLE 9.2

Format of the Referral Register to be Maintained in all Referral Institutions which are Receiving the Patients at Higher Level

Sl. No.	*Registration No.*	*Name of Patient*	*Age*	*Sex*	*Date and Time of receiving the patient at referred hospital*	*Name of Institue where referred*	*Diagnosis*	*Reason for referral*	*Received by whom*	*Feed-back received*

Medical Superintendent upto Rs. 10,000 (Rupees ten thousand only) to meet the emergency.
- The user's charges are to be retained at the site of collection. These are to be used by the Senior Medical Officer Incharge of the hospital.

DEMOGRAPHIC PROFILE OF DISTRICT ROPAR (See Health Map 9.1)

Ropar district came into being on the eve of reorganisation of Punjab on 01.11.1966 and is spread over an area of about 2055 sq. miles. The district has semi-hilly and far flung areas. District Ropar is bound by Chandigarh, on East; District Nawanshahr, on the West; on the North Himachal Pradesh (e.g. District Una and Bilaspur) and on the South by District Fatehgarh Sahib, and Patiala.

The health services are being provided through the Primary Health Centres, Civil Hospital, Rural Hospitals, Subsidiary Health Centres and through a network of sub-centres. Seven secondary level institutions, namely Civil Hospital, Mohali, Civil Hospital, Khera, R.H. Kurali, Civil Hospital, Ropar, PHC Chamkaur Sahib, Civil Hospital, Anandpur Sahib and R.H., Nurpur Bedi have been taken over by the Punjab Health System Corporation for strengthening the services including development of referral system. We are taking up Nurpur Bedi, Chamkaur Sahib to depict referral design. (For zoning see R.H. Nurpur Bedi and Chamkaur Sahib Plan). Maps 9.2 and 9.3.

CRITICAL APPRAISAL

Authors personal visit to Ropar district, discussions with the health staff in various institutions and the staff of Punjab Health System Corporation revealed the following deficiencies, which need immediate attention to ensure the success of referral system. It should be extended to other districts after correcting the problems mentioned below. These are based on personal research.

1. Half Hearted Approach in Introducing Referral System: Provide Full Facilities at each Level

Most of the doctors indicated that they do not have the full facilities as worked out by the working group. How can one expect a good referral system from hospitals which are not well equipped? Even some of the equipments supplied are not functional, creating additional problems of its use. Along with it, there are no technical experts to handle the equipments supplied. It is suggested that before further embarking upon new areas, we should ensure that the facilities are in functional state.

Map 9.1

Rupnagar District

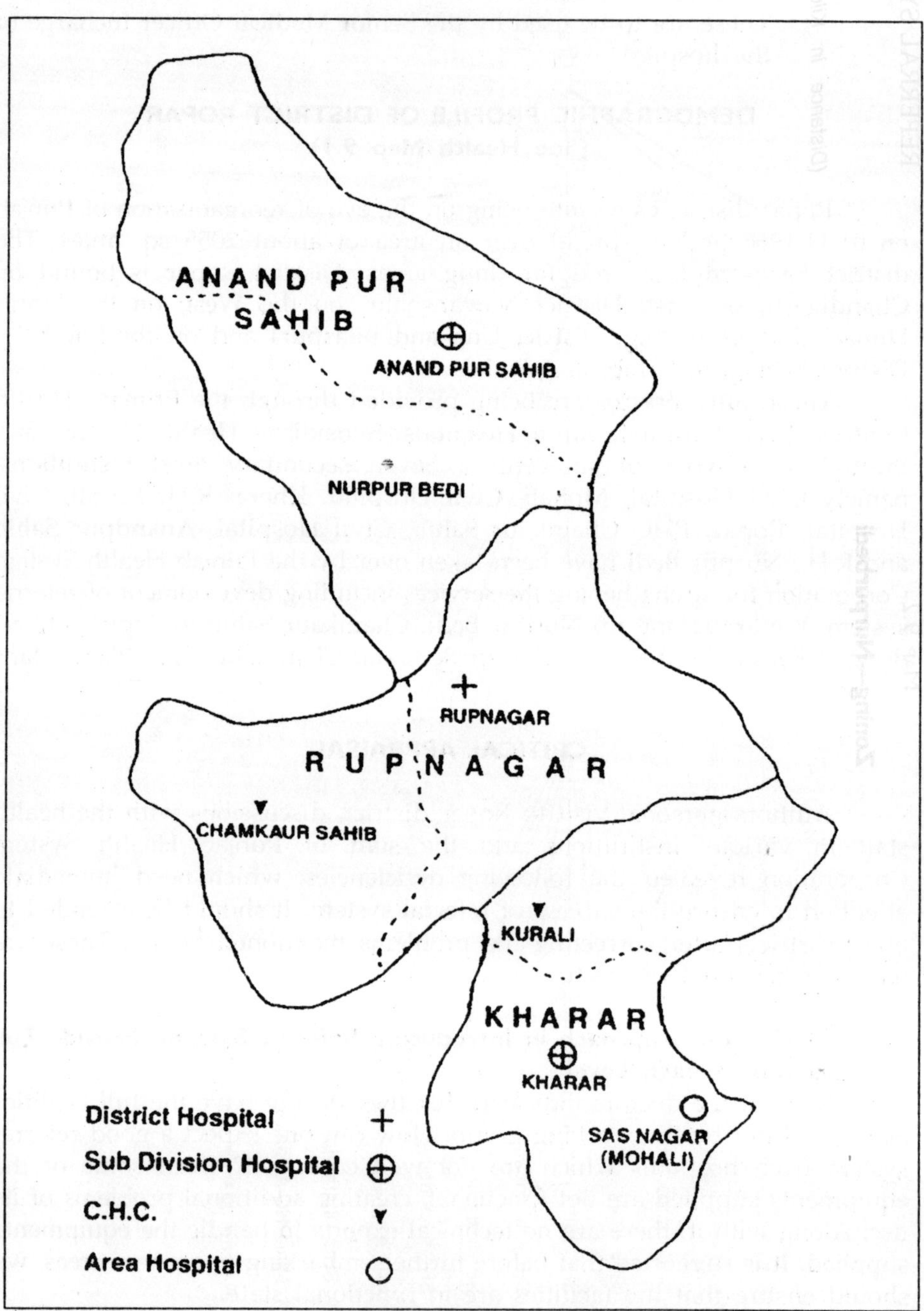

Source: Referral Manual, Punjab Health Systems Corporation, compiled by Dr. H.V. Jindal, p. 86.

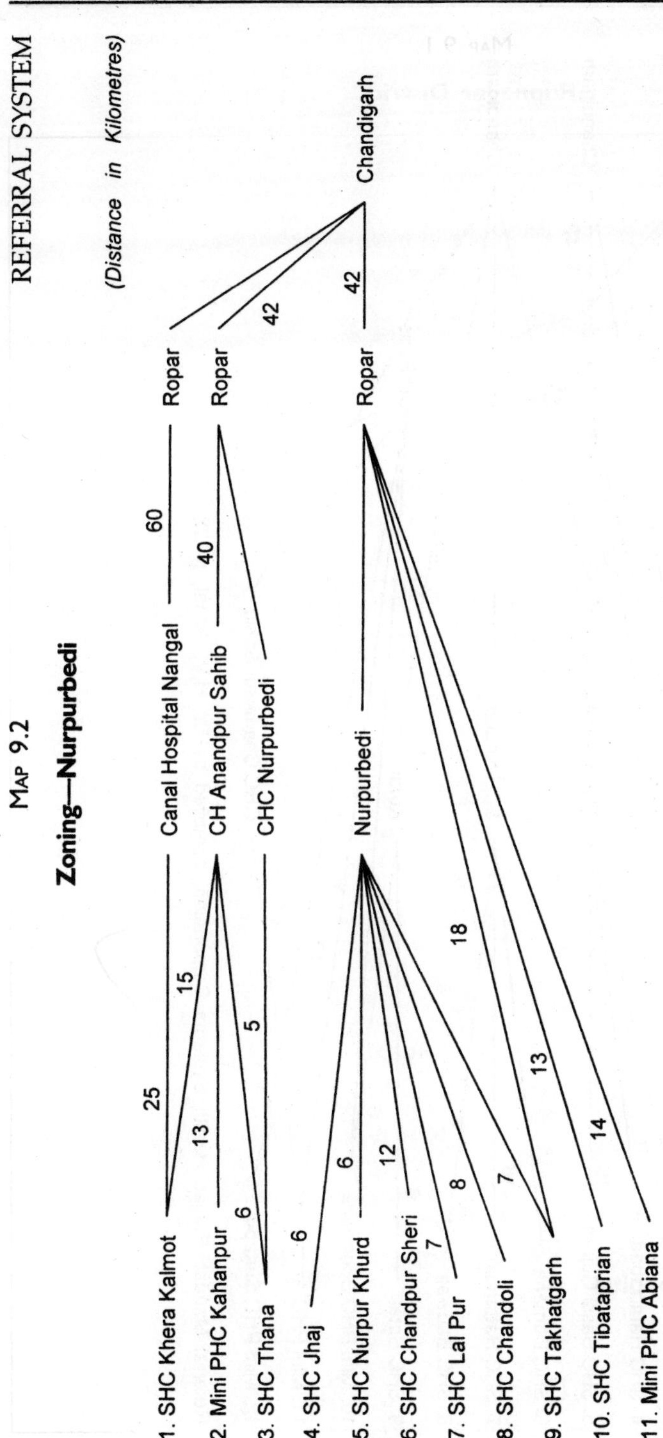

Source: Referral Manual, Punjab Health Systems Corporation, compiled by Dr. H.V. Jindal, p. 28.

REFERRAL SYSTEM

MAP 9.3

Zoning—Chamkaur Sahib

(Distance in Kilometres)

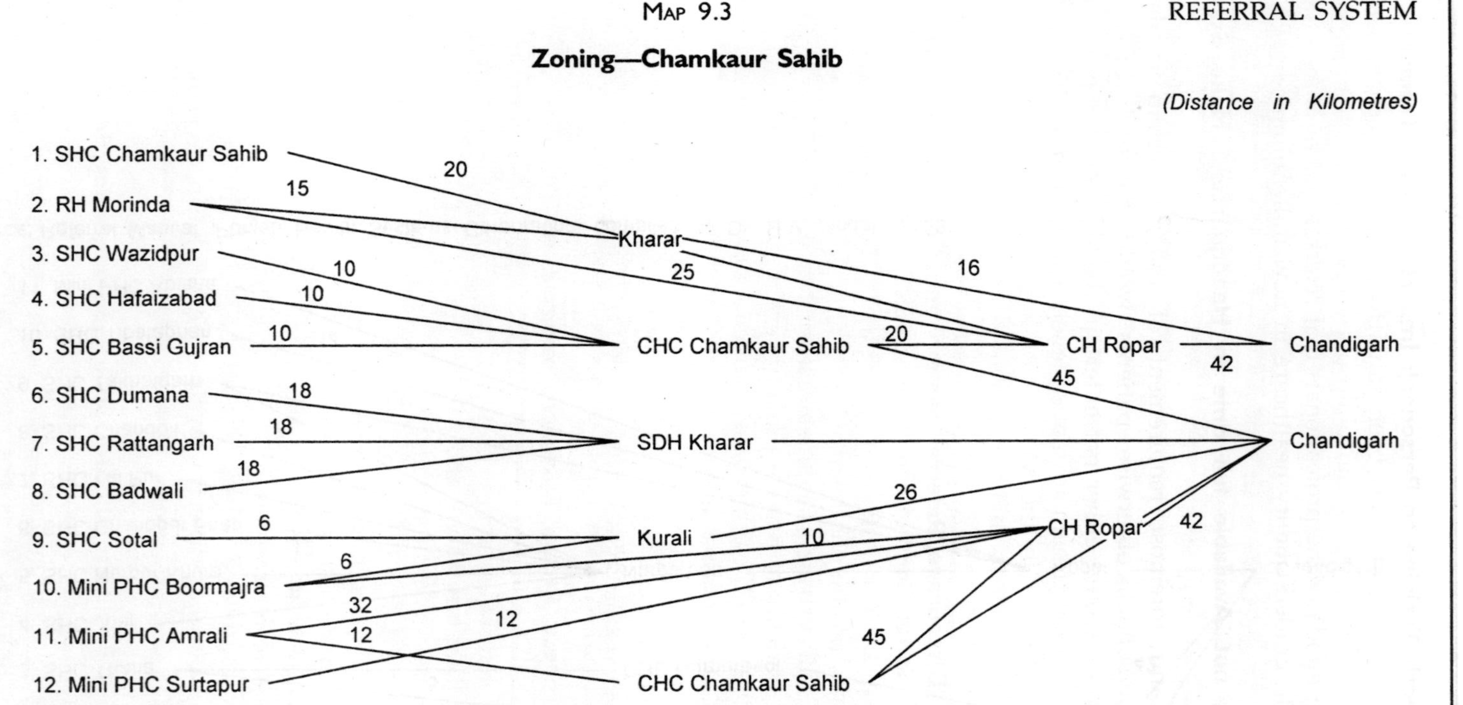

Source: Referral Manual, Punjab Health Systems Corporation, compiled by Dr. H.V. Jindal, p. 28.

2. Lack of Indepth Training to Personnel: Impart Intensive Training

At present, the training has been imparted into the mechanics of referral system but not its rationale, philosophy and utilities. It must be ingrained into the minds of the professionals that referral system is the only answer to provide graded quality healthcare in new millennium.

3. Professionals not Available full time in Headquarters: Make Stay Compulsory

The first and foremost requirement of referral system is the availability of personnel, otherwise patients would approach private nursing homes. They would either not entertain the referred complicated case or would try to shift them to higher level. The government should make the stay of doctors in the Vicinity of hospitals mandatory, with provision for full facilities, to make their stay attractive.

4. Professionals Discourage Referral System and Collude with Private Practitioners: Strict Control over Professionals

Professionals are cheating the Government. They are getting non-practicing allowance on the one hand while on the other hand, they work in off duty hours with private practitioners. In such a situation, they would send the referred patients to private practitioners to get some money and discourage referral system. Referred patients often travel long distances only to be kept waiting in the out-patient department for hours or even days. The out-patient department must be organised to give them priority over other patients. Government should adopt strict measures to check this menace, which is against medical ethics.

5. Lack of Awareness: Proper Publicity through Mass Media

People being illiterate and ignorant do not understand the meaning and procedure of referral systems. They are treated in the same way as other patients resulting into agony and pain. There is a need to educate the people through press, T.V., radio and posters.

6. No Feed-back: Report Back to the Previous Level

It has been found that patients referred to higher level do not come back and report as to what was wrong and how it has been treated. Thus, one of the purposes of referral system, i.e. providing higher knowledge to lower functionary is missed. There should be some arrangements for meetings among experts at different levels, to exchange notes about the referred cases.

7. Lack of Library Facilities: Allocate Sufficient Money for Books

The professionals once appointed rarely read the latest developments in their field of specialisation and general health management. How can they learn new techniques? It is not possible always to send them for training. It is suggested that books and journals may be made available to keep them upto date, different districts can subscribe to different journals, which may be exchanged after some time.

8. Ambulance Van Out of Order or POL is not Available: Ensure that Vans are in Working Conditions

Critical patients are to be shifted immediately but delays occur due to non availability of either vehicle or POL, or Driver. Referral systems requires good transport management.

9. Lack of Effective Communication: Provide Mobile Phone Facilities

It becomes difficult to contact expert as there are no facilities. What is the consequence? Patients reach but the doctor is not available, creating critical conditions. There is a need to provide good communication system among the components of referral systems.

10. Lack of Seriousness among Top Level Functionaries Create Interest in them

It has been seen that the top officials do not take pains to find out the shortcomings in the referral system during their field visits. This lukewarm attitude spreads among functionaries at lower levels. The result is the mushroom growth of nursing homes, which are fleecing the illiterate and ignorant people. Today, medical professionals are mainly interested in making money and not in excellence. There is a need to change this culture, otherwise the whole of Government Medical and Health System would collapse. Under the circumstances, there is no need to subsidize health services, because of its inefficiency and little use to the people.

11. Insensitive to the Needs of Patients: Develop Cordial Relationships

Doctors care very less for the patients. Dr. Iqbal S. Ahuja in his article, "Self-Introspection, 1st January, 2000 (*The Indian Express*, New Horizons! New Hopes) rightly says that there seems to be decline in human relationships. Money has started playing a bigger role in the maintenance of relationship. The soul and body relationship, purity of heart, thought and action have all deteriorated. Time has come for introspection into thyself. Where are the days when the patient treated the doctor like a second God? Why have we deteriorated in thought and action? Why self has come before the service. We all need introspection in our hearts." The teachings of Swami Vivekananda can help the professionals in rejuvenating the system. To quote him, "Let us all work hard, my brethren; this is not time for sleep. On our work depends the coming of the India of the future. She is there ready waiting. She is only sleeping. Arise and awake and see her seated here, on her eternal throne, rejuvenated, more glorious than she ever was—"This motherland of ours."

12. No Assurance of Quality Medical Care: Introduce Medical Audit

Quality assurance means delivery of efficient and effective medical care, which is a *sine qua non* for referral system. The health institutions need to develop standards of quality in a comprehensive and scientific manner. They should not concentrate merely on technical competence, but also ensure effective communication with patients, and develop work culture. Professional quality care can be ascertained by medical audit, which can ascertain the advantage of referral systems. Medical Audit is defined as an evaluation of medical care in retrospect, through analysis of medical records of referred patients. Dr. C. Prakash, as eminent health and medical expert, suggests the need of developing referral index.

The discharge reports and summaries evaluation of referred patients can provide useful indications of quality of healthcare. How well the hospital has passed on the information to the agencies who referred the cases? Similarly, what details the referring agencies have provided to the referral hospital, are these adequate or inadequate, appropriate or inappropriate, etc. Thus, two-way referrals should be functioning. The quality of referrals should be ascertained both-ways to find the gaps for corrective actions. The simple indicators suggested for referral functions are:

1. Number of patients referred to hospital per annum.
2. Nature of referrals made.
3. Agency referring the cases.
4. Feedback system for referrals, i.e. number of referrals for whom the referring agency was informed.
5. Higher level hospital and referrals to district or sub-division hospital for future care or follow up and reports of such follow up if any from the periphery.
6. Similarly, referrals from one unit to another unit of the referral hospital, time lag between the admission and referral, exchange of information between the units and outcome of such referrals can be appropriate indicators for assessment of quality of referrals.[7]

World Bank deserves appreciation for providing both expertise and finances to introduce referral system in healthcare system in sonic of the states of the Indian Union. State governments should take the maximum advantage of this generous aid to improve their health system in the new millennium. World Bank can only provide facilities, but cannot take the place of hundreds of health functionaries, on whose shoulders the success of installation, implementation and utilisation of referral system depends.

In a report submitted to the Governing Council, Paul G. Hoffman, an ex-administrator of UN Development Programme, said:

> "External assistance has a limited but a vital role to play. It will help break the vicious cycle due to the fact that poverty breeds poverty and poverty of opportunity perpetuates it. Poor nations, like poor people, are caught up in the day-to-day fight for survival. Forced to

live a hand-to-mouth existence, they cannot put enough to invest adequately in their own futures, poor because they cannot develop their own resources and unable to develop their resources because they are poor."[8]

Colonel Hla Han, Burma's Minister for Health, while addressing the 24th session of the WHO Regional Committee for South East Asia held in Rangoon, stated:

"The destinies of our nations are now once again in our hands, but as developing nations, the limitations which exist in our economic and social sectors have greatly impeded our endeavours to implement health programmes to full satisfaction. Our economy is anemic. We are also short-handed in trained personnel in the field of health. Furthermore, lack of knowledge of proper techniques and methods has created numerous problems in our efforts to undertake tasks with our capabilities."[9]

Thus, in the less developed countries, with their burden of sickness and the deficiencies in health installations, personnel and education and their scanty resources, the process of development is arduous. It would be impossible for many of these countries to develop with their internal resources.[10]

Multi-lateral technical assistance provided by World Bank can do miracles if it is properly integrated into the health system of the country. Transparency, accountability, ethos, dedication, professional competence should be injected into the health systems in new millennium to make the referral system a success and make the lives of people healthier and happier.

Notes and References

1. Karnataka Health System Development Corporation Project, Deptt. of Health and Family Welfare, Govt. of Karnataka, Bangalore, January, 1996, p. 109.
2. NIHFW, Management Training Modules for Health Assistants, New Delhi, 1987, p. 129.
3. Karnataka Health System Development Project, *op. cit.*, p. 103.
4. *Ibid.*, p. 104.
5. Based upon the Referral Manual prepared by Punjab Health Systems Development Corporation, Chandigarh (Compiled by Dr. H.V. Jindal).
6. *Ibid.*
7. C. Parkash, Quality Healthcare In Hospital Administration and Management, Vol. 111 (Editors S.L. Goel and R. Kumar), New Delhi, Deep and Deep Publications Pvt. Ltd., p. 294.
8. 12th Session of UNDP Governing Council, 7-23 January 1971, pp. 112-14, (UNDP-E/5043-Rev. 1.
9. WHO: SEARO, 24th Session on the WHO Regional Committee for South-East Asia, New Delhi, Nov. 1971, p. 60.
10. *WHO Chronicle*, Vol. 22, No. 7, p. 315. (Statement of Dr. K.N. Rao, Chairman of Executive Board).

CHAPTER 10

PANCHAYATI RAJ AND RURAL DEVELOPMENT

"In the process of rural transformation, the time is now for each person to lend a finger of cooperation if not with mind, then with body; if not with body, then with wealth; if not with wealth, then with encouraging or urging others to cooperate. If each were to lend one small finger, together the mountain would be lifted! And when the subtle ties which join us together in universal brotherhood are recognized as unbreakable, then cooperation will become inevitable, and together we will reach new and greater heights!"

"Panchayats have been the backbone of the Indian villages since the beginning of the recorded history. Gandhiji's dream of every village being a republic has been translated into reality with the introduction of three-tier Panchayati Raj system to enlist people's participation in rural reconstruction. 24th April 1993 is a landmark day in the history of Panchayati Raj in India as on this day the Constitution (73rd Amendment) Act, 1992 came into force to provide constitutional status to the Panchayati Raj Institutions."

—*Author*

Panchayati Raj and Rural Development

The salient features of 1992 Act are:

(i) to provide three-tier system of Panchayati Raj for all States having population of over 20 lakh;
(ii) to hold Panchayat elections regularly every five years;
(iii) to provide reservation of seats for scheduled castes, scheduled tribes and women (not less than one-third of total seats);
(iv) to appoint State Finance Commissions to make recommendations regarding financial powers of the Panchayats; and
(v) to constitute District Planning Committee to prepare draft development plan for the district as a whole.

According to the Constitution, Panchayats shall be given powers and authority to function as institutions of self-government. The powers and responsibilities to be delegated to Panchayats at the appropriate level are:

(a) preparation of a plan for economic development and social justice,
(b) implementation of schemes for economic development and social justice in relation to 29 subjects given in the eleventh schedule of the Cosntitution, and
(c) to levy, collect and appropriate taxes, duties, tolls and fees.

The provisions of the Panchayats (Extension to the Scheduled Areas) Act, 1996 extends to Panchayats in the tribal areas of Andhra Pradesh, Chhattisgarh, Gujarat, Himachal Pradesh, Jharkhand, Maharashtra, Madhya Pradesh, Orissa and Rajasthan. This has come into force on 24 December 1996. All States have passed laws to give effect to the provisions contained in the Act 40 of 1996, except J & K.

Mahatma Gandhi underlined the importance of individuals in the Panchayati Raj Structure. To quote him: "In this structure composed of innumerable villages, there will be ever widening, never ascending, circles. Life will not be a pyramid with the apex sustained by the bottom, but will be an oceanic circle, whose centre will be the individual, always ready to perish for the village, the latter ready to perish for the circle of villages, till at last the whole becomes one life composed of individuals, ever humble sharing the majesty of the oceanic circle of which they are integral units."

Gandhi outlined his concept of the 'ideal' society in an article in *Harijan* in 1946. Indian independence must begin at the bottom. Thus, every village will be a republic or Panchayat, having full powers. It follows, therefore, that every village has to be self-sustained and defending itself against the whole world. It will be trained and prepared to perish in the attempt to defend itself against any onslaught from without. Thus, ultimately, it is the individual who is the unit. But this does not exclude dependence on willing help from neighbours or from the world. It will be free and voluntary play of mutual forces. Such a society is necessarily highly cultured in which every man and every woman knows what he or she wants and, what is more, knows that no one should want anything that the others cannot have with equal labour.

Panchayats have been a vibrant and dynamic identity of the Indian villages since the beginning of recorded history. Experts believe that the concept of self-governance existed during Rig Vedic period (around 1200 B.C.). There were "Village Sabhas" and Gramin (Assemblies of Village elders) who took interest in the welfare of villages. The system of Panchayati Raj is thus deeply rooted in our tradition. From time immemorial, this system has exercised powers, both executive and judicial. This village government took decisions and actions based upon religious values and customs and traditional conventions with respect to various matters.

The census definition of a rural area is as follows: "In India, the smallest area of rural habitation is the village. It generally follows the limits of a revenue village that is recognised by the district administration. The revenue village need not necessarily be a single agglomeration of habitations. It may have one or more hamlets. But the revenue village has a definite surveyed boundary and each village is a separate administrative unit with separate village accounts."

The rural-urban classification is based on a cut-off point of a certain population within an area. Rural is generally comprehended in contrast with the urban, the two concepts having been assigned positions at the opposite poles of a continuum. Excessive attempts to segregate rural and urban problems are actually a dangerous proposition. Besides, all rural areas are not homogeneous and therefore to suggest common solutions to solve rural problems throughout the country is not at all possible. Inspite of common inherent problems, each area is distinct.

Thus, the Constitutional Amendment Act of 1992 envisages

democratically constituted Panchayat Bodies which are entrusted with the task of rural development through a decentralisation of powers, functions and resources.

CONSTITUTIONAL STATUS

Rationale

India: Panchayti Raj Development Report, 2001 (Vol. I) by NIRD, Hyderabad states: The rationale for the Amendment was that the Panchayati Raj Institutions had been in existence for a long time, but they had failed to acquire the status and dignity due to irregular elections, prolonged super sessions, inadequate representation for women and weaker sections, insufficient devolution of powers, and lack of financial resources. These lacunae could not be rectified until appropriate constitutional support to the PRIs was provided by including certain basic and essential features in the constitution itself to impart to them a measure for a mandatory set-up for the Panchayati Raj Institutions, based on holding of periodic elections to these bodies, provision of reservation for the weaker sections including women and a mechanism to provide financial assistance to them on a regular basis (Mukherji and Yugandhar, 1994).

After independence, efforts were made by the States to introduce Panchayati Raj System. To give a boost to the system and to ensure its effective functioning, it became necessary to amend the constitution. The Constitution (73rd Amendment) Act, 1992 (App. I) that came into force w.e.f. 24th April, 1993 conferred constitutional status to Panchayats and government from the village upwards. It was considered by the experts that there is an imperative need to enshrine in the Constitution certain basic and essential features of PRIs to impart certainty, continuity and strength.

The Central Government has shown the political will to constitutionalise the status of PRIs in larger public interest. The Constitutional Amendment Act, 1992 has therefore been cherished as a watershed event for achieving rural development through democratic decentralisation. It has laid down certain mandatory provisions in terms of structural organisation of PRIs while the functional aspects are left to the option of respective states. (See Table 10.1)

The 29 subjects to be assigned under the Eleventh schedule to the PRIs are as follows:

1. Agriculture including agriculture extension.
2. Land improvements, land reforms and soil conservation.
3. Minor irrigation and watershed development.
4. Animal husbandry, dairying and poultry.
5. Fisheries.
6. Social forest and farm forestry.
7. Minor forest produce.
8. Small scale industries including food processing industries.

TABLE 10.1
Provisions of 73rd Amendment

Mandatory	*Optional*
2-3 Tier Structure	Direct election of GP Chairperson
Direct Elections	Role and Scope of Gram Sabha
Reservation for Weaker Section	Powers and functions of the each tier
Fixed Tenure	Financial Devolution
State Finance Commission	Maintenance and Audit of Accounts
State Election Commission	Composition and functions of DPC
District Planning Committees (DPCs)	Reservation to Adhyakshas' posts at GP, TP and ZP level by rotation.

9. Khadi, village and cottage industries.
10. Rural housing.
11. Drinking water.
12. Fuel and fodder.
13. Roads, culverts, bridges, ferries and waterways.
14. Rural electrification including distribution of electricity.
15. Non-conventional energy sources.
16. Poverty alleviation programmes—IRDP, JRY.
17. Education including primary and secondary schools.
18. Technical training and vocational education.
19. Adult and non-formal education.
20. Libraries.
21. Cultural activities.
22. Markets and fairs.
23. Health and sanitation including primary health centres and dispensaries.
24. Family welfare.
25. Women and child development.
26. Social welfare including welfare of handicapped and mentally retarded.
27. Welfare of weaker sections and in particular SCs and STs.
28. Public distribution system.
29. Maintenance of community assets.

The mandatory provisions have helped solve the problems of lack of uniform structure, dominance of upper castes and vested interests, irregular elections and frequent super sessions. The catch lies in the area where each state has to frame its own laws to operationalise the mandate given in favour of strengthening the PRIs.

As discussed above, rural development so far has been characterised by centralised planning with emphasis on macro-level targets than on ground level realities and felt needs of the community for whom these programmes were designed. Huge amounts spent under these programmes were not evaluated against the end objective viz., removal of poverty or improvement of standards of living in the rural areas.

Based on the Directive Principles enshrined in the constitution, various Governments made attempts toward setting up of multi-structured Panchayat Raj system but did not endow it with requisite powers and resources. It is only now after more than 45 years of independence, that 73rd Amendment of the Constitution enables Panchayats to play a substantial role in the local self-government. However, the emergence of PRIs is leading to changes in rural power structure as well as the equation between the officials and non-officials. Within the Panchayat Raj set-up there is a grim fight, directly or indirectly among the political parties to capture power, as it facilitates their political power struggle, at higher levels, as well as among different tiers of PRIs for appropriating maximum resources. PR system has to surmount many challenges by evolving consensus in the long-run, if it has to survive and play an important role in ensuring growth and equity in rural areas.

With the 73rd Amendment to the Constitution envisaging the establishment of Panchayats as units of local government, it is mandatory for the State to devolve adequate powers and responsibilities upon the PRIs. The success of this system essentially depends upon the external as well as the internal polito-administrative set-up. Although political will is said to have been demonstrated by way of constitutional amendment at the centre and through the state legislation, yet it needs to be further reiterated in terms of devolution of funds, functions and approach needs a fresh look. For example, traditional means of Audit and Accounts tell upon the autonomy of PRIs. The PRIs are being subjected to the same out-dated norms of department which are paper-orientated and negative in approach. This has doused the enthusiasm of the elected representatives in being able to show results, utilising local talent and resources. The aspirations and expectations of the community though raised by the PRIs have not been fulfilled to a great extent due to paucity of resources. This has eroded the faith of the common man in the local government. The alienation of people thus shadow their active participation in developmental process.

At the State government level, it is apprehended that non-empowerment of Gram Sabhas with inadequate devolution of powers, finances and top-down approach to planning, monitoring and evaluation, manipulation of the pattern of reservation for the posts of Adhyakshas by the ruling party of the PRIs. Further, vesting of major powers, functions and funds at ZP/TP level could impoverish the GP in reaching the goal of self-reliance or empowerment of the poor and weak. Delay in constitution of District Planning Committees (DPCs) would bring the process of rural-urban synchronization to a stand still. This, in short, may take away the representative character of the PRIs and weaken the instrument of checks and balances in the system.

A Round Table Conference on 'Financing for District Level

Development', 19th May, 2001 suggested the following:

1. Simplify some of the categories and abolish some of the categories, which have become irrelevant like the plan/non-plan distinction.
2. The money that is coming from the center can go directly to the district even if it is mentioned as a figure in the state budget. At least, the transfer be done directly to the district level or to the Panchayat level or the taluk Panchayat level or the Gram Panchayat level because it certainly would eliminate a whole lot of double accounting. Also there is a case for managerial efficiency to talk in terms of a direct transfer of not just central funds, but funds coming from other sources into the Panchayat area.
3. When you talk about Panchayat accountability and transparency to their electorate, in this context, it is essential that every time a fund transfer of this nature takes place to the Panchayat, there should be a mechanism, which is not very difficult in today's electronically linked world, of giving publicity to the people of that area so that they know that this much money has come to the Panchayat from a particular source. Therefore, there is much need and scope to improve the information system all down the line.
4. Then there is the issue of over-engineering of the entire structure. Here you have to move, between what items have to be subject to conditionalities and what kind of conditionalities are actually essential and what extent of freedom of decision-making should be allowed to which level. These are very serious issues and there are no simple answers, e.g., there could be a kind of hiatus in the priorities of let us say the general population and the priorities of the people of a particular Panchayat. Are we going to force certain kinds of conditionalities on them or compel them to do a sectoral allocation, which will suite our requirements.
5. There is also the issue of a whole set of parallel paraphernalia that has developed and which works through the MLA's committees, user committees and a whole lot of other agencies which really are not required to be set-up. And you have the same operation for the central government's schemes also.

Both levels (Centre and State) have to do some hard thinking on this issue and transfer the appropriate responsibilities to the Panchayat. Here the World Bank projects create a special problem when, invariably, they set-up an entire monolithic structure for each project which has worked all the way right down to the bottom without taking note of existing institutions in the field. This has happened for water supply, watershed development.

They want a user committee to decide how the implementation should be done, to manage the maintenance of the project, etc. and they have a point. This is also because there is a certain uneven democratic culture across the country which will result in Panchayati Raj institutions that are not fully responsive to the population. But we cannot have differentiated division of powers across the districts, we should not also be doing that.

But what we can do is—at all times to work through the existing Panchayati Raj agency, because, we have to live within the structure and strengthen and empower the panchayati raj institutions for effective decentralisation.

In order to ensure effective decentralisation to actually lead to development, following steps may be taken:

- Train members of Panchayats to put choices before an elected body so that they are in a position to really explain to the chairperson or the Panchayat, e.g. this is the money that has come, this is the total amount that we have, these are the choices, and you must make a decision on this basis and then leave the choices to the decision-making body.
- Train people in prioritizing issues, in making choices that includes minorities, and other weaker people who feel very uncertain and unprotected within a Panchayati Raj set-up.

The time has now come for the political activists, advocacy groups and development agencies to realise the formidable barriers blocking the devolution of political power and resources to Panchayati Raj Institutions. Unless a powerful pro-PRI constituency is built up, the third tier of government is unlikely to move out of the statute book.

The only way to build up healthy PRIs is to implement, honestly and fully, the constitutional scheme of devolution and to leave the PRIs free to function and learn from experience. This is the way democratic institutions have evolved, over time, in India, at the central and at the state levels. The same model should apply to PRIs too.

For fuller empowerment the disadvantaged groups would have to confront the mainstream centres of power, which relegate the rural areas and poor and vulnerable people to the periphery. In the preoccupation with local development one should not overlook the widening rural/urban gap in incomes and development status—which is the prime source of inequity in the Indian society.

The reports of the committee of Panchayat and Tribal Development Ministers of the Schedule *Vs.* States and the Committee of Chief Ministers under the Chairmanship of the Prime Minister submitted on 1997 have been circulated to the State for appropriate action. The important recommendations of the committee of Chief Ministers include:

1. Selection of beneficiaries under various rural development programmes should be left to the Gram Sabha.
2. Requirement of technical sanction for works upto Rs. 10,000 should be waived.
3. Adequate manpower support to the Gram Panchayats would need to be provided.
4. Delegate total control over such manpower to Gram Panchayats.
5. Zilla Parishad Chairpersons be made the Chairpersons of DRDAs.
6. Provide reasonable opportunity of being heard to the PRIs before suspension/dismissal.
7. Gram Panchayat President to be made accountable only to Gram Sabha.
8. Expeditious constitution of District Planning Committees.

The Ministry had introduced the Constitution (Eighty-seventh Amendment) Bill, 1999 in the Parliament on 17.12.1999 to amend Article 243C(2) and (5) of the Constitution to enable the State legislatures to decide the methodology for election of members and Chairpersons of Panchayats at the intermediate level and the district level. It was decided to have wider consultations with all the political parties and the State governments on the Bill. Accordingly, the comments of all the State Chief Ministers were sought in this behalf. A meeting of leaders of all political parties in parliament was held under the Chairmanship of the Hon'ble Prime Minister on 19th May, 2001 to seek the approval of all Political Leaders in respect of the Constitution (Eighty-seventh Amendment) Bill, 1999. Report of the Task Force on Devolution of Powers, Ministry of Rural Development, GOI, recommended:

ADMINISTRATIVE POWERS

1. The framework for devolution should be appropriately backed by adequate autonomy of three tiers of Panchayati Raj.
2. The State Government, having prepared the framework for devolution, should simultaneously reorganize the existing District Administration, so as to enable the PRIs to have their own identity and role in development process.
3. The State Government should also encourage different line departments to take up appropriate measures to integrate their activities with Panchayati Raj System. Likewise, the departments of the Central Government should review the Guidelines of the Centrally Sponsored Schemes indicating the role of Panchayats in implementation of such schemes
4. In order to ensure harmonious integration of different agencies to the service of common objectives of rural development, the District Rural Development Agency (DRDA) needs to be

integrated with the District Panchayat, DRDA can work as a Unit/Cell of the District Panchayat Administration under the overall supervision of the District Panchayat.

5. Administrative Powers between three tiers should be assigned by the State Governments as per the framework given.
6. Issues regarding convergence of schemes should be further pursued, so that PRIs can have greater flexibility in responding to local needs.
7. Keeping in view the principle of subsidiarity, the State Governments may devolve powers and functions to the three tiers of Panchayati Raj in respect of the 29 Items under the Eleventh Schedule of the Constitution, in accordance with the activity mapping provided in Chapter IV.
8. The State Governments may take appropriate steps to transfer institutions/organizations alongwith the activities to the appropriate tier of Panchayats to facilitate smooth functioning of the Panchayati Raj Institutions.
9. The State may transfer functionaries and funds to the PRIs for implementation of various State and Central Sector Schemes as per the outlines indicated in Chapter V.
10. States may provide freedom to the Panchayati Raj Institutions to constitute adequate number of Subject Committees covering important subjects as suggested in Chapter VI (para 6.15). States may also make provision for constitution of Joint Committee as suggested in Chapter VI.
11. The State Government may prescribe mechanisms for monitoring and supervision of the activities of PRIs by Strengthening of Audit System, Constituting inter-tier Standing Committee, Social Audit by Gram Sabha, enforcing Transparency in the activities of Panchayats and Constitution of 'Ombudsman' as suggested in Chapter VI.
12. The devolution package has to be accompanied by availability of qualified and trained personnel at all levels to assist PRIs in their day-to-day operations. Emphasis needs to be given on providing personnel with financial and technical expertise. For this, Technical and Engineering Personnel posted at the Block may be assigned to a group of Gram Panchayats. Particularly, in States, where the size of the Gram Panchayats is too small to allow independent staff support.
13. An Officer equivalent to the District Collector in seniority and status may have to be posted as the Chief Executive Officer (CEO) of the District Panchayat.
14. All Class I posts may be filled on deputation basis from the State Cadre. Class II officers belonging to Panchayati Raj may be recruited through the State Public Service Commissions or on deputation basis from the State Cadres. In case of Class III and

lower staff, the recruitment may be at the Regional/District level through an independent Recruitment Board. The experience of the States indicates that the process should commence with the deputation of personnel from the departments to the Panchayats. The powers and authority to control and appoint can be taken up in a second phase but within a specific time frame.

ISSUES AND RECOMMENDATIONS

We have examined in this chapter the process of democratic decentralisation in historical context, as a tool for ushering Rural Development to rejuvenate the lives of millions of people living in these areas (Refer Chart 10.1). We examine here some of the problems and issues and suggest remedies.

1. Lack of Genuine will to Decentralise

There are half-hearted attempts made at the Centre, State level to part with their own powers in real earnest, in order to ensure maximum delegation of powers and resources to the Panchayat Raj Institutions.[1] The Statutes by the State Government should be so framed as to facilitate the transfer of full powers and that these are actually observed in practice.

2. Absence of Pressure Groups

The exploitation of natural resources, investment in infrastructural development for income generation, technological extension, accessibility and adaptability of delivery systems could benefit the rural poor only if various interest groups get organised as pressure groups overcoming their inherent cultural and historical weaknesses.

3. Role of Vested Interests

One of the criticisms against Panchayat Raj is that although the structure of Panchayat Raj had been ostensibly designed for community involvement but in practice it has provided protection to vested interests, thereby accentuating the socio-economic disparities and discontent in the rural areas.[2] Empowerment of weaker sections could act as a check against monopolising of PRIs by a previleged few.

4. Weak Base at Gram Sabha Level

Any authority or power needs a countervailing force to ensure that it is not misused and that it is accountable. Such a force lends credibility to power. A political process and a system, which loses credibility, cannot exercise power for long time. The bureaucracy as well as elected members could be made accountable to the people only if there is a participatory spirit in the beneficiaries who are not merely the receivers of the programme implemented by others.

CHART 10.1

Genesis, Growth and Diversification of PRI System

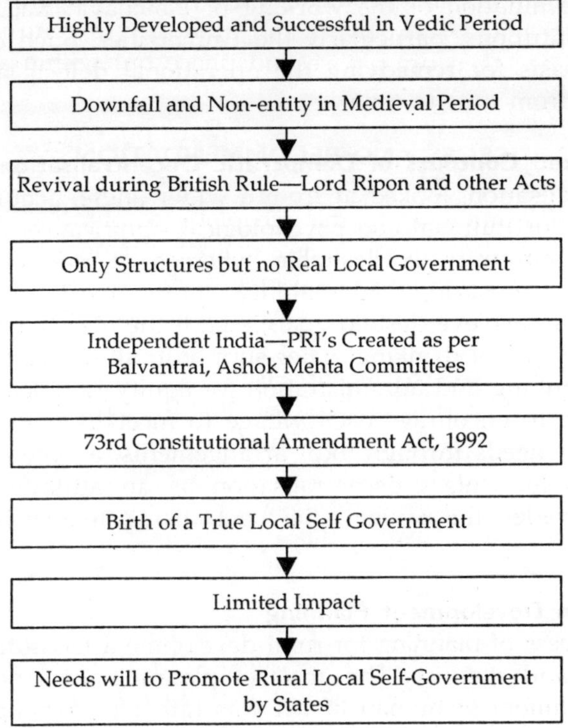

5. Lack of Faith in Decentralisation

The Union and State Governments are passing a number of laws for delegating power to the local level, which the rural masses do not understand. It seems that they are not really convinced. There is a need for educating the masses in various provisions affecting their lives and encourage them to develop self-reliance. People have respect for institutions of the government, if norms and values, which sustain the democratic spirit, inspire those who govern.

6. Inadequacy of the 73rd Constitutional Amendment

In two crucial areas of local government empowerment, viz. local autonomy and local functions and taxation, the provisions of the 73rd Constitutional Amendments are most unsatisfactory. Hence, there is a scope for further constitutional empowerment of local governments, through creation of a separate local list in the Seventh Schedule of the Indian Constitution so that these institutions become viable and self-reliant rather than mere implementation agencies.

7. Need for Strengthening the Evaluation of Democratic Decentralisation

The State Government should arrange for periodic, concurrent and independent evaluation of the working of Panchayat Raj Institutions by competent institutions, particularly the Universities. Such evaluation will provide the basis for remedying the operational defects and suggesting modifications from time to time.

8. Lack of Fixed Contours of Democratic Decentralisation

Decentralisation, looked at from a wider angle, acquires a political, constitutional, institutional and psychological significance. At macro-level, a need for uniformity is desirable whereas at micro-levels, random variations for ensuring adaptability onto local environment is indispensable, to achieve desired goals, e.g., if the objective is to provide a minimum standard of drinking water supply to all the villages in India, a centralised planning and administration for equity is called for. However, if the target is to encourage each village to meet its own perceptions of drinking water needs through local arrangements, a decentralised system alone is suitable. Unless decentralisation as an attitude of mind and approach pervades the system, the centralising tendencies will gather strength.

9. Adhocism in Development Planning

The process of planning for rural development has suffered from lack of continuity and stability. The goals of planning were not spelt out in terms of enrichment of human life. It was rather broken up into material targets, which when achieved were not evaluated in the light of Human Development Index. The planning was macro and centralized while the implementation was done through local agencies, which have not participated in planning. This gap resulted in non-realisation of goals and objectives.

As our democratic objectives are growth with equity, we have to have a truly decentralised socio-economic planning machinery at the Panchayat level. A spirit of co-operative federalism should govern the relationship among the District, State and National level. Uniformity should be insisted only in those cases where the unity and integrity of the nation is at stake, e.g., defence, foreign exchange, technological research and development and policy guidance. The issues of human development should be of a local concern, being handled through the people's institution in the most cost effective and result-oriented manner.

CONCLUSION

The increasing integration of India in the global economy, the budget constraints faced by both central and state governments and inefficiencies in the administrative structure led to the development of a consensus to devolve powers to local institutions to enable people's participation in administration. The 73rd and 74th Constitutional Amendments that conferred statutory status on PRIs and urban local bodies did not have only democratic decentralization as their objective. These institutions were also seen as a process for harnessing and channelising the people's innate abilities to bring about rural transformation in a way that every individual acquired his/her rightful place in the social, economic and political arena.

The Ninth Plan had called for the devolution of functional responsibilities, administrative control on government functionaries dealing with subjects listed in the Eleventh Schedule of the Constitution and financial resources for taking up developmental programmes to the front. Political devolution has taken place. Elections have been held and women, SCs/STs and other marginalized groups have got political representation in the rural areas. Problems encountered in the process of evolution of panchayats has been taken care of with the intervention of courts, civil society organizations and increased public awareness. The strengthening of forces that facilitate political empowerment of rural communities would be an important area of action in the Tenth Plan period. Issues of transparency, accountability and development would require greater attention. States which have lagged behind in devolving functions and finances to panchayats would have to be encouraged to empower the panchayats.

The gram sabhas in most states have been entrusted with only ceremonial functions. The power and functions of gram sabhas need to be enlarged by giving them effective powers of implementation and monitoring of developmental plans. Social audit of all development programmes by the gram sabha would be made mandatory. The committee system adopted in many states to facilitate a more participate decision-making process in the panchayats should be incorporated in the State Panchayat Acts. The powers entrusted to a gram sabha in a Schedule V area could be extended to gram sabhas in non-scheduled areas as well.

Administrative and financial devolution by the states to the PRIs remains an area of major concern. The Constitution has placed onerous responsibilities on PRIs. They require financial resources to discharge the tasks assigned to them and emerge as viable institutions of self-government. Financial devolution is also desirable as the control of investment decisions by local communities leads to better utilization of scarce resources. Panchayats would need greater powers of taxation and avenues for non-tax revenue. States could provide matching grants to panchayats to take up specific projects. Apart from the funds that flow to panchayats for centrally sponsored and state sector schemes, unties grants could also be provided to the PRIs. The PRIs need to raise resources from the local community and end their dependence on government funds. The functional domain of the PRIs can be enlarged only if they pay adequate attention to their resource-base.

The onus for devolving functions, functionaries and financial resources to the PRIs rests with the state governments. Though the state have, slowly, transferred functions and finances to the PRIs, these institutions are hampered by lack of administrative support. PRIs have to be adequately staffed and the functionaries must be trained in planning, budgeting and accounting tasks. An elaborate system for auditing of panchayat finances has to be put in place. At present, adequate safeguards against the misuse of resources by elected functionaries do not exist in many states. These issues need to be tackled on a priority basis.

The 74th Constitutional Amendment Act provided for the constitution of District Planning Committees (DPCs). However, the Constitutional provision on DPCs is rather weak as it provides for the preparation of only draft Plans by the DPCs. State governments have not given adequate attention to the DPCs and the Government of India's guidelines on district planning have not been fully operationalised. DPCs should be set-up and its functionaries must be trained in the basics of planning. The gram sabha/panchayat should be associated with the preparation of villages development Plans based on the felt needs of the panchayat samiti and district-level plans to make the grass-root planning process a reality in the Tenth Plan period.

With a not very encouraging experience gained so far after the 73rd Amendment, it is time to have a sincere introspection in a very dispassionate way. The expereince is not certainly disastrous. Things could improve in years to come with the bureuacracy developing a mind-set to work with the elected representatives and *vice-versa* with the sole objective of consolidating grass-root democracy in the country keeping in view the basic indicators of a strong mindset and a strong political will. The process of devolution has to be based on the cardinal principle that what is appropriate for a given tier should be performed by that tier and not by a higher tier. The issue of autonomy to the PR institutions needs to be assessed in relation to accountability of PR institutions to development administration.

Last but not the least, devoltuion of powers and transfer of subject to the PR institutions should not be made either as a political gimmick or election rhetoric. It shall be prudent for the MPs and MLAs, including ministers and bureaucracy, to consider transfer of powers to PR institutions as mandatory and duty bound with grace and humility. A system cannot die of power. It can die of a death in attitude.

Local Self-Government has the potentiallity to involve the rural poor or the beneficiaires in the planning, implementation, monitoring and evaluation process. Building a simple database for the common people is another vital task for local level planning. Both top-down and bottom-up flow of information is a necessary condition for successful decentralized planning. Development communication, guidelines, finances and local needs, priorities and preferences, feedback on specific policies and plans are needed to keep the decentralized system lively.

Sitakanta Sethi in an Article, "People Planning in Participation in Decentralised", *Kurukshetra* (Sept. 2003) observes: For the structural transformation of a backward economy like India, it has been recognized that investment in education, health and infrastructure, etc. is essential for sustained growth. With a vast number of schemes, it is really a difficult task to direct effectively from the top-central government. Therefore, it becomes essential to devise a system of information flow, financial flow and delegation of responsibilities to the lower level bodies. It organizes participation at various levels through formal and informal methods so that the needs and aspirations of the disadvantaged or excluded groups at the gross-roots level are met.

Mahi Pal in his article, *Yojana* (Aug. 2004), "Panchayati Raj and Development" in *Kurukshetra* observes that PRIs have great potential for promoting development of masses. But this potential has not been fully exploitd. Panchayats should be strenghtenened further and given functional, financial and administrative autonomy in different levels so that the elected representatives have full freedom to play their role effectively.

The Panchayats at village, block and district levels are close to the masses and provide ample opportunities to local people to solve their problems collectively in a participatory manner and thereby strenghten the process of human development. The successful experiment of participatory planning in the implementation of the Ninth Fivey Year Plan in Kerala is an eloquent example of this.

Notes and References

1. T.N. Chaturvedi, *IJPA*, July to Sept., 1978, Vol. XXIV, No. 3.
2. Abhijeet Datta, *IJPA*, Vol. XLII, No. 2, April-June, 1996, p. 150.

CHAPTER 11

EDUCATION FOR WOMEN EMPOWERMENT: VITAL FOR HEALTH DEVELOPMENT AND EDUCATION

"Women's expectations and hopes for a greener, cleaner, responsive and representative politics have gone up. They will send out more clearly and energetically the message of women's empowerment and social development. For that reservation needs to be accompanied by considerable amount of affirmative action programme."

—*India Panchayati Raj Report, 2001, Vol. II, NIRD, Hyderabad, India,* pp. 302-03

"Real change in India will come when women begin to affect the political deliberations of the nation."

—*Gandhiji*

Education for Women Empowerment: Vital for Health Development and Education

Women who number 498.7 million according to 2001 census, represent 48.2 per cent of country's population of 1,027.01 million. The development of women has always been the central focus in developmental planning, since Independence. Though there have been various shifts in policy approaches in the last 50 years from the concept of welfare in the 70s, to development in the 80s, and now the empowerment in the 90s, the Department of Women and Child Development, since its inception has been implementing special programmes for holistic development and empowerment of women with welfare programme, particularly in the sectors of health, education, rural and urban development, etc. Initiatives undertaken in the area of women's empowerment include:[1]

- Welfare and Support Services
- Employment and Training
- Socio-economic Programme
- Swayamsidha
- Swa-shakti Project
- Balika Samriddhi *Yojna*
- Plan of Action to combat Sexual Exploitation of Women and Children
- Declaring 2001 as Women's Empowerment year
- Instituting National Commission for Women
- Rashtriya Mahila Kosh
- National Institute of Public Cooperation and Child Development
- Central Social Welfare Board
- Food and Nutrition Board
- Information and Mass Education

CHART 11.1

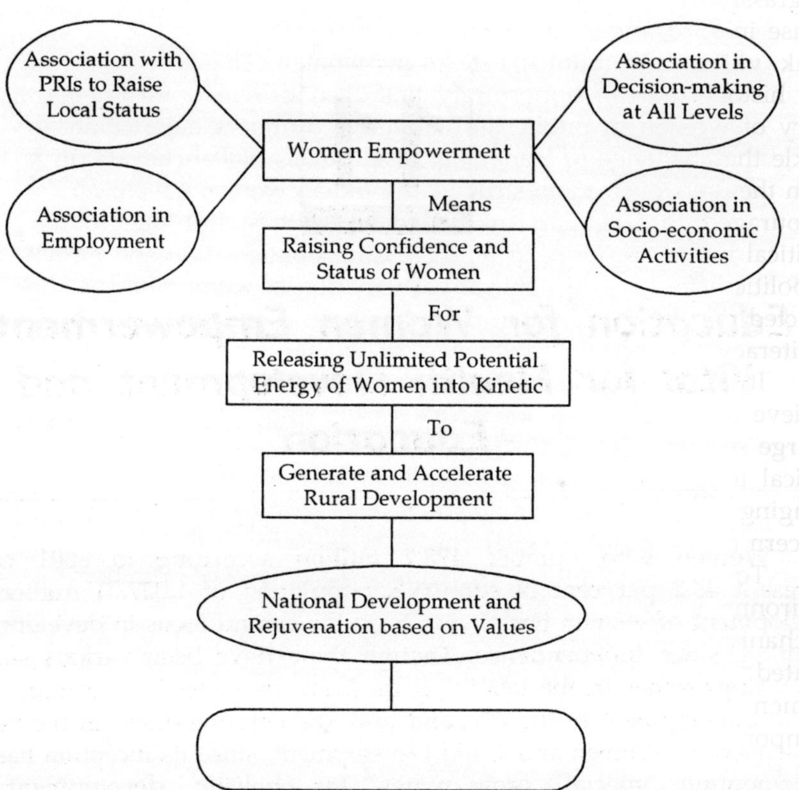

The Constitution of India has guaranteed equality before law and equal protection of law (Art. 14) and prohibits discriminatory provisions for women and children (Art. 15). It has made provisions to prohibit traffic in human beings and provides for just and human conditions of work along with maternity relief (Art. 23 and Art. 42). It is a constitutional duty of every citizen to renounce practices derogatory to the dignity of women (Art. 51A).

To quote J.P. Singh, Indisputably, India is committed to the cause of empowerment of women. However, the journey towards progress is long and arduous. In a world of challenge and competition, both the state and the society have to constantly attune themselves to the changing needs. It is recognized that the development of the country is not possible if women, comprising half of the human resource, as labour force and citizens, stay away from the national development process. Women's participation in the political process of development is of crucial importance from the consideration of both equity and development.

India has heralded the new millennium by pronouncing the year 2001 as Women's Empowerment Year. In terms of political empowerment, nearly seven lakh women occupy positions as members and chairpersons of grassroots democratic institutions in India, following the reservation clause in 73rd and 74th Amendment providing one-third seats at district, taluk, village and municipal level for women. This is for the first time in our history that an opportunity has been provided for such substantial entry of women in public life and large numbers have come forward to tackle the challenge of leadership at all levels of Panchayats. In fact, right from the days of freedom struggle the Indian women have been consistently encouraged to take part in the active politics. But due to the vitiated political milieu, resulting from increasing politicization and criminalisation of politics, the level of political participation of women has been adversely affected despite the fact that there has been a marked increase in the level of literacy and political awareness of women.[2]

It is recognized that the goals of poverty alleviation are difficult to achieve without the full and active participation of women, who constitute a large section of the workforce in the country. Women's empowerment is critical to the process of development of the community and, therefore, bringing them into the mainstream of development has been a major concern of the Government.

Towards this end and in order to empower women, an enabling environment, with requisite policies and programmes, institutional mechanisms at various levels and adequate financial resources has been created. The Ministry of Rural Development has special components for women in its programmes and funds are earmarked as 'Women's Component' to ensure flow of adequate resources for their development.[3]

POLICY FOR THE EMPOWERMENT OF WOMEN

In order to address the concerns of women in society, the Government of India has established the Department of Women and Child Development within the Ministry of Human Resource Development. A National Policy for the Empowerment of Women, 2001, provides the framework for addressing women's issues. The objectives of the policy are as follows:

- Creating an environment through positive economic and social policies for full development of women to enable them to realize their full potential.
- The *de-jure* and *de-facto* enjoyment of all human rights and fundamental freedom by women on equal basis with men in all spheres—political, economic, social, cultural and civil.
- Equal access to participation and decision-making of women in social, political and economic life of the nation.
- Equal access to women to healthcare, quality education at all levels, career and vocational guidance, employment, equal remuneration, occupational health and safety, social security and public office, etc.

- ❑ Strengthening legal systems aimed at elimination of all forms of discrimination against women.
- ❑ Changing societal attitudes and community practices by active participation and involvement of both men and women.
- ❑ Mainstreaming a gender perspective in the development process.
- ❑ Elimination of discrimination and all forms of violence against women and the girl child.
- ❑ Building and strengthening partnerships with civil society, particularly women's organizations.

COMMITMENTS OF THE TENTH PLAN TO EMPOWER WOMEN

The Approach

To continue with the major strategy of 'Empowering Women' as Agent of Social Change and Development

Strategies

To adopt a Sector-specific 3-Fold Strategy for Empowering Women, based on the prescriptions of the National Policy for Empowerment of Women. They include:

Social Empowerment

To create an enabling environment through various affirmative developmental policies and programmes for development of women besides providing them easy and equal access to all the basic minimum services so as to enable them to realize their full potentials.

Economic Empowerment

To ensure provision of training, employment and income-generation activities with both 'forward' and 'backward' linkages with the ultimate objective of making all potential women economically independent and self-reliant.

Gender Justice

To eliminate all forms of gender discrimination and thus, allow women to enjoy not only the *de-jure* but also the *de-facto* rights and fundamental freedom on part with men in all spheres, viz. political, economic, social, civil, cultural, etc.

Programmes

In keeping with its past and present policy objectives, the Government has launched a number of programmes focussed on women. In 1993, the Women in Agriculture programme was initiated which aimed at 'training' women farmers with small holdings, in allied activities such as animal husbandry, dairying, horticulture, fisheries, etc. In 1998, a scheme was started that aimed at empowering women in rural areas. It was called

Swashakti—Rural Women Development and Empowerment Project. In 2001, the government launched *Swayamsiddha*—Integrated Women Empowerment that aims at holistic empowerment of women through awareness generation, economic empowerment and convergence of various schemes. In 2002, *Swadhar,* aimed at women in distress such as destitute widows, women prisoners released from jail but without a family, women survivors of natural disasters was launched. Assistance under this programme includes food, clothing, healthcare, measures of social and economic rehabilitation through education, awareness, etc. In the international arena, India has ratified the International Convention on Elimination of All Forms of Discrimination Against Women (CEDAW) 1993 and endorsed the Mexico Plan of Action, 1975; the Nairobi Forward Looking Strategies, 1985; the Beijing Declaration as well as the Platform for Action.[4]

STATUS OF WOMEN

"That society would be highly developed and prosperous where women have their rightful place", expounds Manu. The Status of women varies enormously from one part of the world to another. However, nowhere do women enjoy equal status with men. In the developing countries like Africa, the Middle-East, Asia and Latin America, the status of women is so low as cannot be imagined by women in the developed countries.

The woman is the pivot around which the family, the society and humanity itself revolves. It is well said that the hand that rocks the cradle, rules the world. Women play a significant role in the development of their offspring. Truly, if a man is educated one person is educated but if the woman is educated, the whole family is educated.

Sumitra Mahajan, Minister of State, Department of Women and Child Development in her message in "Year of Achievements and New Initiatives" mentioned that the women have a high place in our society and this cannot be just an ornamental position. As much as we worship *shakti,* we have to recognize the innate power of women to nurture their families and to build a new community, based on participation and equality. In recognition of this, we have instituted the STREE SHAKTI PURUSKAR named after five eminent women of the Indian history, namely, Devi Ahilya Bai Holkar, Rani Laxmi Bai, Mata Jijabai, Rani Gaidinliu Zeliang and Kannagi and will be given to honour the women who have triumphed over difficult circumstances and fought for and established the rights of women in various fields.[5]

Status is a relative term. In sociological expression, it denotes neither rank nor hierarchy but only position *vis-a-vis* others in terms of rights and obligations.[6] In the ultimate analysis, status is "the conjunction of positions a woman occupies, as a worker, student, wife, mother. The power and prestige attached to these positions and the rights and duties she is expected to exercise."[7]

Women's status can then be analysed in terms of their participation in decision-making, access to opportunities in education, training, employment and income.[8] In recent years, there has been an increasing recognition of the interface between women's ability to control their fertility and their exercise and enjoyment of other options in life.

In ancient India, women enjoyed a high place of respect in the society as mentioned in Rigveda and other scriptures.[9] Volumes can be written about the status of our women and their heroic deeds from the Vedic period to the modern times. But later on, because of social, political and economic changes, women lost their status and were relegated to the background. Many evil customs and traditions stepped in, which enslaved the women and tied them to boundaries of the house. The untold miseries and sufferings of women of the 19th century awakened the conscience of mankind. Many reformers like Raja Rammohan Roy, Swami Dayanand, Justice Ranade, Mahatma Gandhi, and other championed the cause of the emancipation of women. The Constitution of India also prohibits any discrimination on grounds of sex. Many laws have also been enacted by the Government of India to protect the rights of women.

Anna Kajumulo Tibaijuka, Executive Director (UNCHS), says: "Where women are not involved in public decision-making, the quality of services deteriorates. It is time for change from the practice of leaving women to do only the dirty work. We are aware that women have been instrumental in the urban social movements that aim at improving urban poor neighbourhoods. They do this because they want to protect their families' health and create livable communities. These numerous women's initiatives must be recognized by involving them in governance structures by addressing the things they care about, in urban policy, planning and management. Women and men have specific and different needs, in areas such as transport, public spaces, the implementation of by-laws, and security. These must all be addressed."[10]

B.K. Chaturvedi has stated in his foreword: "The need to improve the access of women to national resources and to ensure their rightful place in the mainstream of economic development has been emphasized time and again at various fora at national and international levels. Keeping this in view, the year 2001 will be celebrated as the year of women's empowerment."[11]

Jagmohan, Minister of Urban Development and Poverty Alleviation, GOI, suggests the need of involving women in urban affairs affecting their lives. To quote him: "As we know the problems and challenges facing humanity are global but they occur and have to be dealt with at the local level. Women have the equal right to freedom from poverty, discrimination, environmental degradation and insecurity. To fight these problems and to meet the challenges of sustainable human development, it is crucial that women be empowered and involved in local government as decision-makers, planners and managers.[12]

Women's Empowerment is critical to the socio-economic progress of the community. Bringing women into the mainstream of national development has therefore been a major concern of the Government.[13]

The Members of International Union of Local Authorities (IULA), Representating Local Governments World-wide, firmly believe that:

1. Democratic local self-government has a critical role to play in securing social, economic and political justice for all citizens of every community in the world and that all members of society, women and men, must be included in the governance process;
2. Women and men as citizens have equal human rights, duties and opportunities, as well as the equal right to exercise them. The right to vote, to be eligible for election and to hold public office at all levels are human rights that apply equally to women and men;
3. The problems and challenges facing humanity are global but occur and have to be dealt with at the local level. Women have the equal right to freedom from poverty, discrimination, environmental degradation and insecurity. To fight these problems and to meet the challenges of sustainable human development, it is crucial that women be empowered and involved in local government as decision-makers, planners and managers.
4. Local government is in a unique position to contribute to the global struggle for gender equality and can have a great impact on the status of women and the status of gender equality around the world, in its capacities as the level of governance closest to the citizens, as a service provider and as an employer.
5. The systematic integration of women augments the democratic basis, the efficiency and the quality of the activities of local government. If local government is to meet the needs of both women and men, it must build on the experiences of both women and men, through an equal representation at all levels and in all fields of decision-making, covering the wide range of responsibilities of local governments.
6. In order to create sustainable, equal and democratic local governments, where women and men have equal access to decision-making, equal access to services and equal treatment in these services, the gender perspective must be mainstreamed into all areas of policy-making and management in local government.
7. Women have the right to equal access to the services of local governments, as well as the right to be treated equally in these services and to be able to influence the initiation, development, management and monitoring of services. The provision of services such as education, welfare, etc. governments should aim to see women and men as equally responsible for matters related both to the family and to public life and avoid perpetuating stereotypes of women and men;

8. Women have the equal right to sound environment, living conditions, housing, water distribution and sanitation facilities, as well as to affordable public transportation. Women's needs and living conditions must be made visible and taken into account at all times in planning.
9. Women have the right to equal access to the territory and geographical space of local governments, ranging from the right to own land, to the right to move freely and without fear in public spaces and on public transport.
10. Local government has a role to play in ensuring the reproductive rights of women and the rights of women to freedom from domestic violence and other forms of physical, psychological and sexual violence and abuse.

G. Palanithurai rightly says: Women have come to positions in the local bodies as provision has been made in the Constitution. The outlook of the society towards the women has started changing. But there are hurdles in the process of empowering women. Steps are being taken by the women on their own to overcome the hurdles. It is a long-drawn process. A structure which had been created over centuries to work against the interest of women cannot be altered overnight. To fight against the existing structure, an organised movement involving masses is imperative. In order to make the women achieve result in their positions, a number of interventions are necessary.

The ongoing experiments and experiences suggest that periodical training, orientation and sensitisation can help the women leaders to perform the assigned role in a better way. When the women leaders are responding to the socio-political challenges in this society, they are to be supported by the organisations and institutions which are working for empowerment of women. Wherever such interventions are available, potential and achievements of the women leaders are substantial and impressive. Government will respond to the needs of these women leaders only when they are supported by social organizations and groups.[14]

The 9th Plan working group challenges before elected panchayat women was clear that the component plan had to be hitched to decentralised planning if the promises made to the women were to be actualized. It was no longer enough for plans; programme, allocation and schemes to be made in the government offices at central or even state level. They had to be made by women, where they were situated and where schemes that the women needed and demanded, how much funds were required to be allocated, how they were to be spent, how monitoring was to be done.

Elected women have therefore to fight on several fronts at the same time. They have to fight for their own place in the sun, in the panchayats *vis-a-vis* the patriarchal forces arranged against them—and at the same time, they have to fight the political and bureaucratic state agencies for according a greater role in governance to the panchayats.[15]

Mr. R. Pakhriswamy, Chairperson, Thiruvarur, District Panchayat, Tamil Nadu made the following recommendations in a Round Table Conference (2001) mentioned earlier:[16]

1. Responsibility for ensuring security of Women and Dalits—who face threats from anti-social elements—must be taken by PRIs through the help of political parties. At present, there is absolutely no support to PRIs from these parties.
2. Existing revenue share for scheduled caste and scheduled tribe groups and women must be increased and implemented through Panchayats.
3. 20% of funds allocated to MLAs (Members of Legislative Assembly) and MPs (Members of Parliament) must be transferred to Panchayats for women's social and economic upliftment.
4. Elementary education, up to Std. V, must be entrusted to Panchayats and they should be empowered to appoint teachers at the ratio of 1:10.
5. Local cess must be levied based on land revenue demand.
6. Revenue collection from mines, minerals and royalties from non-conventional energies should be entrusted to Panchayats.
7. Protection of water resources must be entrusted to PRIs. This must include assessment of pollution levels and its impact on water sources, fisheries and the coast—the results of which should be announced in the gazette at the district level. And the 'polluter' must pay compensation.
8. The whole idea of Self Help Groups (SHGs) and the current way of implementing development programmes through them has to be re-looked at. This is because SHGs no longer attempt self-employment for their members. Instead they have become moneylenders—for high interests! Also involving SHGs in development programmes through NGOs has created clashes among village panchayats and gram sabhas, as village panchayats do not have adequate finances for local development.
9. The 3-tiers of panchayats must have inter-linkages, DPC's (District Planning Committees) functions must be strengthened and planning from below must be entrusted to them.

"Indisputably, India is committed to the cause of empowerment of women. However, the journey towards progress is long and arduous. In a world of challenge and competition, both the State and the society have to constantly attune themselves to the changing needs. It is recognised that the development of the country is not possible if women, comprising half of the human resource, as labour force and citizens, stay away from the national development process. Women's participation in the political process of development is of crucial importance from the consideration of both equity and development.

ESSENTIAL STEPS FOR WOMEN EMPOWERMENT

The main efforts required in the context of the Constitution 73rd Amendment is to break the hegemony of male Chauvinism in the rural areas. The rural women cannot achieve empowerment on their own and need support from outside. We must make efforts to ensure the following among women:

- (i) Creating a positive and dignified self-image and self-confidence in dealing with all matters and in all relationships.
- (ii) Ensuring equal participation based on equity and social justice.
- (iii) Developing ability and maturity to think critically.
- (iv) Take part in decision-making and participation.
- (v) Assert when women issues are ignored.
- (vi) Equality and equity for women are non-negotiable.
- (viii) Political power is essential.

Women's entry into the functioning of Panchayati Raj at all levels particularly at decision-making levels will usher an era of equality and prosperity to the villages and empowerment of the women leading to rural development on moral values.

Ultimately, it provides women with the opportunity to transform the legal, political, economic and social system as per the vision of the 21st Century to realize their demand for an equitable, environmentally clean and peaceful world where there would be no difference based on sex, creed, faith, etc. This would make 21st Century really fruitful.

Government, as they stand today would not be able to usher in gender equality in governance as male dominance does not want to yield to promote equality of sex. Women themselves, through their entry into the Politico-legal structures of the nation, must fulfil this task with devotion, determination and without fear. In other words, unless women become government this equality cannot take place. Hence, mechanism by which women can enter effectively, participate and lead the administration, organize and mobilize opinion on national and International issues, and influence policy, are the urgent need of the day. This would then IAY the foundation of equality for the future.

What is needed urgently is interventions at the policy level by women themselves. Why is women's participation in policy and decision-making important and how does one go about improving it? This has to be seen in the present context of women's marginalisation through development policies and the ineffectiveness of constitutional and legal provisions for gender equality.

The formulation of development policies and special programmes for women have the effect of relegating them to a minority category of beneficiaries and not actors and decision-makers for their welfare and improvement. Women, who constitute half of the country's population certainly deserve a better deal than spasmodic doles of mercy. They have to have a say not only in things that concern them directly but in all matters that affect the society in so far as they also have the status of citizens.[17]

The planners, policy-makers and administrators responsible for the improvement of the status of women should not be satisfied only with effective planning and policy-making, but should think of the vehicle or administrative structure through which plans and policies are to be implemented. Myron Weinner has rightly pointed out: "India's forte is one of the crisis management. Instincts of leadership are to cope, rather than innovate, and to work within an existing framework not only of institutions but of ideas as well."

Thus, with the help of well designed administrative machinery using modern management methods we should try to put the policy into action. In this implementation process, women themselves will have to be the most forceful agents for change and active participants in the development effort, wherever they have the opportunity to play a dynamic role. The contemporary social situation of women in India should not be frustrating and disheartening but should be rather challenging and it is the men and women of India, particularly the women have to face the challenge. It has been demonstrated by the women in the field that they are as capable and efficient as men in carrying out various kinds of work and have even much more endurance for hardships than is commonly believed. All of us who are associated with the development of the country in any capacity, must renew our dedication to the cause of women which would lead to national development and modernization.[18]

The National Commission on self-employed women and women in the informal sector has rightly mentioned that although at the Planning level, there is consciousness about women's low status and the need to focus on women's needs in development, but at the implementation level, this awareness percolates very slowly. The delivery system is based on a stereotyped concept of women's development where women are object of piety or welfare and are given some benefits in a sporadic and haphazard manner . . . If the political leadership decides that women's problems have to be tackled on a priority basis, the entire planning processes, implementing mechanism and monitoring system will be geared in no time.

POLICIES AND PROGRAMMES: A REVIEW

Development of women has been receiving attention of the government right from the very First Plan (1951-56). But, the same has been treated as a subject of 'welfare' and clubbed together with the welfare of the disadvantaged groups like destitute, disabled, aged, etc. the Central Social Welfare Board (CSWB), set-up in 1953, acts an Apex Body at national level promote voluntary action at various levels, especially at the grass-roots, to take up welfare-related activities for women and children. The Second to Fifth Plans (1956-79) continued to reflect the very same welfare approach, besides giving priority to women's education, and launching measures to improve maternal and child health services, supplementary feeding for children and expectant and nursing mothers.

The shift in the approach from 'welfare' to 'development' of women could take place only in the Sixth Plan (1980-85). Accordingly, the Sixth Plan adopted a multi-disciplinary approach with a special thrust on the three core sectors of health, education and employment. In the Seventh Plan (1985-90), the developmental programmes continued with the major objective of raising their economic and social status and bringing them into the mainstream of national development. A significant step in this direction was to identify/promote the 'Beneficiary-Oriented Schemes' (BOS) in various developmental sectors which extended direct benefits to women. The thrust on generation of both skilled and unskilled employment through proper education and vocational training continued. The Eighth Plan (1992-97), with human development as its major focus, played a very important role in the development of women. It promised to ensure that benefits of development from different sectors do not by-pass women, implement special programmes and to monitor the flow of benefits to women from other development sectors and enable women to function as equal partners and participants in the development process.

The Ninth Plan (1997-2002) made two significant changes in the conceptual strategy of planning for women. Firstly, 'Empowerment of Women' became one of the nine primary objectives of the Ninth Plan. To this effect, the Approach of the Plan was to create an enabling environment where women could freely exercise their rights both within and outside home, as equal parterns along with men. Secondly, the Plan attempted 'convergence of existing service' available in both women-specific and women-related sectors. To this effect, it directed both the center and the states to adopt a special strategy of 'Women's Component Plan' (WCP) through which not less than 30 per cent of funds/benefits flow to women from all the general development sectors. It also suggested that a special vigil be kept on the flow of the earmarked funds/benefits through an effective mechanism to ensure that the proposed strategy brings forth a holistic approach towards empowering women.

To ensure that other general developmental sectors do not by-pass women and benefits from these sectors continue to flow to them, a special mechanism of monitoring the 27 BOS for women was put into action in 1986, at the instance of the Prime Minister's Office (PMO). The same continues to be an effective instrument till today.

SUGGESTIONS TO STRENGTHEN WOMEN EMPOWERMENT

Women empowerment is not something which can be handed over to women. This is a process which involves sincerity, earnestness and capacity and capability on the part of both men and women. It is a challenging task in village India as even today, if a woman is to travel to her parents house or go somewhere, she must be accompanied by some male members of the family. She cannot take an independent decision. She feels even subordinate to her son. Let us discuss ways and means to improve the process of women empowerment.

1. Low Status: Need of Upgradation

Most of the women in a family feel inferior to male members of the family. From olden times, women act as workers and do not take part in decision-making. This attitude needs change to make women as part and parcel of the family by carving out an important place for her. Swami Vivekananda repeatedly stressed the need for cultivating the faith in one self: "The ideal of faith in ourselves is of the greatest help to us. If faith in ourselves had been more extensively taught and practised. I am sure a very large portion of the evils and miseries that we have would have vanished. Throughout the history of mankind, if any motive power has been more potent than another in the lives of all great men and women, it is that of faith in themselves. Born with the consciousness, that they were to be great they become great.

2. Low Morale: Need of Creating Positive Attitude

At present, women possess low morale which is a depressing situation where she does not get a sense of belongingness. We must develop positive attitude in her by enlightening her about her creative potential for contributing to the overall development of self, family and society.

3. Dependence upon Men since Childhood: Need of Indepenence from Early Stages

In Indian villages, girls remain dependent upon father, brother or cousin and this very feeling continues in their married life. We must give capacity building training to girls in schools to be independent. It does not mean breaking the linkages of family rather it leads to strengthening the bond on an equal platform.

4. Change of Attitude of Men towards Capability of Women

Men have built an impression through observation that women are inferior and they cannot face emerging situations. This attitude has to be changed through positive examples from our country and abroad. Pictures of women doing all types of work need to be screened and shown to both men and women. Though, attitude is changing but it is slow and needs to be accelerated. Face life and its upheavals around you. Be active and tirelessly dynamic. Each exertion undertaken is a shooting spark of "life" from the well of Existence in you. Fearlessly work. With a clear vision, plan and selflessly execute it. Fear not sweat! Hesitate not to face disappointments. Live life, so long as you are alive. Grow through work. Evolve in work. Expand while striving. Make your own life thus rich and sweet. You can. You must. The highest and noblest type of an individual working in the world is known as the "man of achievements" (Yogi). Such men work, neither for the sake of wages, nor for success; they are not after mere sensual pleasures, nor do they aspire to reform the world; they delicately perform their obligatory duties finding peace and fulfilment in their very activity. Their fulfilment consists of doing their duties to the best of their ability without claiming any rights and they are totally unmindful of whether the society commends or condemns their actions.

5. Women Elected Representatives of PRIs give Way to their Men Folk: Need of taking Independent Decisions

Women representatives in PRIs must be trained in the art and science of decision-making so that they are not influenced by extraneous factors. They should discuss among other women and take their opinion. They must develop leadership qualities. K.D. Gangrade in his Article, "Gandhi and Empowerment of Women—Miles to Go" (Ed.) Smt. Savita Singh (International Centre of Gandhian Studies and Research, Gandhi Samiti and Darshan Samiti, New Delhi, "The 74th and 73rd Constitutional Amendments on Panchayati Raj and Nagarpalika with 33 per cent reservation for women has created political space for women. But in most cases they exercise "proxy" power on behalf of men. In reality, women have never been able to get more than ten percent seats in Parliament or other bodies of decision-making. It is hoped that 81st Constitutional Amendment when passed will give 33 per cent reservation of seats in Parliament and State legislatures. This will go a long way to have their say. We should be ashamed of ourselves that after more than half a century of freedom we have neither been able to clothe our women nor able to provide them something as basic as secure and adequate number of toilets and shelter even in the capital city of Delhi."

6. Lack of Interest and Enthusiasm: Need of Enthusiasm

Women lack interest in PRI on account of luke warm attitude to PRIs by State and Union Governments. To make life worthwhile and fruitful, they must generate enthusiasm within themselves. Generation of enthusiasm will take place when they discover for themselves a goal and attach ourselves to the Altar with a spirit of dedication, reverence and love. Once they have surrendered themselves to it, the ideal itself will provide them with the inspiration and strength. Then nothing can hinder the progress of women's march towards that goal and the ideal. The love for the ideal will overcome and vanquish all the hurdles from the ideal, and if it comes to that, life itself will be cast off with a smile, a dedication at that Altar. That was how Bhagat Singh could walk to the gallows with a smile on his face. What is important is that one should choose the right ideal . . . an ideal worthwhile even if it comes to sacrificing one's own life in the endeavour. The ideal should be inspiring, it should arouse the spring of activity in us. Thus, the discovering of the ideal is the secret of generating in ourselves, dynamism and vitality in its fullness.

7. No Forum to Exchange Ideas: Need for All Women Forum

Elected representatives of three tiers should meet once in three months. At present, elected representatives rarely meet at one platform to form opinion upon different activities being carried out at various levels. There is a need to have a quarterly meeting of all the elected representatives to exchange their view points. In this way, they would be more participative while deliberating on important issues.

8. Women MLAs and MPs do not take Interest in them: Need of Motivation by their Own Examples

Women MLAs and MPs should visit frequently the elected representatives of PRIs to solve the problems faced by women members.

9. Women do not Struggle for Employment: Need to Acquire Empowerment

Sarojini Vardappan in her Article, "The Challenge of the 21st Century and Role of Indian Women"—The emphasis now is empowerment. Empowerment is now active process. Power is not a commodity to be transacted, "Power cannot be given away as alms. Power has to be acquired, once acquired it needs to be exercised, sustained and preserved. Women have to empower themselves. It is a multi-dimensional process which should enable individuals or group and individuals to realise their full identity and power in all spheres of life. It consists of greater access to knowledge and resources, greater autonomy in decision-making to enable them to have greater ability to plan their lives or have greater control over the circumstances that influence their lives and freedom from shackles imposed on them by customs, belief and practice. Discrimination of women from womb to tomb is well known, age long traditions and worn out customs are handicaps, women have to struggle, on their way up."

One of India's greatest poets, Rabindranath Tagore, had expressed the pain and inequity of the situation more than half a century ago, thus:

"O Lord Why have you not given
woman the right to conquer her destiny?
Why does she have to wait head bowed,
By the roadside,
Waiting with tired patience,
Hoping for a miracle in the morrow?"

10. Mere Legislations do not keep "Women": Need of Action

Every new legislation has only worsened the position of women. And now their right to property granted by law in a recent judgement by the Supreme Court poses a new threat to her life.

These developments only reinforce the belief that laws alone do not lead to social transformation, unless followed by resolute action and societal awareness of the wrong from time immemorial. And as the eminent jurist V.R. Krishna Iyer rightly says, "The Constitutional provisions are weapons, not victories. Law has to be activated." In short, the struggle for justice—social, economic and political remains to be fought and won. In this scenario, all talk of Women Empowerment is nothing more than empty jargon. The situation demands a revolution of consciousness in the minds of women—in the ways they think about themselves. Women must realize that gender deprivation is inconsistent with their basic human rights. They must realize that they have Constitutional rights to quality healthcare, economic security, access to education, employment opportunities, pay equity and political power.

EMPOWERMENT OF WOMEN: SOME STEPS IN RURAL INDIA

As stated in the Annual Report of Rural Development 2004-05, Women's Empowerment is critical to ensure the socio-economic development of any community. To bring women into the mainstream and to encourage their participation in the process of national development has, therefore, been a major concern of the Government. The various programmes of the Ministry of Rural Development are framed in the above perspective:

- The Ministry of Rural Development is implemetning various poverty alleviation and Rural Development Programmes. These programmes have special components for Women and funds are earmarked as 'Women's Component' to ensure flow of adequate resources for the purpose.
- The major schemes, having women's Component implemented by the Ministry of Rural Development include the Swarnjayanti Gram Swarozgar Yojana (SGSY), Sampoorna Grameen Rozgar Yojana (SGRY), the Indira Awas Yojana (IAY), the Restructued Centrally Rural Sanitation Programme and the accelerated Rural Water Supply Programme.

J. Bhagyalakshmi in his Article, "Women's Empowerment: Miles to Go" in *Yojana* (Aug. 2004) "India as a signatory to the UN Convention has taken several measures to ensure full development and advancement of women. The women-specific progrmames are showing positive results in empowering women, yet, one feels, there are miles to go and promises to keep.

The year 2001 was observed as Women Empowerment Year by UN. The National Policy for the Empowerment of Women was evovled in the same year. The policy recognizes the causes of gender inequality which are related to social and economic struture. The policy underlines the need for mainstreaming gender perspective in the development process. The objectives of the National Policy for the Empowerment of Women include:

(1) Creating an environment through positive eocnomic and social policies for full development of women to enable them to realize their full potential;
(2) The *de jure* and *de facto* enjoyment of all human rights by women on equal basis with men in all spheres—political, eoconomic social, cultural and civil;
(3) Equal access to participation and decision-making in social, politicla and economic life of the nation;
(4) Equal access to healthcare, quality education at all levels, career and vocational guidance, employment and equal remuneration.
(5) Strengthening of legal systems aimed at elimination of all forms of discrimination against women;
(6) Changing societal attitudes and community practices by active participation and involvement of both men and women;
(7) Mainstreaming a gender perspective in the development process;
(8) Elimination of discrimination and all forms of violence against women and the girl child; and
(9) Building and strengthening partnerships with civil society, particularly women's organizations.

Notes and References

1. India 2002, Ministry of Information and Broadcasting, GOI, New Delhi, p. 230.
2. J.P. Singh, Indian Democracy and Empowerment of Women, in *IJPA*, Oct.-Dec. 2000.
3. GOI, Ministry of Rural Development, Annual Report, 1999-2000, p. 66.
4. Ministry of Environment and Forests, 2002, Empowers People For Sustainable Development, pp. 20-21.
5. Sumitra Mahajan, Minister of States, Department of Women and Child Development, Ministry of Human Resource Development, GOI, New Delhi, Message, Deptt. of Women and Child Development, Ministry of HRD, Year of Achievements and New Initiatives.
6. "Towards Equality", Report of the Status of Women, p. 6.
7. Status of Women and Family Planning, C/o No. 6/5/75 Ref. No. E-75, 1975.
8. Worm, Population and Development, *Population Profiles*, No. 7, p. 10.
9. *Rigveda*, 2/17/71; 9/67/10.12.
10. *Shelter*, Vol. III, No. 4, Oct. 2000, XIV.
11. B.K. Chaturvedi, Secretary, Deptt. of Women and Child Development, Ministry of HRD, GOI, New Delhi, Foreword, Year of Achievements and New Initiatives.
12. *Shelter*, Vol. III, No. 4, Oct. 2000, p. IV.
13. Annual Report, Ministry of Rural Development, GOI, New Delhi, 2001-02, p. 60.

14. G. Palanithurai, "The Genere of Women Leaders in Local Bodies: Experience from Tamil Nadu", in *IJPA*, January-March 2001, p. 49.
15. Devki Jain and P. Sujaya, Challenges before Elected Panchayat and Women, in A Round Table on "Financial for District Level Development", 19th May, 2001, United Nations Development Fund for Women, New Delhi, 2002, p. 25.
16. *Ibid.*, p. 24.
17. "Women Participation in Politics: Hard Choice Workshop" by Research Centre for Women Studies, SNDT University, *Economic and Political Weekly*, September 21, 1991, p. 2191.
18. Roopa Sharma, "The Women's Reservation Bill: A Crisis of Identity" in *IJPA*, January-March 2001, p. 66.

CHAPTER 12

HEALTH EDUCATION AT VILLAGE LEVEL: SUB-CENTRE

The first priority should be given to development of right attitudes among people like—

- Acceptance of personal responsibility for health promotion;
- Application of health knowledge and understanding to solve health problems;
- Confidence in scientific health principles/practices;
- Awareness that prevention is preferable to treatment or cure; and
- Conviction that any deviation from normal health status requires immediate medical attention and care.

—*Central Health Education Bureau*

Health Education at Village Level: Sub-Centre

- Reliance on scientific medicine;
- Rejection of superstitutions and quackery;
- Respect for the health of others;
- Willingness to suffer inconvenience for the protection of health of others; and
- Ideal of attaining vigorous high level of health.

—Central Health Education Bureau

Health Education at the village level includes provision of knowledge about communicable and non-communicable diseases in a simple language.

Sub-centre is the most important institution in providing healthcare. The success or failure of healthcare depends upon the attitudes, perception and ethos of health workers and volunteers working in sub-centres. It is a matter of great dissatisfaction that health centres are not doing well and are showing poor performance. This may be attributed to lack of interest about them among union, state and district level health functionaries. Sub-centres are the pivot around which all important schemes revolve. At present, workers in these centres are highly dissatisfied resulting in bad delivery of primary healthcare services. Health centres can really communicate effectively with community, volunteers and the people.

In the new millennium, we must strengthen the health centres to reap the benefits of healthcare. World Health Organisation has also recommended it.[1] The first line health workers are the major work force at the primary level. They provide a substantial part of the primitive and preventive components of the essential healthcare package. They also identify and refer complicated cases and emergencies. However, there are marked variations in their level of training among Member States, with some workers being trained for only

CHART 12.1

Health Education at Village Level

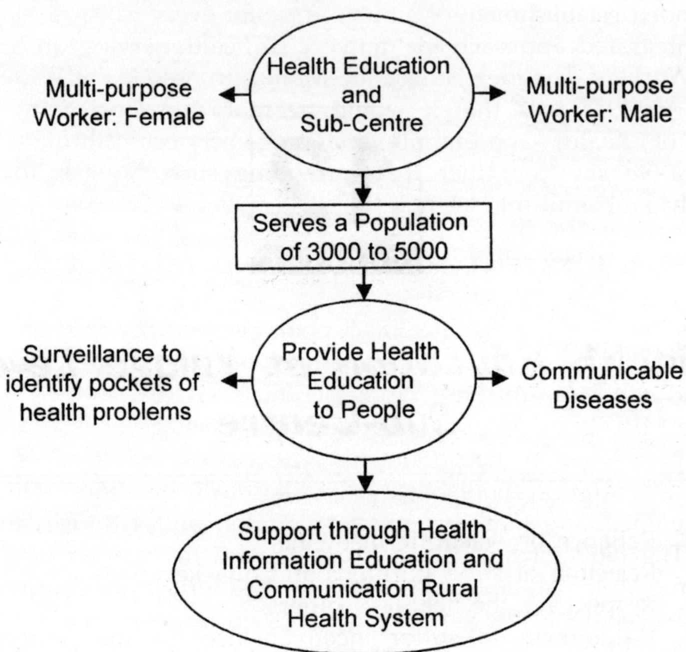

one and a half months. Appropriate training, proper deployment, and basic supplies and logistic support for the first line health workers are important for the delivery of essential healthcare.

The staffing pattern in peripheral health units is an important indicator of the effective functioning of PHC in basic health units, and shortages of personnel are reported from several countries. In the majority of countries of the region, auxiliary health workers are the main providers of care at the first level static health facilities. Medical officers are not usually posted to this level, except in DPR Korea and recently in Maldives.

To overcome the problem of limited access to static health facilities in some areas, many countries have organized outreach services through which health workers regularly visit communities to provide healthcare. Services commonly provided are immunizations, family planning, health education, growth monitoring and advice on nutrition, basic maternal care, vitamin A distribution, and treatment of common ailments such as diarrhoea and acute respiratory infection. Data on disease incidence and vital statistics are also collected during outreach visits in some countries.

I. RATIONALE AND PHILOSOPHY

During the Fourth Plan period, two committees viz., (1) Committee on Multi-purpose Workers (MPW) under Health and, Family Planning

Programme (also known as Kartar Singh Committee) 1972-73, and (2) Srivastava Committee, 1974 were constituted to suggest ways and means to improve the rural health services. The Kartar Singh Committee recommended establishment of a Sub-Centre for every 5,000 rural population and an integrated approach for delivery of health services through Multi-purpose Workers. The idea behind the Multi-purpose Health Worker Scheme launched in 1977 was that it would be more appropriate to provide a package of health and family planning services "through a single administrative set-up, rather than providing such services in a vertical manner through multiple agencies.

2. EXTENT, FUNCTIONS AND TRAINING

It is the most peripheral contact point between the Primary Healthcare System and the community. It is manned by one Multi-purpose Worker (Male) and one Multi-purpose Worker (Female)/ANM.

The MPW scheme aims at providing a package of health services to the rural population at their doorsteps. The main objective of this scheme is to ensure a minimum availability of public health facilities, which include preventive medicine, family welfare, nutrition and curative and referral services. The launching of this scheme marked the merger of the vertical programmes into an integrated health delivery system, thus lending additional strength to the Primary Health Centres.[2]

As per the norms, each Sub-centre is required to be manned by a trained Female Health Worker (ANM) and a trained Male Health Worker known as Multi-purpose Worker (Male). The Govt. of India had initiated a scheme of training and thereby converting the uni-purpose workers under various programmes to multi-purpose workers. However, because of the shortage of MPW's (Male) at Sub-centre level, a scheme of basic training for MPW (Male) was initiated during the 7th Plan period. Under this scheme, 10th pass candidates are selected and trained for one year before they are inducted into services.[3]

The Basic Training of MPW (M) is being done in 56 Training Schools throughout the country under 100% centrally sponsored schemes. The schools have a total admission capacity of 3390.

In order to train the required number of ANMs in the rural areas, there are 477 ANM Training Schools functioning in the country with an annual admission capacity of 16,445. Health Assistants (F) are trained through 42 Promotional schools with annual capacity of 2596. The number of Health Worker (F) under training was 5762 out of which 1871 qualified. The duration of the training is 18 months. 10th pass girls preferably from the local villages where their services will be utilised later at the Sub-centres and Primary Health Centres are admitted for the basic course. These are utilised for providing continuing education/training programmes for ANMs, besides providing the basic training programme of 18 months duration. The purpose of training is that these workers should develop vision, initiative and desire to achieve the goals of Health for all with dedication and perseverance through professional knowledge and behavioural techniques. Jawahar Lal Nehru has rightly said: "No one can really do first class work without a sense of function, without a measure of a crusading spirit, I am doing this, I have to achieve this as a part of great movement in a big cause."[4]

Job Responsibilities of Health Workers (M) (See Chart 12.2)

Malaria

Identify fever cases, make thick and thin blood films of all fever cases and send the slides for laboratory examination, Administer presumptive treatment to all fever cases, Record the results of examination of blood films, refer all cases of positive blood films to the health assistant (male) for radical treatment and educate the community on the importance of blood film examination for fever cases, treatment of fever cases, insecticidal spraying of houses, larviciding measures, and other measures to control the spread of malaria.

Communicable Diseases

Identify cases of notifiable diseases, i.e. cholera, plague, poliomyelitis, and persons with continued fever, or prolonged cough, or spitting of blood, which he comes across during his home visits and notify the health assistant (male) and primary health centre about them and carry out control measures until the arrival of the health assistant (male). Educate the community about the importance of control and preventive measures against such communicable diseases including tuberculosis. Report the presence of stray dogs to the health assistant (male).

Environmental Sanitation

Chlorinate public water sources including wells at regular intervals. Educate the community on: (a) the method of disposal of liquid wastes; (b) the method of disposal of solid wastes; (c) home sanitation; (d) advantages and use of sanitary type of latrines; and (e) construction and use of smokeless chulhas and help the community in the construction of: (i) soakage pits; (ii) kitchen gardens; (iii) manure pits; (iv) compost pits; and (v) sanitary latrines.

Immunization

In the intensive area, administer DPT vaccination, BCG vaccination and wherever available, oral poliomyelitis vaccination to all children aged one to five years, in the twilight area, administer OPT vaccination, BCG vaccination and wherever available, oral poliomyelitis vaccine to all children aged zero to five years, assist the health assistant (male) in the school immunization programmes and educate the people in the community about the importance of immunization against the various communicable diseases.

CHART 2.2

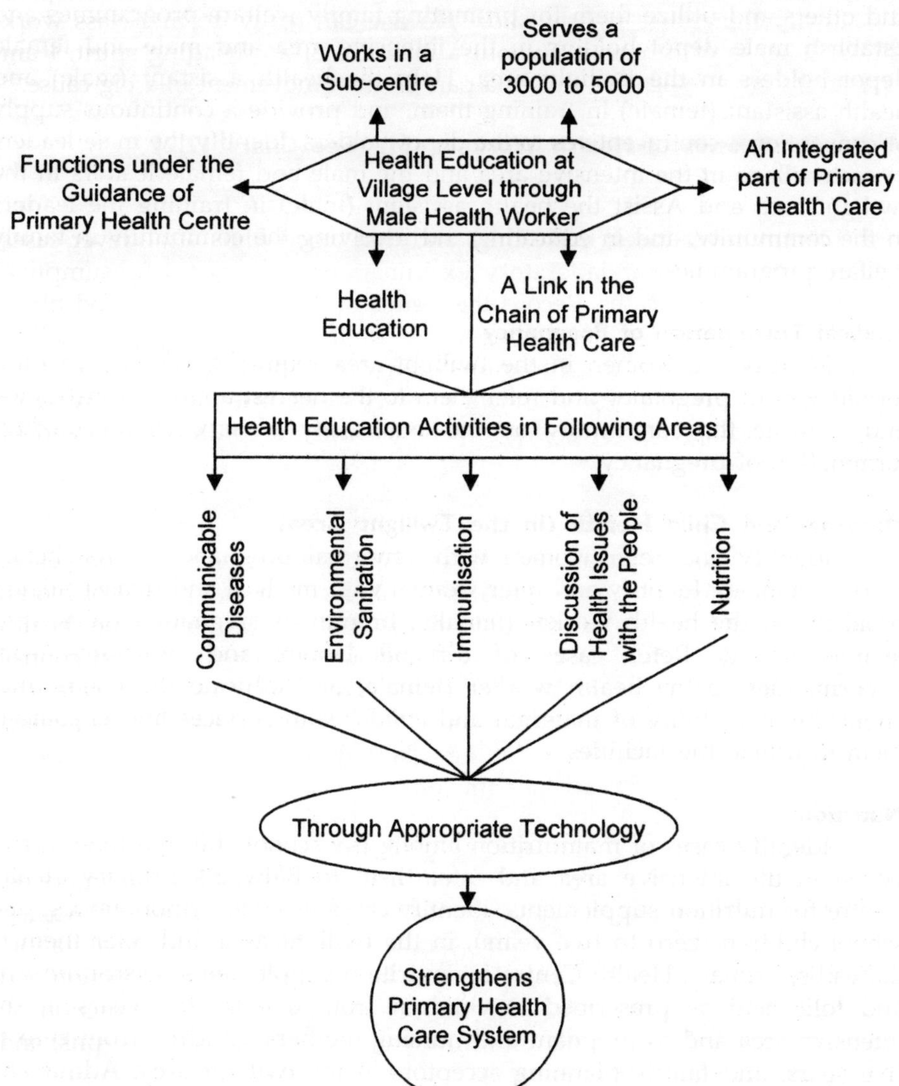

Family Planning

Utilize the information from the Eligible Couple Register for the family planning programme. Spread the message of family planning to the couples, in his area and motivate them for family planning individually and in groups and distribute conventional contraceptives to the couples. Provide facilities and help to prospective acceptors of vasectomy in obtaining the services and provide follow-up services to make family planning acceptors in the intensive area and all family planning acceptors in the twilight area, identify side-effects, give treatment on the spot for side-effects and minor complaints, and refer those cases that need attention by the physician to the *PHCI* hospital, Build rapport with the satisfied acceptors, village teachers and others and utilize them for promoting family welfare programmes and Establish male depot holders in the intensive area and male and female depot holders in the twilight area. Help the health assistant (male) and health assistant (female) in training them, and provide a continuous supply of conventional contraceptives to the depot holders. Identify the male leaders in each village in the intensive area and the male and female leaders in the twilight area and Assist the health assistant (male) in training the leaders in the community, and in educating and involving the community in family welfare programmes.

Medical Termination of Pregnancy

Identify the women in the twilight area requiring help for medical termination of pregnancy and refer them to the nearest approved institution and Educate the community on the availability of services for medical termination of pregnancy.

Maternal and Child Health (In the Twilight Area)

Identify and refer women with abnormal pregnancy to the health worker (female). Identify and refer women with medical and gynaecological problems to the health worker (female). Immunize pregnant women with tetanus toxoid. Refer cases of difficult labour and newborns with abnormalities to the health worker (female) and educate the community about the availability of maternal and child health services and encourage them to utilize the facilities.

Nutrition

Identify cases of malnutrition among pre-school children (one to five years) in the intensive area and refer them to Balwadis Primary Health Centre for nutrition supplements. Identify cases of malnutrition among pre-school children (zero to five years), in the twilight area and refer them to Balwadis/Primary Health Centre for nutrition supplements. Distribute iron and folic acid as prescribed to children from one to five years in the intensive area and to pregnant and nursing mothers, children from zero to five years, and family planning acceptors in the twilight area. Administer vitamin 'A' solution as prescribed to children from one to five years in both the intensive and the twilight areas and educate the community about nutritious diet for mothers and children.

Vital Events

Enquire about births and deaths occurring in the intensive and twilight areas, record them in the births and deaths register and report them to the health assistant (male) and educate the community on the importance of registration of births and deaths and the method of registration.

Record Keeping

Survey all the families in his area and collect general information about each village/locality in his area. Prepare, maintain and utilize family records and village registers, take assistance of the health worker (female) to prepare the Eligible Couple Register from the family records and maintain it up to date. Prepare and submit periodical reports in time to the health assistant (male) and prepare and maintain maps and charts for his area and utilize them for planning his work.

Primary Medical Care

Provide treatment for minor ailments, provide first-aid for accidents and emergencies, and refer cases beyond his competence to the primary health centre or nearest hospital.

Team Activities

Attend and participate in the staff meetings at primary health centre and Taluka Hospital. Coordinate his activities with the health worker (female) and other health workers, including the dais, in the twilight area and meet the health assistant (male) each week and seek his advice and guidance whenever necessary.

3. JOB RESPONSIBILITIES OF HEALTH WORKER (FEMALE) (See Chart 12.3)

Maternal and Child Health

Register and provide care to pregnant women throughout the period of pregnancy and test urine of pregnant women for albumen and sugar and estimate haemoglobin level during her home visits and at the clinic. Refer cases of abnormal pregnancy and cases with medical and gynaecological problems to the health assistant (female) or the primary health centre as well as conduct about 50 per cent of total deliveries in her intensive area and whenever called in the twilight area and supervise deliveries conducted by dais and assist them whenever called in. Refer cases of difficult labour and newborns with abnormalities and help them to get institutional care and provide follow-up care to patients referred to or discharged from hospital. Make at least three post-natal visits for each delivery conducted in the intensive area and render advice regarding care of the mother and care and feeding of the newborn and assess the growth and development of the infant and take any necessary action. Help the medical officer and health assistant (female) in conducting MCH and family planning clinics at the sub-centre and educate mothers individually and in groups for better family health including MCH, family planning, nutrition, immunization, control of communicable diseases, personal and environmental hygiene and care of minor ailments.

Family Planning

Utilize the information from the Eligible Couple Register for the family planning programme and spread the message of family planning to the couples and motivate them for family planning individually and in groups. Distribute conventional contraceptives to the couples, provide facilities and help the prospective acceptors in getting family planning services, if necessary by accompanying them or arranging for the dais to accompany them to hospital and provide follow-up services to female family planning adopters, identify side-effects, give treatment on the spot for side-effects and minor complaints and refer those cases that need attention by the physician to the PHC/hospital. Establish female depot holders, help the health assistant (female) in training them, and providing a continuous supply of conventional contraceptives to the depot holders and build rapport with acceptors, village leaders, dais and others and utilize them for promoting family welfare programmes, Identify women leaders and help the health assistant (female) to train them and participate in Mahila MandaI meetings, and utilize such gatherings for educating women in family welfare programmes.

Medical Termination of Pregnancy

Identify the women requiring help for medical termination of pregnancy and refer them to the nearest approved institution and educate the community of the availability of services for medical termination of pregnancy.

Nutrition

Identify cases of malnutrition among infants and young children (0 to 5 years), give the necessary treatment and advice and refer serious cases to the PHC and distribute iron and folic acid tablets as prescribed to pregnant and nursing mothers, infants and young children (0 to 5 years) and family planning acceptors. Administer vitamin' A' solution as prescribed to children from 1 to 5 years and educate the community about nutritious diet for mothers and children.

Communicable Diseases

Identify cases of notifiable diseases, i.e. cholera, plague, poliomyelitis, and persons with continued fever of prolonged cough, or spitting of blood, which she comes across during her home visits and notify the health worker (male) about them.

Immunization

Immunize pregnant women with tetanus toxoid and Administer BCG vaccination to all newborn infants, and OPT vaccination, oral poliomyelitis vaccine (where available) and BCG vaccine (if not given at birth) to all infants (0 to 1 year).

Dai Training

List dais in the intensive and twilight areas and involve them in promoting family welfare and help the health assistant (female) in the training programme of dais.

Vital Events

Record births and deaths occurring in the intensive area in the births and deaths register and report them to the health worker (male).

Record Keeping

Register: (a) pregnant women from three months of pregnancy onwards; (b) infants zero to one year of age; and (c) women aged 15 to 44 years through systematic home visits in the intensive area and at the clinic. Maintain the pre-natal and maternity records and child care records. Assist the health worker (male) in preparing the Eligible Couple Register and maintaining it up-to-date. Prepare and submit the prescribed periodical reports in time to the health assistant (female). Prepare and maintain maps and charts for her area and utilize them for planning her work.

Primary Medical Care

Provide treatment for minor ailments, provide first-aid for accidents and emergencies, and refer cases beyond her competence to the primary health centre or nearest hospital.

Team Activities

Attend and participate in staff meetings at primary health centre/ community development block or both. Coordinate her activities with the health worker (male) and other health workers including the health guides and dais. Meet the health assistant (female) each week and seek her advice and guidance whenever necessary. Maintain the cleanliness of the sub-centre. Participate as a member of the team in camps and campaigns.

An analysis of duties and responsibilities of Multi-purpose workers: Male and Female indicate very heavy schedule for them. Besides, the problems to be tackled are common, the interpersonal relationships and communications between the two workers need special attention to avoid duplication and wastage of efforts to ensure economy and efficiency. To achieve all these objectives, they need a good working environment, transport facilities and people's co-operation, as this is a challenging and arduous task. It requires determination, hard work, patience, communication skill, dedication on the part of multi-purpose workers to achieve the goals.[5]

4. CRITICAL EXAMINATION

A critical examination of the performance of the scheme reveals dissatisfaction of the villagers. We may mention some of the important aspects which need analysis to improve the existing set-up.

I. Under Utilisation of Time by Multi-purpose Workers

Health services being labour-intensive, the effective delivery of primary healthcare services depends on the availability and efficient utilisation of the available manpower resources. To achieve the objectives of Health for all by the year 2000, through Primary Healthcare approach, Sub-centre staff are expected to work at maximum efficiency to optimise physical resources.

Rapid population growth and limited resources have forced us to a greater recognition of the need to utilise the existing personnel and facilities in the health service system more effectively and efficiently.

Time utilization by health manpower, and their productivity, is expected to be influenced *inter alia* by their attitudes to the job, especially their perceptions of the objectives to be pursued; organizational inadequacies and other constraints; job-related tensions and job satisfaction, etc. The study of Rajneesh Goel found that the utilisation time of MPW (M) and MPW (F) in Karnataka was only 37.5 per cent.

We present here the results of some studies conducted earlier on time utilisation to support these findings.

1. A study of PHC staff Time Utilization pattern was undertaken in a PHC in Uttar Pradesh by S.K. Satpathy *et. at.* (1998). This study included only technical staff (excluding drivers, sweepers, etc.) and the technique followed was a non-participant observation of the staff for several days. From this study, it was found that the non-productive time of such staff was as high as 62%, Services time accounted for 27% and travel accounted for 11%.
2. A study on Cost Analysis of PHCs by M. Kataria and A.P. Srivastava (NIHFW, 1986) included the analysis of allocation of service time at PHC and sub-centre levels. The method used was observation (for field work) and work sampling (at PHC). Besides these two techniques, Delphi technique was also used for supplementing the information collected through the observations.

Three districts from two states (M.P. and U.P.) were selected; one PHC per district was selected. Thus, 3 PHCs from each state were selected and 12 sub-centres (2 from each selected PHC) were selected. The major findings of the study were:

- 50% of the activity time was spent on travelling and unproductive activities;
- Of the other 50% of productive time, 1/5th was devoted to 'Direct Services', the major activity being family planning followed by MCH services (by female workers) and control of communicable diseases (by male worker);

- At PHC, direct services accounted for 47% (UP) and 49% (MP); supportive services accounted for 8% (UP) and 11% (MP); time spent on travel was 22% (UP) and 20% (MP). Thus, only 55-60% of total activity time was spent productively.

Johns Hopkins University conducted studies (1965-68) and came to the following conclusions:

- Only 1/6 of the total health centre effort went into direct service in Punjab, compared to 1/4 in Mysore. Further, in Punjab, supporting activities (33.3%) consumed more than twice as much time than service efforts (15.5%).
- More time was devoted in Punjab to the maintenance of records and preparation of reports than to the provision of services (16.3%), whereas in Mysore a mere 1/3 of the activity time was devoted to records and reports.
- An analysis of the time utilization by service components showed that most of their service time was devoted to family planning activities (per cent of service time devoted ranged from 33-49%) followed by MCH services (22-27%), and immunization (5-15%).

Thus, all MPWS (male and female) were found to devote most of their service time on family planning activities. This could well be attributed to the government's emphasis on target achievement in the family planning programme. Since these workers are given a set target they are forced to spend more time on this activity, and thus neglect other important activities. However, the target approach has been abolished and we would see its impact in later studies.

The main purpose of the scheme was to devote more time on health education, nutrition, inter-sectoral co-ordination, people's participation, which, however, could not be attended to. There is a need to impart training to these workers to make them realise their true role. Only such understanding on their part can change health scene of rural India, otherwise, it would prove to be another institution with liabilities. The main function of MPW is to make people participate in Primary Healthcare activities and get most of the functions performed by them. Besides, they need to devote more time for Inter Sectoral Co-ordination, an essential Component of Primary Healthcare.

The statement that "Time is money" sums up the significance of time management. Though most of the people in Government, Public Enterprises and Private Sector understand the implications of time management but in actual practice, we find that time is wasted and its importance is undermined. Most of the executives and workers in administration complain that they are too busy but still they while away a lot of their time in unnecessary activities. All other resources can be increased whenever required but not time as it is inelastic and therefore, we must make the best use of time. Just to illustrate the importance of time, many studies conducted revealed that persons in administration hardly devote 30 to 40 per cent of their time for the activities they have been engaged for. It means that if proper use is made of time, we can provide services with the existing infrastructure two to three times more and thus the process of development can be accelerated.

Thus, if all the services make the best use of time, we can accelerate the process of development and help the people of the country suffering from abject poverty, ill-health, illiteracy, unemployment, in leading a good standard of life. In developed countries, the most precious resource is time and that is why they are developed but in developing countries, time is unconsciously and consciously wasted in useless activities resulting in underdevelopment or backwardness.

Nation must be committed to utilise even a fraction of second for accelerating the tempo of development to usher in socio-economic democracy as enshrined in the preamble of the Indian constitution and further stressed in Fundamental Rights and Directive Principles of State Policy. How to go about it? How to ensure optimisation of time? How to make the best use of time? The answers to these questions are very simple, i.e. time management at all levels.

If our country can manage time, we can achieve in a year the work of a decade and thus can move fast towards modernisation and development and can say with pride that India occupies a prominent place as in the past in the community of nations.

The aim of time management is not to turn workers into machines who work without interruptions or breaks, nor is it to develop rigid routines. Rather, the aim is to organise and arrange the use of time so that time pressures and overcrowded schedules and wastage are reduced, and that staff can have adequate rest periods without lowering work output.

If forced to work under continuous pressure, people devise means of escape such as by taking a few days off for illness or slowing down their pace and becoming inefficient. These ways of relieving pressure may be observed among staff in an average overcrowded department. It has been repeatedly shown in industry that regular breaks increase work efficiency and work output. We suggest the following methods to optimise time utilisation.

(i) Well Planned Time Table for field Visits

Many of the key personnel have to control a wide network of office. A part of it can be controlled through telephones, or reporting. But, there is a need of personal discussion among the headquarter and the field staff which involves the use of time in travelling and discussion. It has been seen that officials plan their visit in such a way that they waste most of the time in traveling and less in discussion. It is suggested that field/headquarter visits must be well planned so that the discussion can be pertinent and all the issues are discussed to avoid meetings off and on. The headquarter personnel must carry with them a well prepared schedule to guide them in the field while the field people must also come prepared with definite schedule to clarify the vague points.

(ii) Fixing of Time Schedule to Devote Time to Essential Work

Health workers need to design schedule of work to avoid wastage of time and concentrate on only the important items.

(iii) Providing Regular Time for Rest and Recreation to Avoid Fatigue

Health Workers are human beings and thus cannot work beyond their capacity. It is, therefore, suggested that they may observe regular rest periods to feel fresh. However, these rest periods may not be done at will but must be already notified to avoid difficulty to the people until and unless there are compelling reasons for it.

(iv) Brevity

Besides, the workers must learn to be brief and to the point and discourage relatives/friends to visit them in offices. Telephonic discussions must also be brief.

Time management would not only be beneficial to the workers but would also provide more opportunities to the people to share their ideas and views with the workers and this would be able to IAY the solid foundations of people's participation, development and modernisation. It has been observed that workers in health system are not utilizing their time for the assigned job. They are wasting a lot of time in unnecessary activities which are non-productive. We must manage our time purposefully to build modern India otherwise we would remain an under-developed country as time and tide waits for none. We suggest that the health department should provide the following facilities to workers:

(a) We may provide vehicle facility to the workers to reduce time likely to be spent in visiting different places.
(b) We may reduce time spent on record keeping by systematizing records management. We may even think of providing computers to ensure the supply of right information with less time consumption with ready-made software.
(c) There is a need to ensure quality supervision by PHC staff especially Health Assistants to ensure punctuality of health workers.
(d) There is a need for training to make the workers responsive and dedicated.
(e) There is a need to provide accommodation to workers with all facilities in the village to encourage them to stay near the sub-centre and improve rapport with the people.

(f) People may be motivated to come to the sub-centre rather than waiting for the workers visit at their door-steps, after initial meetings.

(g) Advance planning for a month schedule and its wide circulation can optimise time resource utilisation.

2. Low Job Satisfaction

The quality of the Health Institutions run by Government would be dependent to a great extent upon the quality of the employees engaged in their operation. Personnel run the health system. To quote Mrs. Indira Gandhi: "If Government has to do more for the people, its employees must play a more dynamic and more creative role as the instrument for implementing government policies and programmes."[5]

Among the three components required for developmental tasks—men, money and material—it is more the men (or the human element) than any other factor which determine the quantity and quality of the performance and output. After all, even the contribution of money and material to perfonnance depends substantially upon their manipulation by the men in an organization.[6]

There is a general tendency in the organizations to IAY more emphasis on materials and financial management to the utter neglect of the personnel. What are the consequences? It is observed that the process of development takes longer, sometimes even fails. Why?

The main reason for this is that we are not attending to the administration of personnel earnestly and forget that they are the real agents of development and ultimately the beneficiaries of the process of development.

According to Tead: "Personnel Administration is the utilisation of its best scientific knowledge of all kinds to the end that an organization as a whole and the individuals composing it, shall found the corporate purpose and the individual purposes are being reconciled to the fullest possible extent, while the working together of these purposes realise also genuine social benefits."[7]

Dale Yoder defines personnel management as:

"That phase of management which deals with the effective control and use of manpower as distinguished from other sources of power."[8]

Pigors and Myers defines it as:

"A method of developing potentialities of employees so that they get maximum satisfaction out of their work and give their best efforts to the organization."[9]

This dictum also applies to Multi-purpose Workers who are the real providers of healthcare. When they would find job satisfaction or feel congruence with the goals of health for all, they would do their best to achieve the results. It may be made clear that job satisfaction is generated by an individual's perception of how well his job suits him. Job satisfaction may be different at different intervals of time or situations prevailing in an organization.

The words of Ford are the best commentary on job satisfaction. According to him: "Job satisfaction mayor may not be tied to happiness. But we will know that, we are doing something right if we can change the conditions of job so that employees will stay on the work productively. For the older workers the best will be whether they are with us in spirit as well as in body. The way to achieve this end, for new or old employees, is not to confront them with demands, but to confront them with demanding, meaningful work." And the employees will always have the last word as to whether the work is meaningful."[10]

Strauss and Sayles have summarised the significance of 'job' and 'job satisfaction' in the following words:[11]

1. People want self-actualisation.
2. Those who do not obtain job satisfaction, never reach psychological maturity.
3. Those who fail to obtain job satisfaction, become frustrated.
4. The job is central to man's life.
5. Those without work are unhappy. People want to work, even when they do not have to.
6. Lack of challenging work leads to poor mental health. Work-and-Leisure patterns spill into each other. Those with uncreative jobs engage in uncreative recreation.
7. Lack of job satisfaction and alienation from work leads to lower morale, lower productivity, and unhealthy society.

The subject of job satisfaction has been of keen interest for scientific investigation over the years. In the beginning, it was assumed that job satisfaction was related mainly to the amount of money earned. Workers at that time were regarded as part of the machinery to be managed in the most efficient way possible. But Hoppock conducted pioneer research on vocational satisfaction. He interviewed a cross-section of industrial workers and concluded that, 'job satisfaction could not be measured in terms of monetary rewards only. There were many other factors which contributed to job satisfaction, such as the individual's ability to adapt to the work situation, his ability to adapt to his co-workers, his relative status in the socio-economic hierarchy of the group, the nature of work in relation to his interest and abilities and his preparation for the job."[12]

He also conducted the first community-wide study of job satisfaction. He administered a questionnaire and computed an index of job satisfaction. The results indicated that 15% of the sample were not satisfied with their jobs. Robinson and Hoppock collated a number of studies reporting percentage of job satisfaction. They found that two- thirds of the studies revealed dissatisfaction by one third workers.[13]

Job satisfaction does not depend on any single factor but many factors and situations congenial to employees. Conditions of services especially the pay is considered to be the best for job satisfaction.

According to Peter F. Drucker, "The carrot of material rewards has not, like the stick of fear, lost its potency."[14] Gellerman too regards money as an important motivator when he states "money may well turn out to be the costliest motivator of them all, but money may also prove to be the most potent motivator of all, at least in certain circumstances, and when used on a sufficient scale."[15]

Many investigators have pointed out the relative unimportance of money as a motivating factor. Brown goes to the extreme by saying that "of all the incentives known to man, money is the least important."[16]

The Hawthorne experiments introduced the concept of human relations approach to the study of job satisfaction. These experiments highlighted the inter-relatedness of various elements of work, such as working hours, rest, fatigue, incentives, employer's attitudes, as well as formal and informal organizations.[17]

Mayo, concluded that the most important determinant of job satisfaction was group interaction. Mayo was the first author to consider the worker from the psychological perspective and to add the psychological dimension to job satisfaction.

Sajid Iqbal in his Article, "Money cannot buy me love for a job" in *Economic Times* dated 16th August, 1999, says that: "Often managers are not happy with their pay packets because money is not a motivator but a sop for putting up with a rotten job. National Studies of the changing work force conducted by families and work institute, New York, in 1994, found that Open Communication was ranked highest by respondents when choosing their current jobs."[18] We discuss here the factors which can motivate Health Workers and improve their job satisfaction.

4. Factors Responsible for Job Satisfaction

(i) Conditions of Service and Fringe Benefits

Money occupies the most important place in all contractual obligations. The very definition of work declares that it has to be paid for Haire *et al* have rightly pointed out that "pay in one form or another, is certainly one of the mainsprings of motivation in our society."[19]

An adequate and sound salary structure together with other working conditions is the *sine qua non* for the organisational efficiency and effectiveness. Otherwise, as the Administrative Reforms Commission aptly observes, it has been one of the major factors for strikes, agitations, inter-service tensions and rivalries, indifferent attitude to work, poor performance, frustration and low morale of the employees.

However, we must be clear that no compensation plan can satisfy all the employees. The true efficiency in an organisation can be promoted only through dedication and loyalty of its staff members. The Health managers must motivate the employees through no financial incentives. The quality of the health services depends more on the loyalty, the faith and the sense of mission which workers bring in the organisation than on the money expended on them.

(ii) Participation of Workers in Primary Healthcare Delivery System

This can enhance their efficiency. We should encourage workers' participation in the achievement of primary healthcare goals. His participation would build his morale and ultimately his efficiency. An ILO document mentions that the individual worker "is not just a cog in the very big wheel, but that his personal effort is essential for the achievement of the overall production plan."[20]

The research theory in social organisational psychology has also suggested that participation in group decision-making enhances satisfaction among members and removes tensions. Michael R. Copper and Michael T. Wood have shown that satisfaction was greater where participation was complete than where it was partial.[21]

There is a need to practise 'Management by Objectives' to ensure fruitful participation. Management by Objectives shifts the focus to goals, to the purpose of the activity, supervisor and subordinate personnel of an organisation jointly identify its common goals and ensure performance. The PHC staff must encourage the development of such concepts among employees.

(iii) The PHC must Promote Effective Communication between the Workers and the PHC

It is not the official queries or the reservations in the confidential reports that earn staff loyalty. It is the extent that average staff member appreciates the objectives and purposes of the services rendered. The PHC staff should foster in the staff an 'esprit de corps', a spirit of togetherness and dedication to duty.

Changes in methods, organisation or physical facilities that should enhance substantial improvements in efficiency may result in drastically reduced efficiency, if the personnel are suspicious or resentful of the contemplated change. This type of resistance, sometimes referred to as organisational treason, must be anticipated. In order to administer an organisation in a manner designed to induce healthy attitudes among the workers towards the new changes, support should be obtained from the multi-purpose workers before any change is injected. The PHC staff must encourage the workers to participate in developing solution. Under these conditions they will accept their responsibility to co-operate with others, and they will try to perform their assigned tasks in order to avoid a breakdown in the chain of interrelated functions. To quote Ted R. Brannen:

"Only by an understanding of the individual, his habits, expectations, and beliefs, can the administrator know what is needed to induce his spontaneous co-operation for the benefit of the organisation."[22]

(iv) Nature of Job and Professional Growth

The greatest efficiency and productivity will flow from the efforts of those who find satisfaction in their work and conditions of service, who sense an awareness of usefulness of their function, who feel encouraged to move ahead and to meet new challenges, who perceive their working environment as one in which high standards of performance are maintained and rewarded and not one in which indolence and incompetence can be ignored or even protected and rewarded. Motivation can do miracles as a motivated worker can achieve more than an expert with no motivation. Health Managers must, therefore, devote considerable time and effort in planning for and achieving high levels of motivation and morale. In such a situation, we would achieve goal congruence, i.e., identity between the multi-purpose workers, goals and the Health organisational goals.

Living together is a beginning
Keeping together is progress
Working together is success.[23]

5. Co-operation and Support from Public

The people in Health Administration should have a sense of dedication, responsibility and be responsive and alert to the aspirations of the citizens. Citizens on the other hand should also provide meaningful co-operation to Health Administration. Under such an atmosphere, it would be very easy to implement the health tasks to ensure positive health for the people.

6. Participation of Beneficiaries

Multi-purpose Workers (MPWS) must understand that they should learn the art and science of motivating the community to participate their own health programmes. We mention here the following things to be achieved by MPWS:

(i) Creating will and determination among the members of the community for improvement of their present and future health.
(ii) Identification and development of the local resources, thereby generating self-reliance among the community.
(iii) Mobilising the available manpower for productive and useful activities.
(iv) Providing an open forum for the community to discuss its problems and find indigenous solutions which may be efficient and economical.

(v) To develop local leaders who can further educate and mobilise the people in the area.

(vi) Arranging extra-curricular activities to generate social awareness through well designed publicity.

(vii) Encouraging the people to develop themselves rather than depend upon the Government for all activities and thus become self-reliant which is the key to development.

To quote Brook Adams, "Administration is the capacity of coordinating many, and often conflicting, social energies in a single organism, so adroitly that they may operate as a unity."[24] Thus, community participation is the Pivot of the Rural Healthcare System.

(vii) Effective Supervision

Under the new MPW scheme, supervision is regarded as the organic link between the PHC and the grass-root workers/beneficiaries. The major components of the supervisors work include planning and assessment of training needs, checking of records and public relations and supplies. Though most of these functions are carried out by almost all the supervisors, what is conspicuously missing is the sense of competence in the execution of these jobs. In particular, the component of 'assessment of training needs' leaves much to be desired. Also, it is disheartening to consider record checking and surprise field visits—a major method of supervision. Calculated guidance and meaningful monitoring ought to have been integral to their function. But these were not. Prominent among the problems that face the supervisors besides problems such as those relating to the logistics of fieldwork, supplies, transport incentives, etc. is the one relating to fixing up of work priorities and targets to be executed by MPWs. For example, those supervisors who in turn reported to the bosses who subscribed less to FP activities and more to their own specific work/discipline-oriented activities (malaria) or those whose bosses were primarily inclined towards FP invariably found their instructions conflicting in either case with the result that both the supervisors and MPWs, and their work suffered.

At other times, the supervisors themselves tended to exhibit bias in fixing work priorities that by and large reflected their parent departmental work/orientation (e.g. malaria) even at the cost of the other activities. However, the supervisors felt that the programme implementation was good.

The medical officers, regarded as the PHC Health Team Managers, were found suitable from the technical qualifications! work point of view but were found wanting in other equally critical dimensions of the work such as inspiring the staff reporting to them to perform qualitatively better, inculcate in the workers a good tradition of field work and establish rapport with the local population with a view to promoting preventive and rehabilitative healthcare.

(viii) Sound Logistic Support

1. Prompt and adequate drug supply,
2. Provision of a first-aid kit,
3. Regular provision of necessary registers, and
4. Provision of transport facility, at least during emergencies and immunization camps.

(ix) Tapping the Potential

Health workers possess the potential which need be utilised Dr. Suresh Kant in his Article, "Tap That Potential" in the *Indian Express,* Dec. 15, 1999, Chandigarh, rightly suggests that Neuro Linguistic programming suggests that individual behaviour can be changed. Upgrading mental software is the answer. Everyone has the requisite mental resources and potential to produce excellent outcome. The need is to properly optimise the potential of health workers by the leadership at primary health centres and district health system.

(x) Promoting Team Work

District health system should promote team work to avoid unnecessary duplication of effort, increase co-operation, develop ideas, maintain motivation, improve quality of health services and ensure satisfaction of the people. Aankur Uppal in his article, "The High Road" in the *Indian Express,* Dec. 1999, Chandigarh rightly suggests that in an organization it is the team that operates. One has to have trust in that team and empower it to convert ideas into reality successfully. . . . There is no soft route. Hard work is the key to success. Making money should not be the only endeavour of a person.

5. RECENT DEVELOPMENTS

From April 1996, India's Family Welfare Programme has adopted a target free approach. This new approach is known as Reproductive and Child Health Programme (RCH). The RCH is considered to be equivalent to Family Planning + Child Survival and Safe Motherhood (CSSM) Programme + Prevention of RTIISTD and Aids + a client approach in providing Family Welfare and Healthcare Services.[25]

In order to find out the impact of New Approach (Target Free) let us mention briefly the two studies undertaken by Population Research Centre in the Districts of Belgaum and Dharwad. At the instance of the Ministry of Health and Family Welfare, Government of India, New Delhi and as a part of monitoring and evaluation of the performance of the family welfare programme under the new target free approach, the Population Research Centre, J.S.S. Institute of Economic Research, Dharward, undertook a rapid survey in the rural areas of Belgaum District, Karnataka state during the last two weeks of December 1997 and first two weeks of January 1998. Using a simple and short questionnaire, the survey interviewed a total of 1,000 currently married women age 15-44, from 50 villages, at the rate of 20 women per village. The study found:

- Monitoring the weight and blood pressure, and urine tests were not carried out for the majority of women during their pregnancy by multi-purpose workers females.
- Of the births that took place at home, the majority (62 per cent) were attended by untrained persons including relatives, friends and neighbours.
- Little less than one-quarter of women in the rural areas of Belgaum District have an unmet need for family planning, that is, they are not using contraception even though they do not want any more children.
- Among the three registers (Eligible Couple register, ANC register, and Immunization register) examined, the EC register was found to be relatively more complete and accurate than the other two registers.[26]

In another study a rapid research survey was conducted in rural areas of Dharwad district in Karnataka during February-April, 1997 to check the coverage, quality of services and client satisfaction under the new strategy of 'target-free' approach.

The facility survey of 50 sub-centres showed that major problems are lack of housing accommodation for the ANMs (50 per cent), unoccupied official quarters (one-third of the cases), lack of adequate furniture, thermometer, BP apparatus, torch light, uristixl bendix solution and metronidazole tablets. On the other hand, ANMs reported a huge supply of IFA tablets. ANMs also complained about lack of supply of EC, ANC immunization and other registers. Some of the important policy recommendations emerging from the study are:

(a) Improve ANM services, especially make them visit women with unmet need for contraception, and past acceptors of sterilization.

(b) As a large number of sterilization acceptors complain about side effects, a special health campaign for sterilized men and women should be launched by multi-purpose workers. In order to safeguard future levels of acceptance, past acceptors should be made to feel that they are looked after well by programme functionaries.

(c) It should be ensured that such Centres have adequate supply of drugs, and attempts should be made to reduce waiting time and provide free services at primary health centres. The guilty should be punished.

(d) A television set could be placed in PHC waiting room and also a VCP to disseminate information and messages on health and family welfare and facilities in sub-centres.

(e) Concerted attempts should be made to raise immunization levels by workers as they appear to have reached a point of stagnation before acquiring universality.[27]

6. FACTS AND SUGGESTIONS

We give here facts and suggestions to improve the functioning of sub-centres.

(i) Effective Logistic Support

There are enormous logistical problems like perennial shortage of medicines (e.g. wide spectrum antibiotics), non-availability of proper equipments (e.g. oxygen cylinder), storage facilities (cold and ordinary) and most important of all, inadequate transport facilities. For efficient and effective implementation of the MPW scheme, these critically important logistical problems need to be solved expeditiously.

(ii) Demarcating Smaller Areas

The population and the area MPW is supposed to cover intensively appears rather high. Hence, the authorities would do well if they could think of reducing this heavy size of population. This would certainly enhance the qualitative impact of the scheme in terms of greater client satisfaction, improved overall health conditions of the people and consequently, enhanced confidence of the people in the scheme.

(iii) Allocating Family Welfare Activities Exclusively to ANMs

It would be better if female MPWs (ANMs) alone were made to work for family planning and thereby, relieve the male workers of their FP responsibilities so that they can concentrate on their multi-purpose work more rigorously and cover a larger number of clientele.

(iv) Refresher Courses to Create Confidence

Some of the workers, particularly the male, do not appear fully confident and professionally capable of conducting their duties in a manner desired by all. Hence, they need to be reoriented and given refresher/crash courses periodically.

Training is: (a) an action process, (b) by which capabilities of the Health personnel can be improved, (c) to meet the Health workers needs in terms of their knowledge, skills, and attitudes required in performing tasks and functions, and (d) within relatively short period of time.

Training is the well articulated effort to promote competence in the Health service by imparting professional knowledge, by broadening of vision and adoption of correct patterns of behaviour among the Health employees with regard to their existing functional responsibilities. It also enables the Health employees to equip themselves for senior administrative positions in future.

Marshall suggests the development of the following ingredients to promote right and rational attitudes:[28]

(i) development of rational thinking,
(ii) development of objective thinking,
(iii) development of social understanding,
(iv) development of aesthetic responsiveness,
(v) development of practical abilities, and
(vi) development and placement of memory in action.

(v) Leadership Role of PHC

PHC doctors and supervisors should provide leadership and guidance to MPWs. This would hopefully help increase their interest in work.

According to Haimann, "Leadership is the process by which an executive or a manager imaginatively directs, guides and influences the work of others in choosing and attaining specified goals by mediating between the individual and the organisation in such a manner that both will obtain the maximum satisfaction."[29]

To quote Keith Davis, "Leadership is the ability to persuade others to seek defined objectives enthusiastically. It is the human factor which binds a group together and motivates it towards its goals."[30]

(vi) Decentralization of Authority

Towards vesting the privileges and powers with the PHC Medical officers for rewarding the subordinate staff or awarding punishment to them, conferment of authority and delegation of power to PHCs by the district and state level health bodies needs to be effected immediately. This would ensure effective control and supervision at PHC level.

(vii) Transport Facilities

Some transport facilities may be provided to MPWs so that they can save time for productive work especially during field campaigns.

(viii) Strengthening Supervisions

Supervision of Multi-purpose Health workers needs to be strengthened as supervision is considered the link pin between PHC and the grass-root workers/present and potential users.

(ix) Financial Allocation as per Actual Need

The present method of uniformly allocating financial resources to the sub-centres irrespective of their size in terms of population served, disease profiles and geographical/locational consideration, should be changed and a rational method of financial allocation needs to be followed.

(x) Multi-purpose Approach at all Levels

The Multi-purpose Health Workers Scheme aims at as wide a coverage of health problems in as much as it envisages totality of health via integration of both programmes/activities and services. Hence, the role of the MPW is considered pivotal. However, the purported multi-purpose orientation appears to be confined to the MPWs alone as if they alone mattered exclusively. But, what is required is multi-purpose orientation at all levels. However, such a development is rarely found in the implementing agencies beyond the PHC/SC level. The legacy of the uni-purpose health work philosophy and its erstwhile practitioners tends to manifest itself in a variety of forms. For example, at the district level unipurpose-oriented and programmes departments continue to exist. Similarly, the erstwhile Unipurpose Health Coordinators/Supervisors continue to exhibit biases that smack of their parental discipline orientation. For example, those who work in the area of malaria tend to emphasise the component of malaria work more than the others in the multi-purpose work with the result that, willy nilly conflicting and counterproductive instructions are issued. Therefore, one needs to carefully re-examine the concept of multi-purpose work as also reorient both the office and field-based staff to the new requirements and the philosophy of the MPW scheme.

P.H. Rayppa and N. Bhaskara Rao in their study found that there was no proper integration of work under this scheme at the state and district levels. Even at the periphery level, health workers tended to think generally in terms of unipurpose activities rather than multi-purpose work.[31]

(xi) Displaying the List of Available Medicines

The wonders of modern medicine serve no purpose when people have no access to the drugs and vaccines that relieve suffering and prevent death.

Fernandos Rntegana in his article, "Action For Equity" in *World Health* (March-April 1992, p. 7) rightly stresses that primary healthcare can only be more effective if even the most remote health centres can rely in receiving regular supplies of affordable drugs of good quality and if health workers are trained in their use. If medicines are not available at health centre, people loose confidence in the whole system and will seek other remedies, usually from sources unqualified to diagnose or prescribe.

In view of the perennial shortage of medicines at the PHCs and SCs, the doctors/MPWs should arrange to display on information boards about availability of medicines. This would help to erase the wrong notions that people have about the integrity of the PHC/SC staff *vis-a-vis* availability.

(xii) Strengthening Sub-centers

In view of the limited reach ability of PHCs (the servicing zone being by and large confined to a radius of three to five kilometers), there is a strong need to strengthen the sub-centres that MPWs are available for most part of the day and night.

(xiii) Building Morale and Motivation of Multi-purpose Workers

Morale has an individual as well as a group or institutional aspect. It is a self-stimulating incentive within the minds and hearts of the multi-purpose workers. A whole some morale stimulates loyalty, generates cooperation and encourages team work. As these are essential for the achievement of the goals of sub-centre and primary healthcare system. Planning and Scheduling of Work under the multi-purpose workers' scheme, health workers provide integral health services based on targets and directives from district and PHC levels. Health workers at sub-centres need to schedule their day-to-day planning activities for the whole month. The work schedule for health workers is thus a simple management tool that will help deliver better primary healthcare to the rural areas of India.

(xiv) Providing Congenial Organisational Climate

It would be of utmost significance to stress that organisation is not merely a structure; in fact, it embraces a structure as well as the human beings who man and run it in order to realise the pre-conceived objectives. We must always strive through administrative improvements and reforms to remove the irritants which creep into the organizations to ensure an effective organisational climate. We may ensure the following:

(a) Clear definition of objectives.
(b) Systematic grouping of related activities.
(c) Maximum delegation of authority.
(d) Minimum layering.
(e) Proper conditions of work.
(f) Provision for easier communications.[32]

(xv) Creating Ethical Values of Service Among MPWs

Workers must be imbued with the ideal of service. It was rightly held by the Gamer that "No society can reach heights of greatness unless in all fields critical to its growth and creativity there is an ample supply of dedicated men and women." The ideals of ethics enshrined in the valuable scriptures of all religions must be imbibed by MPWs to make Healthcare a success. Swami Vivekananda has put beautifully the ideals of service which must be practised by MPWs with interest and dedication:

> "It is a great privilege
> for all of us to be allowed
> to do anything for the world
> in helping the world.
> We really help ourselves."

In brief, we can suggest the following very important remedies:

(1) Prompt and adequate drug supply.

(2) Provision of a first-aid kit.
(3) Regular provision of necessary registers.
(4) Provision of transport facility, at least during emergencies and immunization camps.
(5) More effective training programmes.
(6) Job Satisfaction.
(7) Recognition of good work.
(8) Promotional opportunities.

We may conclude by saying that the Health Department should give top priority to remove bottlenecks at the sub-centre level and infuse ethical and moral values among MPWs to make a success of the dream of Health for All.[33]

Notes and References

1. WHO: SEARO, Health Situation in South-East Asia Region, 1994-97, New Delhi, 1997, pp. 184-85.
2. Annual Report, 1996-97, Ministry of Health and Family Welfare, Govt. of India, p. 33.
3. *Ibid.*, p. 34.
4. Jawahar Lal Nehru and Public Administration, *IJPA*, New Delhi, 1975, p. 88.
5. Presidential Address by Mrs. Indira Gandhi delivered on October 22, 1971, at the Annual Meeting of *IJPA*, New Delhi.
6. S.L. Goel, Personnel Administration and Management, New Delhi, Sterling, 1996, p. 6.
7. Ordway Tead: The Art of Administration, New York, McGraw Hill, 1951, p. 145.
8. Dale Yoder, Personnel Management and Industrial Relations, New Delhi, Prentice Hall of India, 1972, p. 6.
9. P. Pigor and C.A. Myers: Personnel Administration, Tokyo, McGraw, Kogakusha, 1961, p. 11.
10. Robert N. Ford, Motivation Through the Work Itself, American Management Association, New York, 1969, p. 199.
11. George Strauss and Leonard R. Sayles, Personnel: The Human Problems of Management, Prentice Hall of India, New Delhi, 1971, p. 26.
12. R. Hoppock, Job Satisfaction, Harper and Row, New York, 1935, p. 252.
13. H.A. Robinson and R. Hoppok, Job Satisfaction Resume of 1951, *Occupation*, 10(2), 1952, p. 594.
14. Quoted in S.L. Goel, Personnel Administration and Management, New Delhi, Sterling, 1996, p. 364.
15. Quoted in S.L. Geol, Personnel Administration and Management, New Delhi, Sterling, 1966, p. 304.
16. A. Kornhouser, Psychological Studies of Employee Attitudes, *J. Consult Psychol*, 8, 1944, p. 132.
17. J.A.C. Brown, Social Psychology of Industry, Pelican, London, 1969, p. 193.
18. *The Economic Times*, New Delhi, 16 August, 1999, p. 7.
19. Haire Mason *et al.*, Psychological Research on Pay: An Overview, *Industrial Relations*, 3(1), 1963, p. 3.
20. ILO: International Labour Conference, 33rd Session, Provisional Records, p. 34.
21. Micheal R. Cooper and T. Micheal Wood, Member Participation and Commitment in Group Decision-making on Influence Satisfaction and Decision Riskness", *Journal of Applied Psychology*, Vol. 59, No. 2, April, 1974.
22 Ted R. Brannen, The Organisation as a Social System, a paper presented at the

Midwest Regional Members' Conference of the College on Oct. 23, 1958, on Kansas city, Missourie.

23. S.L. Goel, Personnel Admn. and Management, New Delhi, Sterling, 1997, p. 323.
24. Brook Adams, The Theory of Social Revolution, New York, 1913.
25. Ministry of Health and Family Welfare, Govt. of India (No date), Manual on Target Free Approach in Family Welfare Planning, New Delhi.
26. B.M. Ramesh, S.B. Ganiger and D.G. Satishal, "Family Welfare Programme Under Target Free Approach. A Rapid Survey in Belgaum District, Karnataka, 1998, Population Research Centre, J.S.S. Institute of Economic Research, Dharwad, pp. 56-58.
27. P.N. Marl Bhal, Target Free Approach to Family Planning Programme: A Rapid Survey in Dharwad District in Karnataka, 1997, Population Research Centre, SSS Institute of Economic Research, Dharwad, pp. iii.
28. Hames L. Marshal, Development Teaching, New York, 1949, pp. 190-306.
29. Haimann, Professional Management, Eruasia, New Delhi, 1966, p. 440.
30. Keith Davis, Human Relations at Work, McGraw Hill, New Delhi, 1967, pp. 96-97.
31. P.H. Rayppa and N. Bhaskara Rao: Multi-purpose Health Workers' Scheme in Karnataka: A Study of Malur and Dibbur Primary Health Centres in Kolar District, Bangalore, ISEC, 1982, Mimeo.
32. S.L. Goel, Personnel Administration and Management, *op. cit.*, p. 324.
33. John W. Gardner, Excellence, New York, 1961, Harper and Brothers, p. 154.

CHAPTER 13

HEALTH EDUCATION AT VILLAGE LEVEL THROUGH COMMUNITY HEALTH WORKERS AND TRAINED BIRTH ATTENDANTS

"A dynamic process of change and innovation is required to be brought about in the entire approach to health manpower development, ensuring the emergence of fully integrated bands of workers functioning within the 'Health Team' approach."

—*Health Policy, 1983*

Health Education at Village Level through Community Health Workers and Trained Birth Attendants

It has been realised that health status of the rural population can be improved not merely by increasing the number of doctors or increasing the availability of medicines, but by making each individual realise and appreciate the need of simple steps in sanitation, preventive, promotive and rehabilitative health activities. The Government's new health policy aims at providing adequate medical care, where such care is needed and to educate the people in the matter of preventive and promotive health.

PART A: VILLAGE HEALTH GUIDE SCHEME (See Chart 13.3)

A. GENESIS AND GROWTH

In pursuance of the decision of the government of India to devote special attention to the health needs of the rural population and to ensure people's participation in their own health activities, a number of measures have been taken, the most important of which is the launching of a new scheme, namely, the Health Guides Scheme, in October 1997. Under this scheme, every village or community with a population of 1000 selects one person from among its residents, who is willing to serve the community and enjoys its confidence.

The following criteria is to be observed while selecting community health workers: (a) CHW may be of either sex; (b) The person selected must be a permanent resident of that village itself and may be from any vocation; (c) He may even be a practitioner of one of the systems of medicine, residing in his village; (d) He/She should be able to read and write. However, since

CHART 13.1

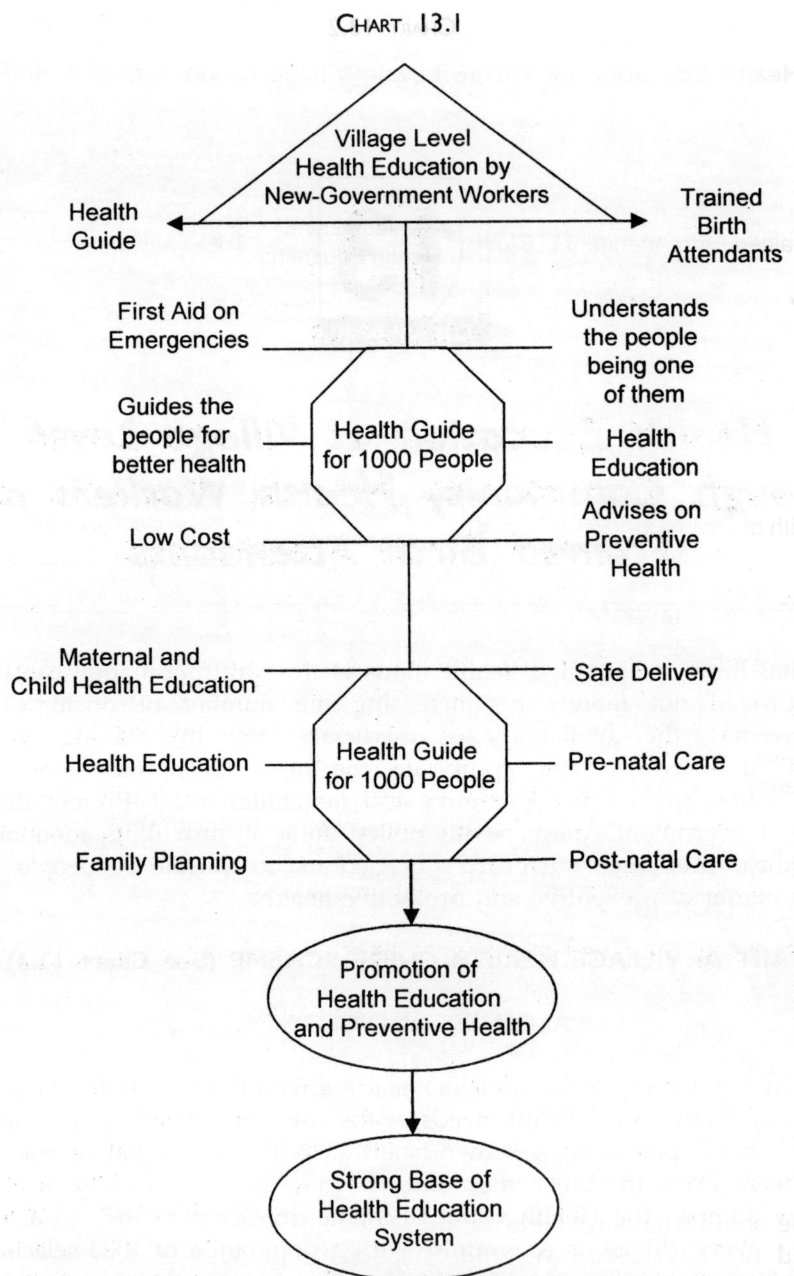

with higher level of education, better quality of service would be available the person to be selected should have had formal education up to the sixth standard; (e) He should be social service minded and be able to spare 2-3 hours every day for community health activities; (f) He should be physically active and willing to serve at least for 3 years as community health worker;

CHART 13.2

Health Education at Village Level—Village Health Guide Scheme

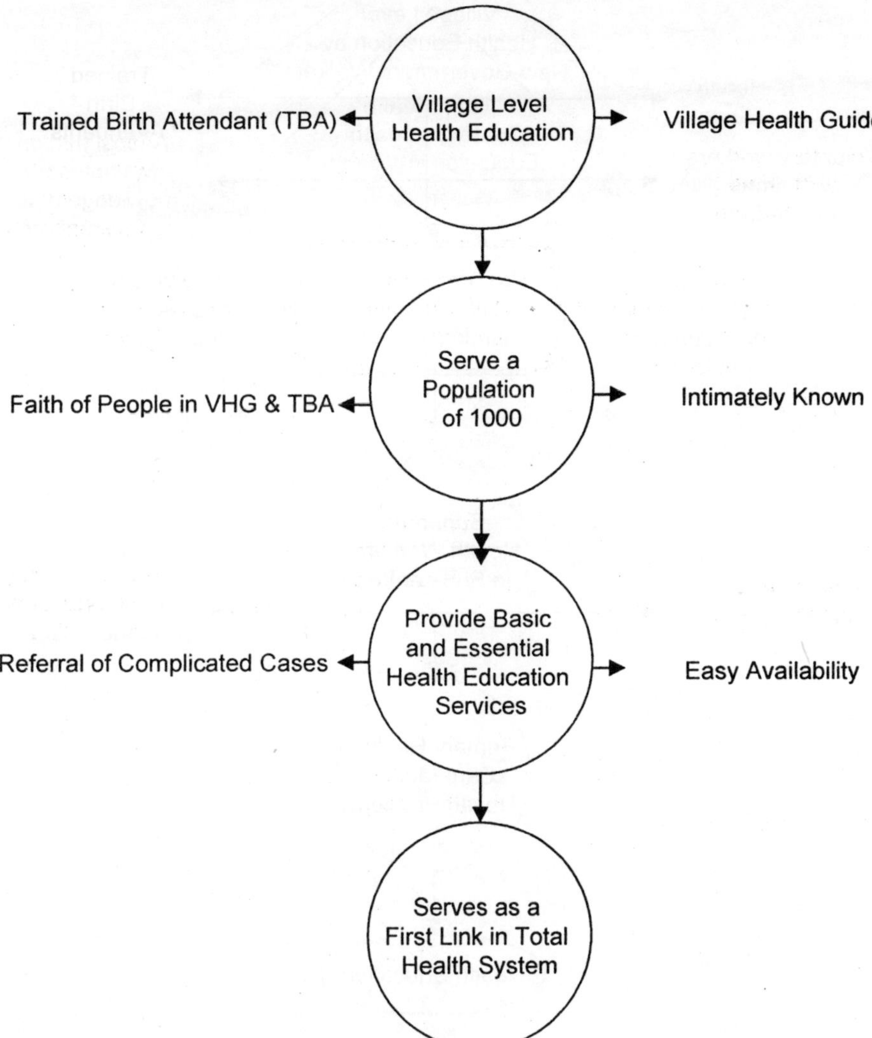

(g) He should be acceptable to all sections of the community; and (h) He should not belong to any group, faction or political organization of the village which may limit his acceptability.

With these guidelines, the village community is requested to recommend 2-3 persons considered suitable by them to be Health Guides. The final selection may be made by the medical officers of the Primary Health Centre jointly after consulting the Block Development Officer and the field staff of various government organisations. The Health Guide is given training in simple and basic health services for three months at the Primary

CHART 13.3

Services a Population of 1000

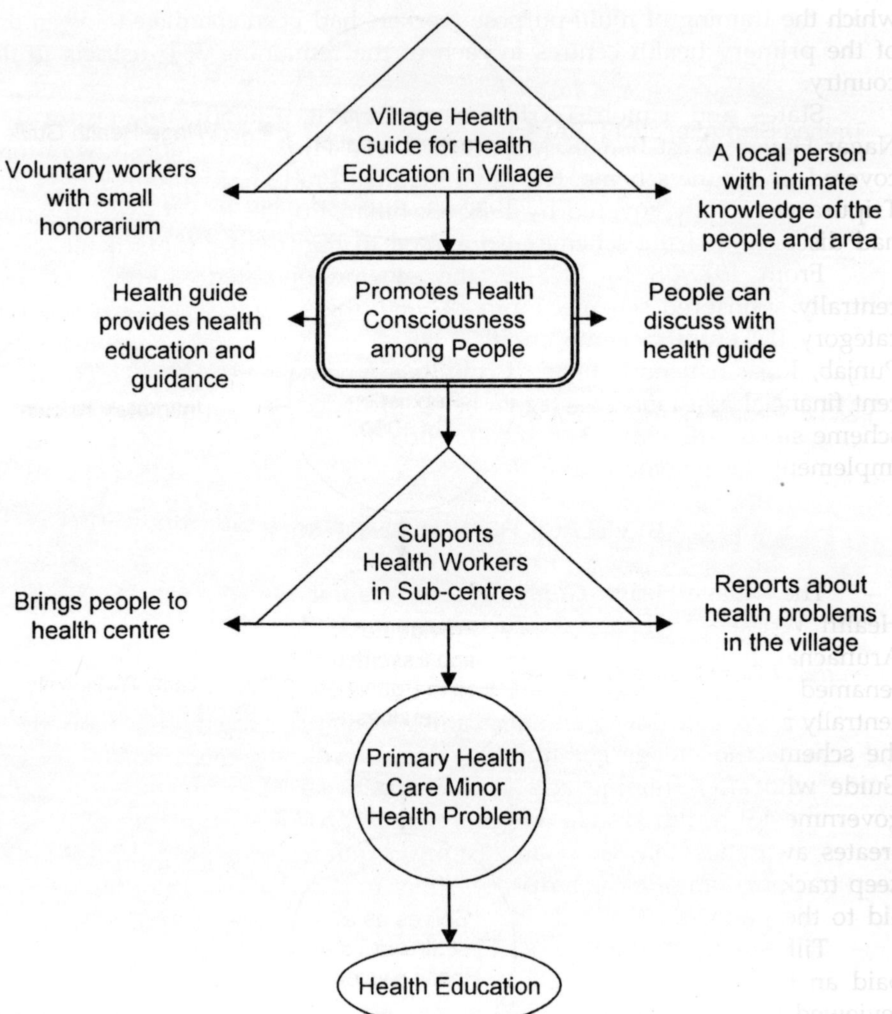

Health Centre to which he belongs. During training, the Health Guide is taught the fundamentals of health and hygiene, treatment of common ailments, maternity and child healthcare, first-aid, etc. After training, the Health Guide goes back to the village to serve the community. He is provided with a kit containing medicines and also a manual. The kit consists of common remedies belonging to the modern system of medicine, besides remedies under the traditional system in vogue in that part of the country. The worker is expected to work in his spare time for two to three hours daily. During the period of training he is paid a stipend of Rs. 200 per month for three months. After training he is given an honorarium of Rs.

50 per month for working with the community and also Rs. 50 worth of medicines per month.

In the first phase, the scheme was introduced in the 28 districts in which the training of multi-purpose workers had been completed and in one of the primary health centres in each of the remaining 364 districts in the country.

States and Union Territories of Gujarat, Chandigarh, Dadra and Nagar Haveli, West Bengal, Maharashtra and Himachal Pradesh were fully covered under the scheme. Haryana, Madhya Pradesh, Manipur, Orissa and Tripura were fully covered by 1982-83. Bihar, Punjab and Rajasthan which had discontinued the scheme also agreed to reintroduce the scheme. .

From 1977-78 to 1978-79, the scheme operated as 100 per cent centrally sponsored scheme. From 1979-80, the scheme was converted into category II Central Scheme on 50:50 basis, as a result of which States like Punjab, Rajasthan and Bihar discontinued the scheme. However, 100 per cent financial assistance was again being provided for implementation of the scheme since 1-12-1981. As a result, Punjab, Rajasthan and Bihar agreed to implement the scheme again.

B. VILLAGE HEALTH GUIDE SCHEME

The Village Health Guide Scheme was initially started as Community Health Workers' Scheme on 2nd October, 1977 in all the States except Arunachal Pradesh, J & K, Kerala and Tamil Nadu. The Scheme was renamed as Village Health Guides' Scheme in 1981 when it was made 100% centrally sponsored scheme under Family Welfare Programme. According to the scheme the village community selects a volunteer as a village Health Guide who after training acts as a link between the community and the governmental health system. He/She mainly provides health education and creates awareness on MCH and Family Welfare Services. He/She has to keep track of communicable diseases, treat minor ailments and provide first-aid to the patients.

Till March 1999 about 3.23 lakh VHGs were working. Each VHG is paid an honorarium of Rs. 50 per month. The Scheme has recently been reviewed by a committee of experts which has looked into various aspects of the scheme such as the usefulness of the scheme, the work done by VHGs, capability of VHGs in the context of institutional arrangements available in the country, enhancement of honorarium and other facilities available to VHGs, etc. The committee obtained feedback from the states and visited some of the states to get first-hand information and it has submitted its final report/recommendations and the same is being examined in the Ministry.

Jagdambi Prasad Yadav, in his presidential address delivered at the Twentieth Convocation of IIPA (Bombay, 15 July, 1978) defined the philosophy of the VHG as "The philosophy of the community health workers' scheme is to place people's health in people's hand. It is well-known that in most parts of rural India even rudimentary public health facilities are lacking from times immemorial. The CHW's scheme is designed to take healthcare to doorsteps of people. It is hoped that the community health workers will bridge the gap between rural community and healthcare—preventive, promotive and curative."

Speaking on the new health policy, Shri Morarji Desai, former Primer Minister of India, said, "Whatever development we want to do in the country depends upon the capacity of the people to do their work efficiently and to go on increasing their productive capacity in any field of work, that they can take up. And if this is to be done, health becomes a very primary condition. Unless a person enjoys fairly good health, it will not be possible for him to do work efficiently. It is, therefore, necessary for us to see that the people of the country are enabled to maintain their health in a fairly good manner, so that they are able to follow their work and profession efficiently and live also a healthy life."

C. ACTIVITIES OF HEALTH GUIDE

Let us now mention in detail the activities of Health Guide so that we can appreciate the assessment of the scheme.

The Health Guide receives technical guidance from the Health Worker (Male/Female). After training, the Health Guide is supposed to carry out the following health activities. (based on Module prepared by NIHFW)

1. Malaria

Identify fever cases, make thick and thin blood films of all fever cases. Send the slides for laboratory examination. Administer presumptive treatment to fever cases. Keep a record of the persons given presumptive treatment. Inform the Health Worker (Male) of the names and addresses of cases from whom blood slides have been taken. Assist the Health Worker (Male) and the spraying teams in spraying and larvicidal operations. Educate the community on how to prevent malaria.

2. Communicable Diseases

Inform the Health Worker (Male) immediately if an epidemic occurs in his/her area; take immediate precautions to limit the spread of disease and educate the community about the prevention and control of communicable diseases.

3. Environmental Sanitation and Personal Hygiene

(a) Chlorinate Drinking Water Sources at Regular Intervals

Keep a record of the number of wells chlorinated. Assist the Health Worker (Male) in arranging for the construction of the following:

Soakage pits, Kitchen gardens, Compost pits, Sanitary latrines, Smokeless chulhas.

(b) Educate the Community about the Following

Safe drinking water, Hygienic methods of disposal of liquid waste, Hygienic methods of disposal of solid waste, Home sanitation, Kitchen gardens, Advantages and use of sanitary latrines, Advantages of smokeless chulhas, Food hygiene, Control of insects, rodents and stray dogs.

(c) Educate the Community about the Importance of Personal Hygiene

4. Immunization

Assist the Health Worker (Male/Female) in arranging for immunization, Educate the community about immunization against diphtheria, whooping cough, tetanus, smallpox, tuberculosis, poliomyelitis, cholera and typhoid.

5. Family Planning

Spread the message of family planning to the couples in his/her area and educate them about the desirability of the small family norm. Educate the people about the methods of family planning which are available. Act as a depot holder, distribute nirodh to the couples, and maintain the necessary records of nirodh distributed. Inform the Health Worker (Male/Female) of those couples who are willing to accept a family planning method so that he/she can make the necessary arrangements. Educate the community about the availability of services for Medical Termination of Pregnancy (MTP).

6. Maternal and Child Care

Advise pregnant women to consult the Health Worker (Female) or the trained dai for pre-natal, natal and post-natal care. Advise pregnant women to get immunized against tetanus. Educate the community about the availability of maternal and child care services and encourage them to utilize the facilities. Educate the community about how to keep mothers and children healthy.

7. Nutrition

Identify cases with signs and symptoms of malnutrition among pre-school children (one to five years) and refer them to the Health Worker (Male/Female). Identify cases with signs and symptoms of anaemia in pregnant and nursing women and children and refer them to the Health Worker (Male/Female) for treatment. Assist the Health Worker (Male/Female) in administering Vitamin A solution as prescribed to children from one to five years of age. Teach families about the importance of breast-feeding and the introduction of supplementary weaning foods. Educate the community about nutritious diets for mothers and children.

8. Vital Events

Report all births and deaths in his/her area to the Health Worker

(Male). Educate the community about the importance of registering all births and deaths.

9. First-Aid in Emergencies

Give first-aid in the following emergency conditions, refer these cases to the Primary Health Centre as necessary and inform the Health Worker (Male/Female). Drowning, Electric shock, Heat stroke, Snake bite, Scorpion sting, Insect stings, Dog bite, Accidents, carrying out procedures in dealing with accidents, keep a record of first-aid given to each patient.

10. Treatment of Minor Ailments

Give simple treatment for the following signs and symptoms and refer cases beyond his/her competence to the Sub-centre or Primary Health Centre.

Fever, Headache, Backache and pain in the joints, Cough and cold, Diarrhoea, Vomiting, Pain in the abdomen, Constipation, Toothache, Earache, Sore eyes, Boils, abscesses and ulcers, Scabies and ringworm. Keep a record of the treatment given to each patient.

11. Mental Health

Recognize signs and symptoms of mental illness and refer these cases to the Health Worker (Male/Female). Give immediate assistance in emergencies associated with mental illness. Educate the community about mental illness.

D. EXPERIMENTS ON PHC IN DIFFERENT PARTS OF THE WORLD

In this section we would review (on the basis of case studies conducted by the health experts in different parts of the world) the progress of the implementation of primary healthcare in different parts of the world. After this we shall discuss the progress of primary healthcare in India.

Experiment of the Soviet Union (Kazakhstan)[1] (Before Split of USSR)

Before the Russian Revolution of 1917, Soviet Kazakhstan was one of the most backward and neglected provinces of Tsarist Russia. Not more than two per cent of the total population could read and write. In the field of health, there was not a single medical institution and the number of medical personnel was negligible.

Today, this region enjoys all the health facilities. Five medical schools and 26 junior medical colleges have helped to train some 40,000 doctors and more than 130,000 intermediate level medical workers. The bed population ratio is 12:4.

After the revolution, primary healthcare formed the basis of the health system. It provided service through out-patient clinics and posts staffed by mid-wives and fieldscher (medical auxiliaries). Each post is staffed by a nurse as well as a fieldscher and a mid-wife and covers about five hundred people. Those posts list the support of the population to carry out health activities. These also train "assistants", voluntary health workers from the Red Cross Society. The posts are also helped in their work by members of the rural workers' councils, by school teachers, by students, by rural youth groups, and by the managements of collective and state farms. The function of each post is to organise and carry out primary preventive health measures, i.e., immunisation, home visiting of patients and new "born babies, sanitary inspection of land and installations, primary epidemic, central measures, health education, etc. In addition, the post-carries out primary curative measures including treating patients, carrying out instruction of the rural or district physician, or referring patients to the physician for medical advice and treatment. There is a medical store attached to every post.

Primary Healthcare in Kazakhstan as in all the Republics of the Soviet Union is closely integrated with socio-economic plans of the rural districts and also with the overall medical care system.

Soviet Kazakhstan has 60 years' experience in the organisation and successful development of a national public health system and of primary healthcare. The conditions under which the people of the Republic were able, virtually from scratch, to build up a public health service closely resemble conditions in developing countries that are still experiencing the aftermath of colonial oppression. The study of Kazakhstan's public health experience should therefore prove useful for all public health administrators particularly for representatives of the developing countries.

Experiments of Columbia[2]

The problem of health in Columbia is typical of the situation in most developing countries. In fact, mortality rate is very high, 45 per cent of the rural population have no access to safe drinking water. The former health system has not been meeting existing demands of the population. Thirty-six per cent of the population in rural and urban slums never or rarely use doctors or hospitals. They are organising a new mode, called M.A.C. system (Modulo de Amplication de Cobertura). Dr. Norberto Martinez explained the thinking behind it: "We were aiming at people who had been inaccessible, culturally, economically and geographically to formal health provision. There were rural people and rural migrates living in belts of misery around the cities, not participating in modern economic and social life. These people were not using the health services, so we needed to build a bridge between them and the services by using auxiliaries drawn from their own communities. High technology was not appropriate because it cost much and our resources were limited. Moreover, most people were dying of a few basic diseases that could be cured or prevented by using a fairly simple technology without the need for highly qualified personnel."

The key to the new system is Columbia's own brand of the barefoot doctor selected from the area to be served. These workers are trained for four months and receive an allowance of US $ 50 a month. They serve 3,000 people in the fringe urban areas or 1,000 in the more scattered rural areas. Each group of 6 workers is backed by a MAC health centre to which they can refer difficult cases.

"It is perhaps too soon to judge just how effective the MAC system will be. But even in its two years, it seems to have reached out to a section of the population previously untouched by the health services. It has made a start on the crucial vaccinations and environmental health campaigns that will prevent so much disease. Above all, it has begun to get people out of their traditional fatalistic attitudes to diseases which lead them to suffer patiently, believing that basically nothing could or should be done about it unless they were at death's door. The marginal millions of Columbians are becoming actively interested in doing something individually and collectively to improve their own health."

Experiments in Thailand[3]

More than half of Thailand's approximately 7500 graduate physicians live and practice in Bangkok. The doctor-population ratio was 1 : 22,070 for the provinces and 1 : 84,000 for the countryside. The people in the countryside did not have any access to medical care. WHO (UNICEF assisted) provincial healthcare project was formulated whereby it is planned to train 22,400 village health volunteers, about 200,000 village health communicators, 2800 tambon doctors and 8400 granny mid-wives during the next five years.

"Although Thailand still has a long way to go before healthcare reaches all its citizens, the adoption of Primary Healthcare programmes will do much to alleviate the feeling of hopelessness that many villagers had thought was their inevitable fate."

Experiments of Costa Rica and Mexico[4]

There were no organized health services available in these two countries. The shortage of health workers hampered the development of health services. In 1972, WHO and other agencies began collaborating in a local development effort (PRODESCH) to identify and stimulate the type of activities that could be meaningfully undertaken by the community itself. The progress is going on. They are both examples of how communities with outside support can resolve their own problems and thus can generate enough confidence in themselves to go ahead with other socio-economic efforts.

Most of the countries in Asia, Africa and Latin America have either introduced or are planning to introduce Primary Healthcare system to provide healthcare to the unprivileged section of their countries. This is a challenging task which requires constant, continuous and persistent efforts of their governments and especially the health departments. All these countries may learn from each other's experiences and improve the mechanism of primary healthcare programmes. If such programmes are successful, it is sure that the healthcare would soon be available to all the people in the world.

E. CRITICAL APPRAISAL OF THE HEALTH GUIDE SCHEME IN INDIA

Health Guide Scheme in India has not made much impact so far. It was initiated to provide healthcare for the people and by the people. A seed can flourish and develop into a full-fledged plant only in a congenial soil and environment. Similarly, Health Guide Scheme can be successful if a sound organisational set-up is provided for its growth. Let us analyse the reasons which are responsible for its failure in the areas where the scheme was introduced. If we want to put the scheme on a sound footing, we may keep the following facts and suggestions in mind.

Lack of Commitment on the Part of Health Experts and their Associations

There persists widespread negative and unhelpful attitude among health personnel towards the healthcare of the poorest strata in the rural and urban population. They are not aware of the social responsibility to the society. If the doctors at the primary level are not mentally convinced of the scheme, changes at the grass-roots are unimaginable and impracticable. Most of the doctors and health experts contacted by the writer pointed out that, "Such schemes are unworkable as the community health workers cannot learn much during such a brief training. Instead of being an asset to the healthcare system, they may reverse the trends and these may create more problems than solutions." Others remarked: "They are already too busy with their routine functions. They are already overworked. They do not find any time to have intimate contacts with the community." A few remarked that "the present healthcare system cannot meet the needs of the society. The new system may be given a trial but the care may be taken to plan the scheme effectively before its introduction." The Medical Association has been vocal enough and described this scheme as a "cruel joke." The major hurdle is the opposition to change. Established health associations, institutions and organisations find it difficult to come out from their ivory towers and adjust to change and accept new challenges and responsibilities. Their resistance may be an attempt to defend their false prestige or traditions. Thus, there is a need to convince and train the health experts and their organisations before launching such schemes. We may cultivate a change in their attitudes in the interest of the programme.

At the recent Golden Jubilee celebrations of the Indian Medical Association, its President, Dr. J.Y.R. Sarma, said that the IMA had not been consulted by Planning Commission in the matter of evolving an effective pattern of rural healthcare and a national policy on health. He complained that various Governments had instead devised schemes arbitrarily to "suit the fancies and philosophies of changing personalities." If the entire medical manpower could be involved through their professional organisations he was confident that it would be possible to achieve the objective of the scheme. There is an element of truth in this criticism.[5] The government should not only consult experts before formulating any scheme but should also be able to energize, enthuse and develop a rapport with the professional organisations and, through them, their individual members to take an active part in the community health programmes.

Opposition from the Personnel of Traditional System of Medicine and Local Allopathic Practitioners

The scheme is being opposed by the established personnel of traditional system of medicine and local allopathic practitioners. They view this scheme as an encroachment on their authority and prestige. Most of the community health workers interviewed by the writer remarked, "practitioners of all the systems of medicine are making a lot of money by exploiting the illiterate poor in the villages. They think that if the scheme becomes successful, their future existence is uncertain. Besides, they have a strong hold on their clients and through them they spread propaganda against the utility of this scheme." One of the workers went on to the extent, "These practitioners would warn community that those people who would consult the community health workers would be in trouble as they knew nothing." Thus, there is need to educate these practitioners properly and associate them in the planning and implementation of the scheme.

Insufficient Training to Community Health Workers

The training imparted to the community health worker is quite inadequate. He has a very weak educational base. Dr. C. Parkash, Senior Medical Superintendent, Medical College, Rohtak, remarked about this scheme to the *Tribune.* "The scheme is conceptually sound. . . . Since the success of the scheme will largely depend on the quality of personnel chosen for the job. . . . A bare three months' training to a person who had schooling up to sixth standard is not likely to adequately equip him for the job."[6] The same opinion was expressed by Prof. S.P. Gupta, Professor of Medicine in Medical College, Rohtak.[7] The Indian Medical Association suggested that the qualification for a CHW should be matriculation and that he must undergo at least 15 months' training to acquire the fundamental knowledge needed for his work. He is to be trained in medicine, art of communication, leadership, etc. The people pointed out that the community health workers do not have much education and training to discharge the responsibilities entrusted to them. The success of the scheme would depend upon the confidence of the community in these workers. There is need for screening these workers so that we retain only those workers who can really be effective. Besides, it has also become apparent that the process of retraining is essential in order to fill the gaps in the initial training or to refresh the health and medical knowledge imparted on a poor educational base.

Absence of Positive Rural Bias in Medical Education

There is national commitment to reorient medical education profession and health services, so as to serve the needs of rural people. All the expert bodies have agreed to modify the syllabus of undergraduate medical education as to produce a basic doctor who would have the ability to cater to the needs of the rural area. It is necessary to make the medical colleges act not as ivory temples in majestic isolation but take on the responsibility for providing total healthcare for specified segments of the rural population.[8] The aim of medical education should be to promote happiness through better health of most of the deprived hundreds of millions of human beings. With the contemplated changes in the contents of the undergraduate course, the students would be in a position to appreciate the problems of rural people and would develop proper motivation to help them.

Lack of Proper Health Education of the Village Community

Rural people lack functional literacy which is *sine qua non* for any endeavour towards community development. This requires a great effort on the part of the State Governments; voluntary institutions and the health administrators should properly educate and enlighten the people. Properly planned programmes of health education would go a long way in propagating the ideals of a primary healthcare. It was observed by the writer that no regular efforts are being made to educate the public either by the health department or by the CHW. CHW devotes most of his time in providing curative care rather than laying much emphasis on educational approach. We must provide elementary and simple health education to the community. It should be based on indigenous technology. According to Dr. Mahler, the required new type of health education should be, "neither over-sophisticated for condescending but that gains the confidence of the individuals and communities by explaining health technology in a language they can understand so that they can participate genuinely in taking decisions concerning their health. In short, a replacement of passive health education by active health learning." Besides, the beneficiaries should be asked to contribute to the cost of Primary Healthcare. Everyone should realise his responsibility towards the health coverage of the community. When the rural people would be contributing, they would like to participate and take interest in its functioning. Some nominal contributions may be taken from the people themselves depending upon their income.

Absence of any Mechanism to Involve the Community

Community participation is the way to development but how to go about it ? In the field of primary healthcare, it was pointed out by the workers that, "It is impossible to educate all the people by them. They have to carry out their own work, and this is only their part time duty. At present, there is no system to involve the community." It is suggested that we may involve teachers, Panchayat members and other influential men and women to diffuse the health education in the community. The constitution of Youth Clubs, Mother's Clubs, etc., as has been done in Democratic Republic of Korea, may promote functional literacy and health education among the community.

Exploitation by Community Health Workers

Community health worker is the pivot of the whole scheme. The success or failure of the scheme would depend to a great extent upon the attitudes, perception and ethos of the workers. It has been mentioned that "These workers are not being selected properly. The selection of a Community Health Worker has become a political patronage." Such a scheme would have no chance to grow and ultimately survive if we do not find workers who are committed to bring about a social change in the villages. They must have missionary zeal. Their enthusiasm should not be dampened by unfavourable local conditions. They must have zeal and perseverance to reorient the attitudes of the people, otherwise the whole scheme would be a failure. Some people went to remark, "These community health workers have become the agents of the political parties. They are making a lot of money. They want to pose as doctors. They are not easily accessible. They are exploiting the poor people." A section of medical practitioners apprehends that, "half-backed and semi-literate persons masquerading as barefoot doctors will play havoc with the health of the masses." What is the difference then between the private practitioners and CHW workers. It is high time that we select, train and develop our community health workers properly. We must get a system by which we must be able to assess the work of these workers. The *Tribune* editorial dated 17 July, 1975 had rightly commented that, "If picking good men is the most important of them all, dumping the bad one is the next most important." We know that even poorly devised machinery may be made to work if manned with well trained, intelligent, imaginative and devoted staff. On the other hand, the best planned organisation may produce unsatisfactory results if it is operated by medicore or disgruntled people. So, we must find out workers who are committed, willing to accept hardships and prepared to work in a spirit of dedication.

Absence of Political Support/Interest in the Problems of Rural Areas

The political elite in the country are not sensitive and responsive to their duties. They are busy with manipulation of politics and find hardly anytime to look into the problems of the people. Because of instability in politics, there is no continuous, concerted and consistent effort to weed out the obstacles in the path of development. What is required is a strong political will and determination to make these schemes successful. Political elite at all levels must support the cause of the rural poor and help them to enjoy the good standards of life which were promised to them at the inception of independence. Political powers and wisdoms are constantly required in a democratic set-up to resolve any problem arising out of the policies and implementation of the scheme. The political elite may have to take bold and unpleasant steps to re-allocate the resources between urban and rural sectors.

Improper Administrative Set-up to Implement the Politics of Community Health

A revolutionary scheme of this type can be successful only if there is proper administrative set-up to implement it. Most of the health experts are of the view that the scheme has been rushed through without examining its requirements. It is suggested that some experts in Public Administration may examine the organisation and procedures which are being used to implement the scheme. They may also examine the problems of coordination, control, supervision and headquarter-field relationships. In the light of the suggestions, the existing scheme may be modified to suit the requirements and the scheme in new areas may be set-up according to new recommendations. One of the very important problems is the poor quality of supervision of the scheme. Multi-purpose health workers who are supposed to be their immediate supervisors lack proper orientation and training themselves. It is suggested that the multi-purpose workers may be given refresher courses to discharge their duties efficiently.

Absence of Proper Evaluation

Evaluation is one of the most important components of any scheme. The good evaluation is to measure the impact of this scheme on health, the process of operations and scheme replicability. When the writer contacted the health experts, they pointed many difficulties. Most of them observed, "No evaluation machinery has been designed. No methodology has been designed to measure the output. There is no simple information system by which the assessment of the scheme implemented so far can be made." This situation leads to failure in taking timely decisions and lack of feedback. Without an appropriate feedback, the health workers of the PHC level feel frustrated and their function as agents for information becomes meaningless to them. This lack of feedback is probably one of the most important problems in the development of primary healthcare which needs solution. It is suggested that a simple information system may be designed to suit the conditions prevailing in a particular area.

Insufficient Supply of Drugs

The drugs are very costly. Most of the workers mentioned that "The amount of Rs. 600 per year for drugs is too small to meet the demands of the people." It is suggested that:

(a) The Government must strengthen the drug industries in the public sector and manufacture essential drugs at cheaper prices.
(b) The indigenous medicine may be standardized and used to provide cheaper services.
(c) Beneficiaries may be asked to contribute two to five rupees per head per year to make the scheme viable and effective. This would also encourage more participation.

(d) Researches to exploit local flora and fauna as medicine may be encouraged.
(e) More treatment may be suggested through the control of diet and naturopathy which would lead to better health.
(f) The supply of drugs may be made in time to keep the morale of the workers high and win confidence of the people.

F. CONCLUSION

The experiment of Community Health Workers Scheme in India has not gone on long enough to reveal all the problems inherent in it. Besides, it has not acquired the sophistication and expertise that one associates with already existing health programmes. There has been great opposition from many quarters. They consider this system as inferior and primitive. But their opposition is based on superficial thinking. There is no substitute for a poor country like India where the people cannot afford the costly medical care system. It may be noted here that even highly industrialized societies are depending upon such schemes to provide effective healthcare to the community. There is no denying the fact that this is theoretically sound and can help the unprivileged people and deprived communities to take care of their health problems which otherwise would remain unattended to because of financial and professional constraints. The scheme is a vital link in the country's health schemes. The weakness of the scheme is because of the poor design of the implementation machinery which may be streamlined to provide the health facilities for all.

Let us redesign this scheme in new millennium after the receipt of the assessment report by Government of India and derive benefits out of this low cost scheme. There is no need of abandoning this scheme. We should rather optimise the use of village health guides after giving them fresh training.

PART B: TRAINED BIRTH ATTENDANTS (See Chart 13.4)

A. IMPORTANCE OF REPRODUCTIVE AND CHILD HEALTH

Care of mothers and children—the most vulnerable sections of our society—occupies a paramount place in our health services delivery system. This is reflected from the fact that 9 out of the 17 goals listed in the National Health Policy (1983) related to Maternal and Child Health. Trained Birth Attendants can play a vital role in the promotion of health of mothers and children.

Dai Training Programme

Maternal and Pre-natal mortality rates in the country are high due to lack of even the basic maternal and newborn care, to more than half the women at the time of labour. The SRS data for 1993 indicates that proportion of deliveries attended by untrained hands is still very high in the country.

Currently, about one out of two women do not have access to trained personnel and deliver under conditions of high risk both for women and the newborn. Training of dais is a part of the overall effort to improve basic maternal and newborn care to ensure clean delivery practices, and to increase early referrals of high risk/complicated cases.

The National Health Policy (1983) envisaged that 100% deliveries will be conducted by trained personnel by the year 2000 A.D. This would mean training/retraining of at least one Dai for each of six lakh villages in the country.[9]

Under the CSSM Programme, training of Dais is being undertaken in all the states. The training with emphasis on 'hands on' skill development for the Dais is imparted for 6 days in identified health facilities which have enough case loads.

During 1994-95 and 1995-96, and 1996-97, 31,260, 21,755 and 1,58,459 Dais have reportedly been trained. After completion of training each Dai is provided with a Dai kit (Centrally procured) to help her in conduct of safe and clean delivery.

Prevailing ill-health among women is a major concern. These are being addressed through several programmes, such as nutrition, RH, MCH and RCH. Accordingly, investment in women's health has been one of the actions identified in the Declaration for Health Development in the South-East Asia Region in the 21st Century. It has been recognized in the Declaration that since women's health is integral to development, a multi-sectoral approach would be needed through the development of partnerships with other relevant sectors.[10]

Too many women still die needlessly due to complications during pregnancy and child-birth and too little attention is given to other aspects of women's health. Data clearly shows the link between low maternal mortality and a high proportion of deliveries by trained personnel, well established primary healthcare infrastructure and good referral systems.

Findings from research in the early 1980s and the International Safe Motherhood Conference in 1987 drew the attention of the world community to maternal mortality. During this decade countries adopted various tools for safe motherhood, including the district team problem-solving approach, the partograph, safe delivery kits, and the Mother-Baby Package—a strategic tool for planning safe motherhood programmes.

Yet many problems remain. Most are due to socio-economic and cultural factors, and the failure of the health system to provide good quality services. The training and deployment of large numbers of auxiliary health workers and volunteers in the community contributed to significant reductions in infant mortality but did not substantially reduce maternal deaths. During the past decade, midwives who were trained to provide care to pregnant women and to assist in deliveries were used as multi-purpose health workers in some countries. The focus on their mid-widely role was thus diluted, and maternity care was neglected. Efforts should be made to ensure that all deliveries are attended by Trained Birth Attendants so that high rates of maternal mortality can be reduced.[11]

CHART 13.4

Honorary Workers (TBA)

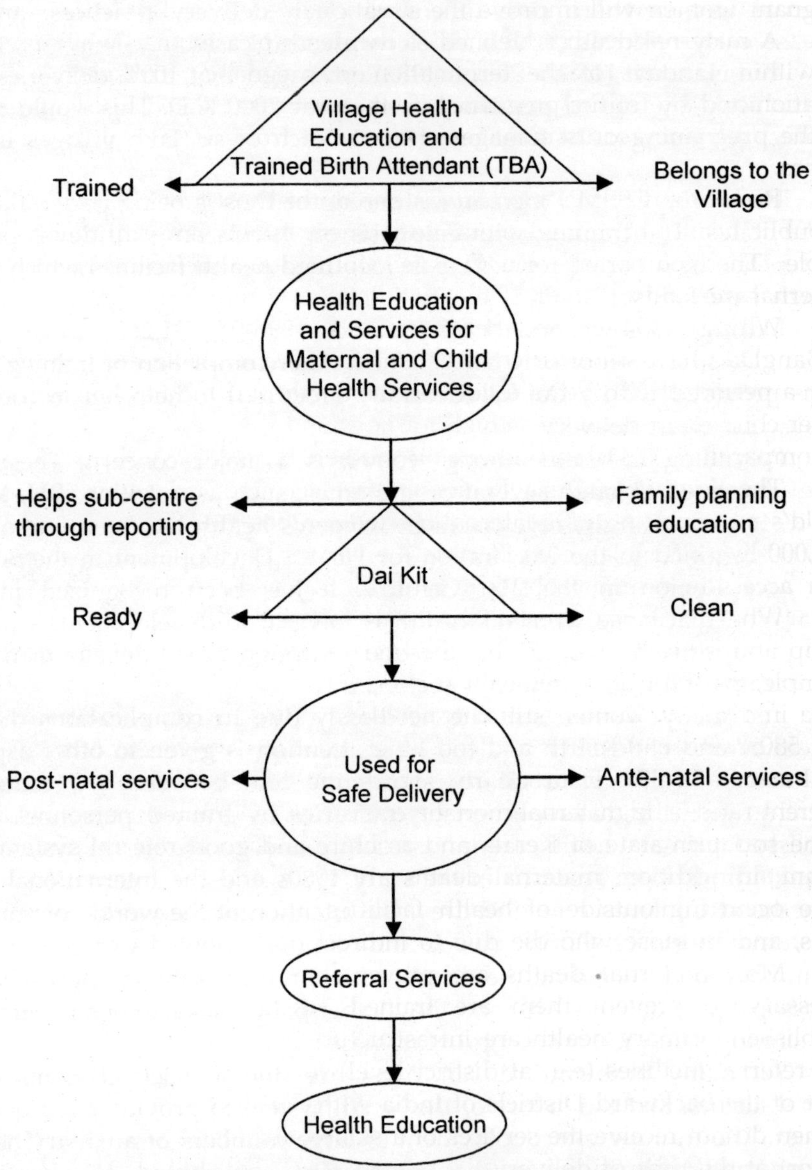

Besides social cost of maternal deaths is very high. The impact of maternal mortality on the individual, the family and society at large is like a pebble dropped into a pond, where the ripples of action and reaction reach out to all. Maternal mortality is therefore now recognized as a symptom of neglect and failure, the society's neglect of women's and girl's health, and failure of the healthcare system to meet their health needs. This situation has to change. A high level of political commitments, strengthening of the health infrastructure, and generation of societal, community and family support to pregnant women will improve the situation.[12]

A maternal death is defined as the death of a woman while pregnant or within 42 days of the termination of pregnancy, irrespective of the duration and site of the pregnancy, from any cause related to or aggravated by the pregnancy or its management but not from accidental or incidental causes.

Reducing maternal mortality is one of the most cost effective strategies in public health, bringing benefits to women, infants and communities as a whole. The goal of the WHO Safe Motherhood Initiative is to reduce maternal mortality to half of the 1990 levels by the year 2000.

When a mother dies, the effects on the family are often devastating. In Bangladesh, a study of children under 10 years of age has shown that over a period of two years following the death of a mother, mortality rates in her children were twice as high for boys and three times as high for girls, as compared to children with living mothers.[13]

The South East Asia Region in fact accounts for about 40% of the world's maternal deaths. Maternal mortality ratios range from 40 to 539 per 1,00,000 live births, largely reflecting the varying social status of women and their access to essential obstetric care.

Where maternal mortality data are not segregated by socio-economic group and other relevant factors, national statistics can be misleading. For example, there are considerable variations between urban and rural areas. In India in 1995, an indirect estimate for the national maternal mortality ratio was 580, with 638 maternal deaths per 1,00,000 live births estimated for rural areas and 389 for urban areas. Different parts of the country also had different rates—the maternal mortality ratio was reported to be as low as 247 in the southern state of Kerala and as high as 1068 in the eastern state of Assam. In addition, maternal deaths are often under reported, especially those occurring outside of health facilities, in early gestation, in remote areas, and in those who die due to indirect obstetric causes.[14]

Most maternal deaths are preventable. The medical interventions necessary to prevent them are trained assistance at delivery, a well established primary healthcare infrastructure with a good referral system, and referral facilities (e.g. at district level) for managing complications. In most of the backward Districts of India with high maternal mortality, most women do not receive the services of a skilled attendant (mid-wife, nurse or doctor) at the time of delivery.

For example, the report of a three year study covering a population of 686,000 in a rural area of India showed that "delay in seeking care and too many and inappropriate referrals through lower levels of the health system not capable of dealing with the problem significantly increased the risk of dying. Similarly, residence in the village proper (which has better transport facilities) as compared to the hamlets had a protective effect. A trained attendant at delivery, presence of an ANM (Auxiliary Nurse Midwife) in the village, an educated husband (the usual decision-maker) and the social custom of migrating to the natal home for delivery, all had a protective effect."

B. NEED AND ACTIVITIES OF TBA[15]

India can not afford highly sophisticated maternal and Child Health Services. The Birth Attendants, if adequately trained and supported can really help in mitigating high maternal and infant mortality rate.

The Dai is an important person in her village. She serves as a link between the families in her village and the ANM. These are some of the things she can do to improve maternal and child health in her village.

1. She should contact every pregnant woman in her area and see that she is registered at the sub-centre or primary health centre.
2. She should attend the weekly pre-natal clinic and assist ANM.
3. She should try to ensure that every pregnant woman in her area attends the pre-natal clinic at least three times, i.e., after the third month to confirm pregnancy during the seventh month and during the ninth month.
4. She should try to ensure that every pregnant woman is immunized against tetanus (two doses—the last dose at least one month before the delivery and the first dose one month before the last).
5. She should try to ensure that every pregnant woman takes iron and folic acid tablets as prescribed.
6. If any abnormal pregnancy is detected she should show the case immediately to the ANM or LHV or refer the case to the PHC.
7. She should ensure that preparations for delivery are made either at home or at the PHC or hospital.
8. If she finds any abnormality during labour she must seek medical aid without delay.
9. When she receives a call for delivery:
   - She should take her kit with her,
   - She should watch the progress of labour carefully,
   - She should allow labour to progress normally without any unnecessary interference, and
   - She should observe aseptic techniques while conducting the delivery.
10. She should see that her kit is always replenished, clean and ready for use during a delivery.
11. She should make the mother and baby comfortable and attend to the nutrition of both.
12. She should instruct the mother and the relatives as to when she should be called immediately, e.g., in case the mother has excessive bleeding or there is bleeding from the baby's cord.

13. In the post-natal period if she finds any complications in the mother, e.g., fever or foullochina, or in the baby, e.g., cord infection or jaundice, she should immediately inform the ANM or refer the mother or baby to the PHC.
14. She should try to ensure that all infants in her area are immunized with BCG, OPT and poliomyelitics vaccine.
15. She should motivate the eligible couples in her area to use a contraceptive method or to undergo sterilization.
16. She should distribute nirodh, foam tablets, and jelly to those couples who require these contraceptives.
17. She should report all births and deaths in her area to the health worker (male) or health worker (female)/ANM.

National Health Policy has also stressed the role of TBAs. A vicious relationship exists between high birth rates and high infant mortality, contributing to the desire for more children. The highest priority would, therefore, require to be devoted to efforts at launching special programmes for the improvement of maternal and child health, with a special focus on the less-privileged sections of society. Such programmes would require to be decentralised to the maximum possible extent, their delivery being at the primary level, nearest to the doorsteps of the beneficiaries. While efforts should continue at providing refresher training and orientation to the TBAs, schemes and programmes should be launched to ensure that progressively all deliveries are conducted by competently trained persons so that complicated cases receive timely and expert attention, within a comprehensive programme providing ante-natal, intra-natal and post-natal cares. Care of mothers and children—the most vulnerable sections of our society—occupies a paramount place in our health services delivery system.[16]

C. FACTS AND SUGGESTIONS

1. Low Status of Trained Birth Attendants

Trained Birth Attendants are doing a good work but their status is very low. They are paid very less and treated like domestic servants. It is high time that the health department should treat them well and support them in their endeavour of safe delivery.

2. Illiterate and Poor Background

At present, most of the women engaged are both illiterate and belong to poor backgrounds. The health department should encourage young educated girls to take up this profession and fix good honorarium for them for delivery of safe babies as well as involve them in other national health programmes.

3. Inadequate Training

Training arrangements are not adequate. They are not trained properly. They attend the programme simply to get an honorarium. The training may be extended to at least 6 months.

4. Trainees Lack Interest

Most of the trainees lack interest and thus do not take interest in training. It is a simple formality that the PHC staff want to complete.

5. No Support from Above

The health functionaries presently provide a casual supervision, support and guidance to the TTBAs. All levels of health system should ensure adequate supervision, support and guidance so that the TTBAs could help the Health Department in achieving the objectives of HFA by 2000 AD.

6. No Arrangements for Refresher Training

Keeping in view inadequate basic training, the importance of regular and repeated retraining cannot be overemphasized. A mechanism should be evolved, whereby, the TBAs receive at least one to two exposures per annum and the retraining should be arranged/organized as near to the residence of TBA as possible. During the retraining the TBA should be adequately compensated by way of per diem, etc.

7. No Interest shown by Voluntary Organizations

Voluntary organizations such as Mahila Mandals, Youth Clubs, FP Clubs, etc. should play enlarged role in propagating the importance of Dai training programme and utilization of the services of the TBAs. They should also cooperate in all the activities organized by the TTBAs.

8. Dai Kit not Replenished

Dai kit is not supplied in time and not replenished in time. Dai kit is very useful but this is not provided during the training causing difficulties in learning. It is not replenished in time. There is a need to develop a fool proof mechanism to ensure the availability of the kit with the Dai.

9. Old Manuals out of date

Manuals need updating. All Dais find the usefulness of the manual. However, all of them do not get it during the training period.

It must be made available to them before training so that it can serve as a reference material. The manual also needs thorough rewriting and revision to accommodate latest developments.[17]

D. CONCLUSION

Despite extensive development of health infrastructure in the rural areas, maternal health is still, by and large, being looked after by the TBAs (both trained and untrained).

We can increase their performance through a well designed training programme which can be a real weapon to improve the existing status of maternal and child health services.

Traditional mid-wives were once thought of as poor relatives in the family of health workers, but now, with training, they are slowly but surely winning favour with health administrations in developing countries, and WHO is advocating their use as one way of meeting basic health needs.

With good reason too, for traditional birth attendants—TBAs as they have come to be known—deliver from 60 to 80 per cent of all babies in the Third World. They also care for mothers before and after birth, and, if need be, help with household chores as well.

Not only are they being counted upon to perform traditional tasks, but also to take on new duties. In some countries they are charged with dispensing oral contraceptives, and with bringing mothers who wish to regulate births to clinics for counselling. In others, they promote breast-feeding.

Today TBAs are appreciated as never before, and people who formerly were sceptical of their worth now accept them as valued members of the health team, according to a report on ten-year trends carried in a recent issue of WHO's Chronicle.

The acceptance is reflected in the number of countries formally recognising the skills of traditional birth attendants through schemes of registration, certification, or licensure. It is also seen in the increase of training programmes run by health administrations for mid-wives.

To encourage training, many countries offer mid-wives incentives. Some pay stipends, and a few provide uniforms. UNICEF gives them a mid-wifery kit, which is prized most.

Above all, the most telling indication of the newly-won respect of TBAs is seen in the change of attitude towards them. In 1972, the majority of 37 administrations replying to a questionnaire thought of them as replaceable, and their services as an unavoidable interim measure.

Today that view is held by a minority, with 56 of 64 countries surveyed considering them as irreplaceable in the decades ahead. "While expanding professional training, countries are also expanding the training of traditional birth attendants," according to a report recently published that describes experiences in seven countries.

All of which makes good sense, for approximately half a million women dies every year, not of disease, but of the complications of child-bearing. And over 10 million children a year die before reaching their first birthday.

TBAs will continue to deliver most of the world's babies, whether they are trained or not. Training however is relatively inexpensive, costing, for instance, US $ 92 in Nicaragua, and $ 17 in Samoa, including the price of the mid-wifery kits.

It is thus a sound investment, for TBAs, by virtue of the service they render to communities, hold a high place in village societies, and thus can influence others. But even more important is their willingness to work with their people living in rural areas.

We can increase their performance through a well designed training programme which can be a real weapon to improve the existing status of maternal and child health services.[18]

Notes and References

1. Based on the article, "A land transformed" written by Prof. T.S. Shardmanow, Ministry of Health of the Kazakhstan Soviet Socialist Republic, and Corresponding Member of the Soviet Academy of Medical Science, in *World Health*, May 1978, pp. 4-6.
2. Based on the article, "Building a Bridge" by Paul Harrison, British Journalist and Photographer in *World Health*, May 1978, pp. 7-11.
3. Based on the article, "Medicine Man" by John Loftus, a Journalist, *World Health*, Oct. 1976, pp. 17-19.
4. Based on the article, "Generating Self-confidence" by Manual Carballo, a member of file unit of maternal and child health division of Family Health WHO Headquarters in Geneva, *World Health*, May 1978, pp. 26-29.
5. *Sunday Standard*, Oct. 1, 1978.
6. *The Tribune*, Oct. 25, 1978, Chandigarh.
7. *Ibid.*
8. India: National Plan for Healthcare Services in the Rural Areas.
9. GOI, Ministry of Health and Family Welfare, Annual Report, 1996-97, New Delhi, p. 25.
10. WHO: SEARO, Highlights of the works of WHO in the South-East Asia Region, New Delhi, 1998, p. 37.
11. WHO: SEARO, Regional Health Report, 1997, New Delhi, 1997, pp. 27-28.
12. *Ibid.*
13. *Ibid.*, p. 13.
14. National Institute of Health and Family Welfare, Management Training Modules for Dai (TBA), New Delhi, Year Not Mentioned.
15. Annual Report, 1996-97, Ministry of Health and Family Welfare, Govt. of India, New Delhi, 1997, pp. 29-30.
16. *Ibid.*, p. 30.
17. *Ibid.*, p. 8.
18. *World Health*, December 1982, p. 30.

CHAPTER 14

WORKING OF PRIMARY HEALTHCARE: PROMOTION AND EDUCATION—A CASE STUDY OF PUNJAB

> "Punjab is the richest state of India with highest malnutrition causing many health problem due to lack of health education."
>
> —*Author*

Working of Primary Healthcare: Promotion and Education— A Case Study of Punjab

We have discussed in the earlier Chapters the essentials of Primary Healthcare. We now examine its working with the help of a case study, i.e. "Working of Primary Healthcare in Punjab." Before we discuss about Primary healthcare, let us examine the demographic profile, health infrastructure and current health status in Punjab State.

DEMOGRAPHIC PROFILE

Punjab is one of the richest states of Indian Union consisting of 17 districts. It is situated in the North-Western region of the country, approximately between 29°32′ and 32°32′ latitude and 73°54′ and 76°56′E longitude. It is bound in the North by Jammu and Kashmir, in the East by Himachal Pradesh, in the South by Haryana and in the West by Pakistan. The river Ravi marks the Western boundary of the state with Pakistan. The state covers an area of 131,015 Sq. Kms. with a population of 21.9 million (1991 census). The percentage of rural population to total population is 70.45%. The state has a higher proportion (28.3%) of scheduled caste population as compared to the country (16.5%). The sex ratio in Punjab is less than the national average. It is 882 females per 1000 males in Punjab, while it is 927 females per 1000 males for the country. The age at marriage for females is 21.07 years as compared to 18.33 years for the country. The average literacy rate of Punjab is 58.51 as against 52.51 of national figure, the female literacy rate is 50.41 as against 39.29 of national figure. The male literacy rate is 65.66 as against 64.13 of national figure. The per capita income at current prices is Rs. 8,423 as compared to national average of Rs. 4,934. Only about 7% of the population is below poverty line as compared to the national average of 30%. In the upper Bari Doab and rural Southern Malwa regions the population that live below poverty line is 30% and 25% respectively.

Administrative Structure

Divisions	3
Districts	17
Sub-Divisions	55
Tehsils	55
Sub-Tehsils	69
Blocks	136
No. of inhabited villages	12,352
No. of towns	120

One of the significant things that happened during the Sixth Plan was the adoption of National Health Policy. Healthcare Programmes were restructured and reoriented for achieving objectives of the policy. Priority was given to extension and expansion of rural health infrastructure through network of Community Health Centres, Primary Health Centres and Sub-Centres on a liberalised population norm. Efforts were made to develop promotive and preventive services along with the curative services.

High priority has been given to the development of Primary Healthcare located as close to the people as possible. The approach and strategy for developing healthcare delivery system in rural areas initiated in the Sixth Plan was pursued vigorously during the 7th Plan to consolidate the health infrastructure and making up the deficiencies in training of personnel, equipment and other physical facilities. Coordinated efforts are being made under various programmes to provide effective and efficient rural health services to the people.

Current Health Situation

We present in brief the current health status of the people in Punjab in Table 14.1.

Analysis of the Table reveals that the health status of the people of Punjab is better than the all India Average. However, it is still not impressive.

In the Punjab State, all policies and programmes as laid down in the National Health Policy, 1983, are being implemented in all earnestness to achieve the national health goals. This is evident from the table. The state has achieved couple protection rate of 65.63%, an infant mortality rate of 53/1000 live births and immunization coverage of over 90%. Yet the health of people in Punjab poses challenge of non-communicable diseases such as cardiovascular diseases, blindness due to cataract, dental caries, trauma, psychiatric problems, addictions, cancers and degenerative conditions. The infant deaths are largely due to neonatal causes, while maternal mortality still is a cause of concern.

TABLE 14.1

Target of Health Indicators by 2000 A.D.

Sl. No.	Indicator	Target	Current Status India	Current Status Punjab
1.	Birth Rate	21.00	28.06	25.00
2.	Death Rate	9.00	9.2	7.6
3.	Infant Mortality Rate	Below 60	73	53.0
4.	Expectation of life at Birth (1990-96):			
	Male	64.00	60.6	66.6
	Female	64.00	61.7	66.6
5.	Percentage of eligible couples effectively protected upto 31st March, 1995	60.00	45.4	65.63
6.	Annual growth rate of population	1.2	2.39	2.08
7.	Family Size	4.3	5.6	5.1
8.	Immunisation Status:			
	(i) T.T. Pregnant Mothers	100%	69	91.3%
	(ii) D.P.T.	85%	82	90.9%
	(iii) B.C.G.	85%	89	88.2%
	(iv) Polio	85%	82	90.4%

Source: Ninth Plan Year Plan, 1997-2000, Govt. of Punjab, pp. 256-57.

HEALTH INFRASTRUCTURE

Punjab has a vast network of Public Healthcare facilities comprising of 217 hospitals, excluding three tertiary level hospitals, 104 community health centres, 484 primary health centres and 1462 subsidiary health centres, dispensaries. The tertiary care facilities in Punjab consist of three Govt. Medical Colleges, two private medical colleges, i.e. Dayanand Medical College and Christian Medical College, Ludhiana and a prestigious Post-Graduate Institute of Medical Education and Research (PGIMER), Chandigarh.

OBJECTIVE OF THE POLICY PROVIDING PRIMARY HEALTHCARE

The National Health Policy aims at providing Primary Healthcare for all by the year 2000 A.D. The National Health Policy IAYs stress on Primary Healthcare, which ensures essential Healthcare to be made accessible to the community in an acceptable and affordable manner and with the community participation. Accordingly, the perspective long-term plan of the Health Department has been proposed, which *inter alia* aims at:

(1) Correcting the existing imbalance in the availability of medical facilities and manpower between Urban and Rural areas.
(2) Providing total health coverage to the rural population.

(3) To provide more and better medical facilities in urban areas to remove regional imbalance.

To achieve these objectives, the long-term health plan envisages the provision of following health infrastructure facilities:

Rural Areas

In rural areas at the village level, there are some voluntary village health functionaries such as trained indigenous Dais and Health Guides. They function as contact persons between the Health Department staff and the village community. In addition, they are providing certain basic health services to the village community under the guidance and support of local MPWs stationed at the sub-centres.

Primary Healthcare Services in the rural areas of the State are provided through a network of Medical Institutions comprising of Sub-Centres (2852), SHCs (1462), PHCs (484), Rural Hospitals (53), Urban Slum Area Dispensaries (252) and CHCs (104). In addition, 40 Mobile Dispensaries have been provided for Intensive Healthcare to serve the population living within 16 Kms of the International Borders of the State. (Refer Table 14.2)

Table 14.2 examines the growth of institutions from 31.8.88 to 1.4.95. The figures indicate that there has been more expansion in 7th Plan as compared to 8th Plan.

TABLE 14.2

Medical Institutions Functioning as on 1-4-1996

Category Institution	*Nos. Exist as on*	*7th Plan 1985-90 Target*	*Achieve-ment 1985-90*	*Achieve-ment 88-89*	*Achieve-ment 89-90*	*As on 1.4.95*
Sub-centre 5000 population	2602	250	150	50	50	2852
Subsidiary Health Centre (dispensaries)	1576	—	—	—	—	1246
(a) Prime Health Centre (Old) at block level	130	—	—	—	—	130
(b) Prime Health Centre (New) at 30,000 pop. level	Nil	330	150	85	95	354
Rural Hospital	54	—	—	—	—	53
Community Health Centres	10	60	36	12	12	104
Urban Slum Area Dispensaries	221	25	10	—	2	252

Source: *Ibid.*, p. 27.

Table 14.3 examines the comparative picture indicating the national norms and level of achievement by Punjab.

An analysis of the Table indicates that Punjab still lags behind the norms. For example, a Community Health Centre should cover a population

TABLE 14.3

Health Department

Sl. No.	Parameters Indicators	National Norms	Level of Achievement
1.	Trained Dais	Atleast one for each village	22276 Dais trained 0.5 villages covered by each Dai
2.	Village Health Guide	One for each village on 1000 Population	One for 1135 population. Total 11657 Trained VHG, i.e., 1196 female 10461 male
3.	Population served Health Workers (M&F)	M 3000-5000 F 3000-4500	5545 Approx. 4638 Approx.
4.	Ratio of HA(M) to HW(M)	1:6	1:5:4
5.	Ratio of HA(F) to HW(F)	1:6	1:4:8
6.	Population covered by Sub-Centres	3000-5000	4648
7.	Population covered by PHC/SHC	20,000-30,000	6499
8.	Population covered by Community Health Centres	About I lakh	1.94 lakh
9.	No. of sub-centres for each PHC	6 sub-centres	6 sub-centres PHC at 30,000 Population
10.	No. of PHCs for Community Health Centres	4 PHCs	6 PHCs

Source: *Ibid.*, p. 255.

of 1 lakh, while in Punjab, it is 1.94 lakh. There is deficiency in many indicators.

The State Government should expand its health services to fulfil the norms. Table 14.4 discusses the norms for setting up these institutions and the finances required for setting up and running these institutions.

Primary Healthcare in Urban Slums

Opening of New Dispensaries in Urban Slum Areas

The purpose of opening new dispensaries in Urban Slum Areas/ other suitable places is to provide medical facilities to the growing urban population and to take-off the work load from the bigger hospitals, so that

TABLE 14.4

Norms for Various Health Institutions

Sl. No.	Type of Institution	Land required	Population to be covered approx.	Non-recurring		Recurring per annum			Total
				Building	M&E	Medicines	Salaries	Misc.	
1.	Health Guide	—	1000	—	0.002	0.006	0.006	—	0.012
							Honorarium		
2.	Sub-Centre	1-2 Kanal	5000	4.20	0.03	0.02	0.06	0.02	0.64
3.	Subsidiary Health Centre	1-2 Acre	8000	12.00	0.10	0.10	2.00	0.052.15	
4.	Primary Health Centre (Old)	2-3 Acre	Block	30.00	1.20	0.15	6.50	0.08	6.73
5.	Primary Health Centre (New)	1-2 Acre	30000	3.00	0.15	0.12	3.00	0.10	3.22
6.	Community Health Centre	3-4 Acre	100000	60.00	5.00	0.20	15.00	NA	15.20
7.	Border Areas Mobile Teams	3-4 Acre	20000	—	—	—	—	—	
8.	25 Bedded Rural Hospitals	3-4 Acre	25000	60.00	4.00	0.25	7.00	0.25	7.50
9.	50 Bedded Hospitals	5-7 Acre	Sub-Division	100.00	10.00	0.50	14.00	0.50	15.00

* The latest information has not been supplied by Health Department. These figures are tentative.

Source: *Ibid.*, p. 276.

staff working there could spend more time in attending to serious cases. Such dispensaries are opened in those parts of the towns which are predominately inhabited by poor working class/economically weaker sections of the society on the recommendation of District Planning Boards, so that people living in such localities may derive maximum benefit from such Institutions. Opening of such dispensaries will also help in providing medical facilities to the slum dwellers near their home.

There are 232 dispensaries functioning in the State in urban areas. 8 Dispensaries were opened in urban slum areas during Eighth Five Year Plan. There is a target of establishment of 40 urban slum area dispensaries @ 8 per year during Ninth Five Year Plan.

NINTH PLAN PERSPECTIVES

Establishment of new PHCs/Upgradation of existing SHCs (Dispensaries) to PHCs

During the 7th Plan period, 330 SHCs were upgraded to the level of PHCs, raising the total Number of PHCs to 460, i.e. one for approximately 30,000 rural population. During 1990-91 and 1991-92, 12 SHCs per year have been upgraded to PHCs. The SHC upgraded to PHC will be provided with one Community Health Officer, one staff nurse, one lab technician and two Class IV employees. The amount on revenue side is meant for salary, purchase of machinery and equipment and material and supply, etc. During the Ninth Five Year Plan it is proposed to establish 50 new Primary Health Centres @ 10 PHCs per year in the State.

Providing Telephone Facilities at 460 Primary Health Centres (PHCs)

In order to establish proper referral system from PHC (at 30,000 population level) upwards, Government of India under the scheme has provided funds on non-recurring basis for the provision of telephone facilities at all the PHCs (except where already existing) in the rural areas of the State. The purpose of this scheme is to give prior information to the higher institution for taking suitable preparatory action for care of the patients being referred from the lower level in case of emergency.

Establishment of Community Health Centres

As per the decision of Cadre Review Committee taken in 1989, it is proposed to establish one CHC for approximately every one lakh population. It has been further decided by the Cadre Review Committee to provide each CHC with a specialist in Medicine, Surgery, Gynae and obstetrics, Paediatric, Anaesthesia 70 CHCs have been established during 7th Five Year Plan. 16 CHCs during 1990-91 and 18 CHCs during 1991-92 were opened, thereby raising the total number to 104.

During Ninth Five Year Plan, besides continuation of 34 CHCs opened during 1990-91 and 1991-92, there is a target for the establishment of 50 new Community Health Centres @ 10 CHCs per year and the emphasis will be given on providing the buildings to those CHCs, which are without buildings.

Continuing Education of PHC/Rural Health Staff (50:50)

Under this scheme, medical and para medical staff working in the PHC/Rural areas of the State is proposed to be given reorientation training in batches, after every 3-5 years, at selected training schools Centres, in order to update their knowledge and improve their skills. The recurring expenditure on salaries, stipends, etc. is shareable on 50:50 basis between State Government and Government of India.

Provision of Additional Lab. Technician at each PHC (50 : 50)

Under the scheme, the posting of Additional Laboratory Technician in each Primary Health Centre, has been provided so that the Blood slides under N.M.E.P. are tested immediately and radical treatment can be given in time. Uptil now, 130 posts of Additional Laboratory Technicians have been created and transferred to non-plan side. The laboratory equipment like Microscope and glass slides, Pricking Needles, Bikers, Stove and blood slides in the laboratories all over the State are also being provided.

Opening of New Dental Clinics at the Level of PHCs/CHCs/RHs and other Suitable Places

It has been found that more than 83% School children in the age group of 6-12 years were suffering from one or more than one dental diseases. Also this incidence was as high as 90% in other age groups.

In order to provide one dental clinic to serve a population of 30,000, 354 new dental clinics have been proposed to be opened in a phased manner at all the PHCs and other suitable places. Already 90 dental clinics have been established under the scheme during 8th Five Year Plan and 125 Dental clinics are being established in a phased manner during Ninth Five Year Plan.

Homoeopathy

For the Development of Homoeopathic system of Medicines in Punjab, 105 Homoeopathic dispensaries and one 10-bedded Cancer and Skin Hospital are functioning in the State.

The Homoeopathic system of Medicines proves very effective, particularly for children diseases, female diseases, skin diseases, chronic diseases and so-called incurable diseases like Asthma, Rheumatism, Arthritis, Psoriasis, etc. In recent years, this system of medicine is becoming more popular.

Some of the Homoeopathic dispensaries in the State have shortage of machinery, medicines and other equipments, so it is proposed to give emphasis to equip these dispensaries with adequate medicines and equipments for providing better services for the suffering people.

Ayurvedic System

For the development of Indian System of Medicine (ISM) in the State, 507 Ayurvedic/Unani dispensaries, 17 Ayurvedic Swasth Kendras, 6 Ayurvedic Hospitals and one Government Ayurvedic College at Patiala are functioning in the State.

At present, existing 507 Ayurvedic/Unani dispensaries functioning in the State are ill-equipped so far as essential furniture/equipments and medicines are concerned. For want of these essential requirements, the suffering people of the State cannot be properly and usefully provided medical facilities. These are being taken care of in the Ninth Plan.

An essential requirement of Primary Healthcare is to ensure potable water supply and safe sewerage system. 65% population is covered with water supply and 50% population is covered with sewerage system in the urban areas of the State. Priority has been fixed to cover 100% urban population with water supply, 80% coverage of sewerage system during the 9th Five Year Plan.

Rural Water supply is in bad shape—Rural Sanitation and Sewerage is almost lacking. There is a need to give top priority to these areas to ensure good health to the people.

CRITICAL APPRAISAL

We have examined the primary healthcare system in Punjab, based on personal discussions with the staff working at CHC, PHC, SC, Health Guide and TBA on random basis and also soliciting the views of beneficiaries. Besides, the discussions with District and State headquarter health staff was also held to get their view points. In addition, the study of documents relating to health in Punjab was also undertaken. We give here the facts and suggestions, which can help in providing decent primary healthcare in the new millennium.

1. Insufficient and Badly Maintained Buildings

Despite rapid expansion, majority of Institutions are without proper buildings. More than 2000 out of 2852 Sub-centres, more than 900 out of 1246 Subsidiary Health Centres, more than 300 out of 484 Primary Health Centres and 60 out of 104 CHCs are without proper buildings and residential accommodation. Similarly, 985 out of 1246 SHCs and 25 out of 53 Rural Hospitals also are without proper buildings. The total number of Institutions without proper buildings and estimated cost per institute is indicated in the following Table 14.5.

Table 14.5 reveals that the task is highly difficult. The cost is very high. Punjab Government has to devise ways and means to raise resources for this challenging task. Without proper buildings, healthcare becomes difficult for both the pioviders and receivers.

In addition, the existing buildings are not fit for provision of healthcare services. These need to be renovated with adequate provision for facilities like bathrooms, drinking water, electricity, etc.

TABLE 14.5

Sl. No.	Type of Institution	No. as on 1.4.95	Institutions without proper building	Cost per Institutin average (Rs. in lacs)
1.	Sub-Centres	2852	2000	4.20
2.	Subsidiary Health Centre	1246	985	12.00
3.	Primary Health Centre	484	300	30.00
4.	Community Health Centre	104	60	60.00
5.	Rural Hospital	53	25	60.00

Source: *Ibid.*, p. 256.

2. Lack of Effective Training of Medical and Paramedical Staff

It is observed that after basic professional training, Officers/Officials have not been exposed to reorientation courses for improving their knowledge and updating their skills, there is also dire need for imparting induction training to the Medical Officers and the para medical staff at the time of their first entry into Government Service. In order to cover this gap, it is proposed to provide reorientation training to all medical/para medical staff after every 3/5 years of service in the State Training Institution, Kharar and Health Family Welfare Training Research Centre, Amritsar. We suggest below the need of training for various categories of personnel.

A. Medical Officers' Training

(i) Fresh medical graduates may be given induction training for a period of at least three months with special emphasis on field training before posting them to Primary Health Centres.

(ii) As a part of undergraduate medical education curriculum, management training programme comprising of financial management, materials management and personnel management, in particular, may be incorporated.

(iii) Periodic in-service training programmes may be instituted.

(iv) Training in medico-legal aspects for medical graduates may be duly stressed.

(v) Training of interns at Primary Health Centre may be done through a well conceived programme based on practical and field experiences. Interns may be posted to Sub-centres to enable them to learn the management of a Sub-centre Independently under an overall composite supervision of Primary Health Centre Medical Officer and members of the faculty from medical, surgical, obstetrics and Gynaecology and paediatrics disciplines of medical college.

(vi) Appropriate training to develop proper and positive aptitude towards primary healthcare may be imparted to medical faculty as a part of training to trainers' programme.

(vii) VOs/NGOs may also be involved in such training programmes by making use of training material and journals produced by them.

(viii) Adequate physical and residential facilities for trainees may be created so that they are ensured of a place to stay in Primary Health Centres for training.

(ix) Medical officer should be trained at P.S.M. Department for implementation of national health programme at least one week in every year.

(x) Medical Officers should be trained in the process of planning, control and monitoring.

B. Training of Para-Medicals

(a) M.P.W.

(i) New recruitment training must be done at PHC level and that should be done mainly through field orientation training.

(ii) There should be on the spot refreshing of knowledge of female M.P.W. at the time of supervision by medical officer/block extension educator as well during monthly and sector meeting.

(iii) They should be given training in the art and science of People's participation.

(iv) They should be trained at in the Sectoral coordinations processes.

(v) Multi-purpose Worker (MPW) should be taken for field practice in Primary Health Centre areas, as the present training is more hospital-oriented.

(vi) MPW training manual does not have a chapter on "understanding the community." This may be got included.

(b) Supervisor

(i) Training must be practical and field-oriented rather than class-oriented training. At least three months field training should be done before promotion.

(ii) Supervisors should refresh their knowledge from time to time during supervision.

(iii) Supervisor should be trained in the art of interpersonal relationships.

Policy regarding training of Supervisors needs to be modified because at present Supervisors and Male Health Workers receive the same training. Being of a different level, Supervisor requires a separate curriculum of training. Training in education methodology and techniques of supervision is to be given. Supervisors have to be trained in problem-solving techniques and not indulge in fault finding.

(c) V.H.G. and Dai

V.H.G. and dai should be oriented about their work at least five days every three months. It should be done seriously.

(d) Training Tutors

Refresher training of tutors of training school should be organized and it should be practical training.

In Resolution WHA 37.31, member-States were urged to support universities in conducting the education and training of workers in health and related fields towards the attainment of health for all. Universities were invited to provide the kind of education and training for students and post-graduates in the health and related disciplines that will prepare them technically and attune them socially to meet the health needs of the people they are to serve. They were also encouraged to conduct biomedical, epidemiological, technological, social, economic and behavioural research required to prepare and carry out strategies for health for all.

Medical and health professions have increasingly been required to break out of their traditional boundaries to encompass emerging developments: increased emphasis on the humanization of care, integrated care, more consumer participation, equal access to care, assessment of technology, cost containment, consideration of the population perspective in planning healthcare, protection of the environment, promotion of health lifestyles, etc.

Advances in the patterns of health development cannot proceed unless the human resources that lead, plan, staff, monitor and evaluate health-related services and programmes are enlightened and enabled to define and respond to societal needs. Given the evolving understandings of health problems and the changing dynamics of health system development, there must be a close and continuous interaction between educational, research and health system development to ensure relevance of education to need.[1]

Too often, the training of health personnel follows a pattern of yesterday's view of healthcare, or even of only the clinical care, and falls seriously short of meeting today's and tomorrow's requirement for personnel who can lead or participate in effective health services responding to people's needs.[2]

3. Lack of Intra-Sectoral Coordination

Health is not the sole concern of health personnel, but there are several related sectors, namely, water supply, and sanitation, nutrition, education, economy and information whose cooperation is equally important but these are never taken care of by Primary healthcare system in Punjab has the Public Health Department of Punjab ever discussed the nutrition content of our food, inspite of the fact that the major problem in Punjab is nutritional deficiency although the food is available in plenty.

The International Conference on Nutrition in Rome in 1992

crystallized awareness about the causes and consequences of malnutrition, and of the ways in which the international community can combat them. It stressed the importance of incorporating nutrition objectives into development programmes and issued recommendations on seven major nutrition strategies. These include: improving household food security; protecting consumers through improved food quality and safety; caring for the poor and nutritionally vulnerable: preventing and managing infectious diseases; promoting appropriate diets and healthy lifestyles; preventing specific micro-nutrient deficiencies; and assessing and monitoring nutritional status.[3]

Shri B.K. Chaturvedi, Secretary, Department of Women and Child Development in his article, "Malnutrition: An Obstacle to National Development", in *Hindustan Times* dated 3rd September, 2000 advocated that time has now come for all agencies working in the development sector to launch a multi-pronged strategy to eradicate malnutrition. We realise that it is complex public health problem, resulting from a combination of factors such as poverty, illiteracy, superstition, social custom and lack of awareness. We already have a National Nutrition Policy which covers all aspects relating to malnutrition with sound prescriptions for combating this problem. We must implement it in full measure. To achieve quicker and more permanent results, malnutrition must be addressed inter-generationally namely through ensuring proper nutritional care of the infant from 0-2 years, adolescent girl and the pregnant and lactating mother.

Some Consequences of Malnutrition are:

- Higher Child mortality,
- Impaired brain growth and development in children,
- Higher maternal mortality,
- Life long physical disability,
- Compromised immunity, easy susceptibility to infections, and
- Increased risk of chronic diseases.

What we can do?

- Nutrition advocacy, sensitisation, capacity building and awareness generation, especially at the grass-root level.
- Preventing onset of malnutrition among 0-2 year old children by promoting complementary feeding of infants at six months, using home-based foods.
- Preventing low birth weight of the newborns and breaking the intergenerational cycle of malnutrition by addressing the nutritional needs of the girl child, adolescent girls, pregnant and lactating women.
- Preventing calorie and micronutrient malnutrition by promoting community-based production of low cost nutritious foods, and consumption of fruits and vegetables.

- Involvement of women's groups in advocating and practising proper nutritional practices.

Present understanding of inter-sectoral coordination invariably means only what the other sector does for the health sector, not what health sector does for the other sectors. It should be understood in the proper perspective to achieve mutual coordination.

4. Lack of Community Participation

In some states of the Indian Union like Karnataka, planning, implementation and evaluation of primary healthcare has been entrusted to Panchayati Raj Institutions. However, in Punjab, there is still the control of bureaucracy over primary healthcare system. In such a situation, how the people can participate in this process? Therefore, there is a need to empower the people, so that they can participate effectively in the affairs affecting their lives.

One of the major problems of primary healthcare is the absentism and lack of punctuality among the health personnel. People are highly agitated over the non-availability of health personnel to provide health services. Realising the feelings of people, the Punjab Government passed an order that the Panchayats would mark the attendance of the doctors. There was great agitation and resentment among health and medical staff. They resorted to strike. As a result, the Government had to withdraw its order. It is high time that the people, especially the disadvantaged sections of the society, should be empowered to usher in true democracy.

Under such an ideal atmosphere, the Government through health experts, can motivate the local people to help in mobilising resources for improving primary healthcare system. WHO suggests the ways and means of mobilising resources. To quote:

The resources available for healthcare, particularly in developing countries, are limited. Community involvement in primary healthcare makes it possible to mobilize community resources that might otherwise remain unused. Examples of such involvement are given below:

- *Action by the people*: This could include the provision of physical labour for building a health centre or constructing a safe well or sanitary latrine; the provision of transport, to take a woman in labour or a sick person to hospital; the organization of a special day for immunization and for indentification of children at special risk.
- *Provision of facilities*: A building owned by the community might be allocated to the community health worker for treating patients or storing medicines and records.
- *Provision of goods and materials*: The following could be provided: food such as grain, fruit, and fish for cooking demonstrations or for distribution to malnourished children; agricultural

implements to boost community food production; or building materials, such as wood and bricks, to be used in self-help construction schemes.

- *Money or contributions*: Money donated for primary healthcare in a community may be used to purchase medicines, to purchase equipment such as agricultural implements, or to pay the community health worker. Methods of obtaining financial resources are many and varied; examples include:
- A fixed payment for each service provided.
- Payment for each service, depending on ability to pay.
- Payment that varies according to the type of service provided.
- Payment for drugs or a prescription, which may vary according to the type of drug and/or ability to pay.
- Payment through an insurance scheme, in which individuals or families make continued regular payments to provide for services when they are sick.
- Donations for services, the amount depending on the patients willingness or ability to pay.
- Payment through an insurance scheme covering preventive and promotive activities as well as individual illnesses in the community.
- Periodic donations (for example, by the local cooperative).
- Periodic fund-raising campaigns, which may include athletic or cultural activities organized by communities.

Partnerships with the community involve attitudinal changes and a new approach to health development. Healthcare providers need to be convinced that illiterate communities are not unintelligent or uncreative. They need to understand that the problems affecting the poor are best understood by the poor; that, therefore, the community must be involved in conceptualizing, planning, implementing, monitoring and evaluating healthcare. In this respect, NGOs and voluntary sectors have a better record than the public sector.[5]

5. Low Utilization of Primary Healthcare Services Inspite of Good Availability and Accessibility

Utilization of services—or actual coverage—is expressed as the proportion of people in need of a service, who actually receive it in a given period, usually a year; for example, the proportion of children at risk who are immunized, or the proportion of pregnant women who receive antenatal care or have their deliveries supervised by a trained attendant. In some cases facilities exist but lack of drugs or poor quality care results in the people not using the services. Other reasons for non-utilization are that facilities may be open at hours of the day when people will not come because they are occupied in the fields or factories. Also, people may be attracted by the prestige of a more distant hospital, and may use it for care that could have been provided by local primary healthcare facilities.[6]

The utilisation of primary healthcare services is very low because of the following reasons:

(i) lack of interest and enthusiasm among health functionaries.
(ii) Lack of infrastructural facilities and public health facilities.
(iii) Non-availability of drugs and medical equipment.
(iv) Lack of faith of the people in the rural health system.
(v) Lack of effective supervision and control.

Thus, we have to introduce reforms at all levels to ensure the optimum utilisation of health services, otherwise it would become an example of clear-cut wastage of resources collected from the hard earned money of the people through various taxes.

6. Lack of Availability of Potable Water Supply and Sewerage Disposal System

Sanitation is a composite concept, which involves waste disposal system, water supply, sewerage and prevention of environmental pollution. It has been variously described by different sanitation experts to finally settle down to the concept of human waste disposal.[7]

Safe drinking water has been one of the felt needs of the people. While making development plans, it was, however, not adequately realised that the absence of sanitary conditions may cause as much harm to health as can polluted water, which is now being contaminated by effluents and chemicals discharged into water. No wonder, sanitation has been given a low priority.

Sanitation is not only the problem of keeping clean; it is a development issue without which a healthy society is not possible. It is the problem of raising production and productivity. In India alone, 15 lakh children below the age of five years die each year of diarrhoeal diseases. As many as 50 diseases are caused due to lack of proper sanitation. And over 80 percent of sickness is caused by human excreta and water-related diseases. The most common of these are intestinal parasitic infections, diarrhoea, typhoid and cholera. Very clearly, major causes of deaths in poor countries are sanitation-related diseases, while cancer is the prime killer in the West.[8]

Let us mention the various diseases due to insanitation:

By Bacteria

- Cholera
- Diarrhoea
- Bacillary dysentry
- Typhoid and para-typhoid

By Protozoa

- Amoebic dysantry

By Virus

- Infective Hepatitis
- Poliomyelitis

By Intestinal Worms

- Hook worm
- Round worm
- Thread worm
- Tape worm, etc.

By Polluted Air

- Eye diseases
- Respiratory diseases
- Skin and hair problems

By Liquid Waste and Stagnant Water

- Malaria
- Kalazar
- Filaria
- Dengue
- Japanese encephilis
- Skin diseases
- Eye problems

By Airborne Micro-organism

- Chicken Pox
- Measles
- Deptheria
- Pneumonia
- Whooping Cough
- T.B.
- Mumps, etc.
- Other respiratory diseases

Reasons for Unsatisfactory Sanitation Status in Urban Slums

- Overcrowding

- Lack of ownness of land
- Lack of safe drinking water
- Insanitation due to open defecation, stagnate water, dirty heap of garbage
- lack of awareness and facilities regarding Health, Hygiene and Sanitation
- Poverty and unemployment
- Make shift shelter and uncertainty about habitat ownership.

The population of India as per the 1991 Census is 844 million, of which 627 million (74.3 per cent of the total) lives in 5.83 lakh villages. At the time of commencement of the International Drinking Water Supply and Sanitation Decade (1981-91), the coverage with sanitation facilities was less than one per cent in the rural areas. By the end of 1990-91 the coverage increased to 2.81 per cent. However, the National Sample Survey Organisation in its Report No. 376 on "Housing Conditions" issued in September 1990 shows that only 1.06 per cent of rural households have flush toilets, 3.70 per cent septic tank latrines, 1.62 per cent service privies and 4.37 per cent other types of latrines. Thus according to this survey, 4.76 per cent of rural households have access to sanitary latrines and 89.25 per cent do not have latrines of any type; they resort to open air defecation. By the end of the Eighth Five Year Plan, the target was to cover 10 per cent of the rural population.[9]

Let us discuss the potable water supply situation in Punjab:

There are 12,428 villages in the state according to 1991 census. out of which 8579 are identified as problem villages as per the criteria laid down by GOI for this purpose. The details of criteria laid down by GOI for identification of problem villages are as under:

(i) Those not having an assured source of drinking water within reasonable distance (0.05 km) or within the depth of 15 meters.

(ii) Which suffer excess of salinity iron, fluoride or other toxic elements hazardous to health.

(iii) Where sources of water are liable to risk of cholera or guinea worm infestation.

Broadly speaking, the State of Punjab has two types of scarcity. Firstly, where the existing drinking water sources in the villages are health hazards, i.e. where the water contains fluorides, total solids, hardness in excess of the permissible limits prescribed by Government of India. Most of such villages are located, in the districts of Patiala, Mansa, Moga, Muktsar, Sangrur, Bathinda, Faridkot, Ferozepur and a part of Amritsar district. In the second category the existing drinking water sources are either deeper than 16 meters (50 ft.) or are situated beyond a distance of 0.05 km from the population. Such problem villages are mostly located in the sub-mountainous areas in the districts of Ropar, Hoshiarpur, Nawashahar and

Gurdaspur. In the case of first category the water is provided after treatment through slop and filters or by installing deep tubewells where there is underground deeper strata yield potable water. In the second category, i.e. where the existing source of deep water is at a distance, the schemes are based either on tubewells or percolation.

The details of Rural Water Supply Scheme are given below:

TABLE 14.6

Sl. No.		No. of villages (in lacs)	Population covered	Expenditure income in (in crores)
(i)	Total No. of villages in Punjab State	12428	141.89	—
(ii)	Problem villages identified as per 1980 list	3712	48.99	
(iii)	________ as per 1985	2475	25.04	
(iv)	________ as per 1992	2292	30.94	
(v)	Total problem villages in the state (ii+iii+iv)	8579	104.97	
(vi)	Problem villages covered upto			
	(a) Sixth Plan	2482	33.15	80.39
	(b) 7th Plan	1416	51.18	.03
	(c) Villages covered with potable water supply upto 31-3-97			
	(a) Problem villages	6716	88.40	416.96
	(b) Non-problem villages	287	5.23	8.04
(vii)	Villages yet to be covered			
	(a) Problem villages	1863		
	(b) Non-Problem Villages	3476		
(xi)	Target during 1997-98	142		
(xii)	Target during 9th Plan	1863		

As far sanitation is concerned, the position is highly unsatisfactory, as only negligible number of villages are covered under the sewerage disposal programme.

Reasons for unsatisfactory sanitation status in rural set-up:

- Lack of sufficient political and administrative will.
- Lack of priority to sanitation and health.
- Absence of uniform administrative structure in states and lack of uniform code and guidelines to NGOs.
- Lack of community perception in sanitation.
- Inadequate information dissemination to rural folks.
- Absence of awareness regarding health, hygiene and sanitation.
- Lack of involvement of target groups like women, youth, school teachers and students, panchayats and NGOs.
- Lack of options for sanitation measures and local trained personnel.

There is no denying the fact that inadequacy of safe drinking water, improper disposal of human excreta, solid and liquid waste leading to unfavourable environmental conditions and lack of personal food hygiene in the rural areas have been the major causes of many killer diseases. According to an estimate, more than 1.7 lakh children are affected by polimyelitis, 2.5 lakh die of tetanus and 15 lakh die of diarrhoea and dehydration every year. This high infant mortality rate is attributed largely to poor sanitation.

7. Maternal and Child Health Services not Effective

It is estimated that each year, at least half a million women die from causes related to pregnancy and childbirth. Over 99% of the maternal deaths take place in developing countries, which account for 86% of the worlds births. In the poorest countries of the world, when a woman becomes pregnant, her chances of dying as a result are between 100 and 200 times higher than those of a pregnant woman of affluent countries.

In India, women in the reproductive age groups and young children contribute about 62% of the population. These groups of the population are also regarded as most vulnerable because of special health problems. Despite our efforts over the last 35 years, the attention given to pregnant mothers, to mothers postnatally and to children has not been adequate to reduce mortality and morbidity.

India has a very high maternal mortality (500-800/100,000 live births) and infant mortality (100-110/1000 live births). The average woman in India can expect to have around 5 to 6 live births and may have 7 to 8 pregnancies. Her lifetime chance of dying from pregnancy- related causes is about 1 in 20. Some of the important causes of maternal mortality are sepsis, hemorrhage, taxaemia, illegal abortion, malnutrition and repeated childbirths. The important causes of deaths among infants and young children are prematurity, tetanus neonatorum, diarrhoea, malnutrition and respiratory infections. Several factors, such as inadequate care of mothers at risk, poor maternal health, lack of referral services, etc. contribute to this mortality.

Respondents Contact with Health Worker and Perceptions about Government Services: A Study (100 Respondents in Ropar District)

One of the important functions of the health workers is to provide healthcare services to the people in their homes. About 36 per cent of respondents were visited by health workers at home. Among them, about 85 per cent of the respondents were visited by ANMs, 37 per cent by male health workers and 5 per cent by anganwadi workers in rural areas. Majority of the respondents (63.5 per cent) were satisfied with the time spent by ANM in discussions with women respondents about their health problems. However, only 22.5 per cent respondents reported that ANM counselled their unmarried adolescent girls and not even a single respondent received Iron and Folic Acid tablets for their adolescent girls.

Currently married women in 15-44 age group, who had visited a government health facility like Hospital, Community Health Centre (CHC), Primary Health Centre (PHC) or Sub-Centre (SC) were asked whether they were satisfied with the services provided and the way the facilities functioned. Twenty-six per cent of them reported that they were satisfied with the services and would recommend it to others. An equal proportion of women reported that the working time of the facilities and their locations are convenient, staff explains how to take prescribed medicines and are friendly with patients. However, women felt no waiting time (26.5 per cent), treatment free (30.3 per cent) and treatment at centre effective (40.3 per cent) as positive factors.

We mention the following problems which need the attention of the persons responsible for primary healthcare.

Knowledge of the female multi-purpose worker is poorer than expected. Female multi-purpose worker does not use her kit during field visits. Female M.P.W. does not visit all the villages regularly and does not visit some villages at all because they are not approachable. Antenatal care through sub-centres is roughly 15 to 20 percent, and internatal and postnatal services are also poor. Multi-purpose supervisors knowledge is the same as that of male and female M.P.Ws., so they are not in a position to check work and train them in field situations. Supervision by them is also very irregular.

Medical officers did not visit the sub-centres, nor are they interested in national health programmes other than family planning. Moreover, B.M.O. does not have adequate administrative powers to take action against workers, who are slack or defaulting. Information education communication (I.E.C.) material supplied to P.H.C. is not utilized usually at sub-centres. Health education posters are usually made for the literate. Illiterate persons are not able to understand messages contained in the posters.

8. Lack of Effective Supervision and Control

Considering the rise in population size, the continuing constraint of resources and the pressure for higher priority to develop other sectors of the national economy, it appears absolutely essential to make the fullest and most efficient use of the available allocations, ensuring against underutilisation, misutilisation and diversion of resources. This objective can be achieved through appropriate administrative reforms, devolution of decision-making power and introduction of relevant managerial techniques. Bimal Jalan says that "the most important organisational reform that deserves to be implemented is to decentralise delivery of government health services." Centralisation of financial powers is a major cause of delay and inefficiency as even the slightest deviation in specification of drugs or service requires approval of a number of departments, with several layers of bureaucracy at state headquarters. Decentralisation of financial powers with performance monitoring can greatly improve the healthcare delivery system in rural areas and strengthen accountability of local institution.[10]

Recommendations

(i) Medical officer and supervisor must pay regular visits to sub-centre and supervise working pattern of M.P.W. as well as support TBAs.

(ii) Block extension educator should devote maximum time on training and reorientation of workers and TBAs.

(iii) Registration of infants should be a continuous process; it should not be done on a fixed month of the year. There should be the same register for infants and for immunization.

(iv) Community must know that dai is not a government servant; she should get compliments from community.

(v) There should not be rigidity in working time of worker; it should be modified according to the availability of the villagers in the houses.

(vi) All administrative powers should be delegated to block medical officer.

Most maternal and infant deaths are preventable, provided M.C.H. and family planning programmes are given equal status and importance, supported by, I.E.C. activities for demand generation and community participation at sub-centre level and below through TBAs.

9. Lack of Effective Evaluation and Monitoring

Monitoring is the process of measuring, coordinating, collecting, processing, and communicating information to assist management in decision-making.

The sources of information used in monitoring health activities include monthly, quarterly and annual reports from health centres and hospitals, data on notifiable diseases, and special surveys.

Good information systems are required for effective monitoring. There is a practice to collect unnecessary information resulting in wastage of human and material resources. It must be emphasized that the problem is not a shortage of data. However, there is often too much data, but the fact that little useful information can be gleaned from them.

We suggest the following to achieve evaluation

1. Primary healthcare in Ministry and Secretariat should have a separate cell to coordinate the activities of nodal officers connected with primary healthcare, namely, Maternal and Child Welfare, Immunization, Health Education, etc.
2. Independent evaluation must be done in every State to improve the quality of services.
3. Improvement in existing information system is needed.
4. Lessons must be learnt from successful NGOs.

5. Services of medical colleges may also be utilised to perform independent evaluation.
6. Every Primary Health Centre should develop one model Sub-centre and one model Primary Health Centre in every district and these should serve as examples for other sub-centres and Primary Health Centres to follow.

10. Limited Coverage of Health Activities

At present, primary healthcare services are not available to all because of mismanagement and lack of available resources. There is a need of optimisation of available resources to spread planned healthcare to all. We suggest the following to achieve this:

(i) The preparation of daily work/tour plan should be done at PHC with participation of the medical officer, block extension educator, supervisor and workers for a month so that all are clear. This programme should be given to all at sub-centre as well as in each village so that everyone in PHC knows when the worker is visiting the village. Both male and female workers should visit a village on the same day to have full impact.

(ii) Unapproachable village should be covered by four team members (2 supervisors and 2 M.P.Ws.), at least once a month. Medical officer should check implementation of plan during monthly meeting as well as a surprise check. Vehicles should be provided for this purpose.

(iii) Workers may identify 3 to 4 informants who are influential in each village and give responsibility of some exceptional families to them. They will give back information to M.P.W. on their visit, like antenatal case, child birth, death, immunization problem, so that worker need not visit each house every time.

(iv) All the national health programmes should be treated equally. More attention should not be given to family planning. Even in family planning attention may be given to sterilization.

(v) Detailed history of patients is to be taken immediately after registration so that the worker can identify high risk cases. This needs sufficient educational training of workers.

(vi) Urine examination, haemoglobin and weight record must be done at sub-centre during antenatal clinic.

11. No Provision for Educating the Community about Health For All

How can one provide rational choices to people in order to modify their healthcare behaviour and practices? In 1997 the RGF came up with a communication strategy focusing on group discussions, and Communications Needs Assessment (CNA), aimed at designing and developing a community-based primary healthcare model of 'Health For All'. To quote the report:

This model uses the concept of social marketing. We organised training workshops for Rural Health Communicators and Primary Health Workers, who put up 96 performances of street plays, 'nautankis', puppet shows, folk songs, 'qawaalis', and 'kajari' in 32 villages of Amethi Tehsil. Through these performances, the RHCs disseminate information about primary healthcare and services available to the community. Mobile health vans provide services like maternal and child healthcare, Immunisation, and treatment of common diseases and injuries, at the doorstep. The community's awareness of hygiene, sanitation, safe drinking water, communicable diseases, diarrhoea, STDs/AIDS and immunisation has been greatly increased, and more people now know the benefits of family planning and birth spacing. The success of the pilot project has encouraged us to continue and expand it all over Amethi Tehsil to achieve the goal of 'Health For All'.

12. Insufficient Funds and Encouragement for Indian System of Medicine

True primary healthcare involves self-sufficiency and empowerment in the long-run. The RGF encourages traditional health practices with a view to making primary healthcare services available in rural areas in Anantapur District, Andhra Pradesh. Forty Community Health Workers have been trained in traditional methods of treatment with ayurvedic and herbal medicines. They have established Health Centres in their villages, selling herbal medicines such as Aloe Jelly, Ashta Churan, Neem Ointment, and Setropaladi, favoured by villagers because they are low cost and have no side effects. We hope not only to promote traditional methods based on local material and expertise, but to document and publish this valuable knowledge. Punjab should try such experiments.

13. Doctors and Paramedical Staff Display Bureaucratic Culture

P.D. Sharma in his article, "Administrative Culture" in *IJPA*, July to September 1990 (pp. 620-21) rightly says that medical doctors and paramedical staff in all cultures have to work and behave like professionals. This professional culture implies a professional comraderie and professional ethics with a high sense of professional skills and pride. The Indian doctors are fairly competent and knowledgeable about their job, but it is a sad commentary on their professional ethic that they behave like 'medical feudals' in the hospital wards and glory in bossing over nurses and attendants. The District Collector or the Superintendent of Police is their 'power model' and the Indian society also evaluates their professional competence in terms of private practice money, which they mint by abusing the public facilities in government hospitals. They seldom find time to read or conduct their own researches. Obviously, they exploit popular ignorance and refuse to share their outdated knowledge or its absence with their colleagues, juniors, patients and society at large.

The general democratic culture of American society keeps the medical professionals constantly on their toes and often showing them their place also. They work under constant surveillance of the legal profession and face social audit in the press. Money minting does not earn a special kind of social status for the American doctor. Rather, the professional competition keeps pushing the fake ones out of circulation. No wonder, my doctor George was a mere doctor. He was George to us all, because he was not a Doctor Sahib. The nurse could disagree with him in the open and he won't mind sitting on the patient's bed and tasting a sample of food from the hospital kitchen. As a professional, he enjoyed tremendous reputation, but he will come to his patients in utter humility, confessing that his treatment was an experiment, based on certain hunches and researches on which the patient should also reflect and comment.

CONCLUSION

More than twenty years after the health-for-all policies and strategies were adopted, it was realized that it was not possible to reach the goal unless concerted efforts were made to reorient the provision of healthcare through appropriate reforms. This involved a complex process of change in health sector policy and institutional arrangements which needed to be carefully initiated by analysing the present situation, the future goals and how these goals could be reached.

The following points should be kept in mind while suggesting health reforms based upon facts and observation:

(1) In view of the differences in the socio-economic and overall health status in different states of the Indian union, health sector reforms should be initiated with the overall national development framework as well as within the framework of the explicit national health policies, which provide the fundamentals such as health for all, equity, social justice and partnership.

(2) The organization of managerial changes in the health systems need to be appropriately monitored and evaluated in order to identify the implications of these changes, not only in terms of efficiency, quality and sustainability, but also in terms of equity.

(3) We should explore effective strategies for the political and administrative management of the process and content of health sector reforms and to make such reform changes known to policy-makers, healthcare providers and the general population.

(4) We should make full use of national institutions and other mechanisms, including WHO collaborating centres, to plan and manage health sector reforms effectively.

(5) Efforts should be made to promote and exchange experience on health sector reforms through appropriate consultations, documentation, use of information technology, including use of

technical forums, with a critical assessment of the positive and negative impact of reforms.

(6) Government of India should provide technical and other support to States to pursue their own health sector reform measures and to coordinate with other research institutions in pursuing and supporting national efforts for health sector reforms.

(7) Existing human resources for health may require reorientation to new goals and tasks in pursuit to the PHC approach. The majority of existing health workers do not possess the appropriate skills or conceptual awareness of the PHC approach. The training they received often emphasized clinical skills, rather than work within communities. Then, too, the skills required for PHC at all levels go well beyond technical competence. For example, if health is understood in broader terms, health workers will be able to identify the social and economic factors that are the main contributors to ill-health in a given situation or among particular groups, for example, young children of families in certain occupational groups. They should be able to communicate with community leaders and other sector professionals in the search for solutions. Skills are required in management, community development, and epidemiology, as well as in integrating different programme tasks.

(8) Primary Healthcare Planners and Policy-makers should achieve the following to make a success of PHC programme.

Bibliography

Anita, N.B. and Bhatia, Kavita, Peoples Health in People's Hand- A model for Panchayati Raj, FRCH, Mumbai. 1993.

Basch, P.E., Vaccines and World Health, New York, Oxford University Press, 1994.

Bhatnagar, S. and Goel, S.L., Development Planning and Administration. New Delhi. Deep & Deep Publications (P) Ltd., 1992.

Bhattacharjee P.J. and G.N. Shashtri, Population in India, A Study of Interstate Variation, New Delhi, Vikas, 1976.

Bosh, Ashish, From Population to People, Delhi, B.R. Publication, 1988.

Brown, Esther, Newer Dimensions of Patient Care, Russell Sage Foundation, New York, 1961.

Cartwright, A., Patients and their Doctors, A Study of General Practice, Routledge Kegan Paul, London, 1961.

Chanawongse Krasal, Rural Development Management, Research and Development Institute, Khon Kaen University, Thailand.

Chandra, R.C., A Geography of Population, Concepts, Determinants and Patterns, New Delhi, Kalyani, 1987.

Chauhan, Devraj, Anaita, N.H. and Ramdan, Sangita, Health Care in India: A Profile, FRCH, Mumhai, 1996.

Das, K., Civil Service Reforms and Structural Adjustment, Oxford, Delhi 1998.

Duggal, R., Nandaraj, S. and Shetty, Sahana, State Sector Health Expenditure-A Database All India, FRCH, Mumbai, 1992.

P. Jurfelds, G. and Lindbergs, Pills against Poverty—A Study of Introduction of Western Medicine in a Tamil Village, Curzon Press, London, 1975.

FRCH, Panchayati Raj Information Resource Book, Mumbai, 1996.

Ghai, Sandhaya, Bursing Services Administration: A Case Study of Nehru Hospital, PGI, Chandigarh (Doctoral Thesis, Panjab University, 1998).

Ghosh, Brindra Nath, A Treatise on Hygiene and Public Health, Scientific Publishing Company, 1970, Calcutta.

Gill, Sonya, Health Status of the Indian People, FRCH, Mumbai, 1987.

Goel, S.L., Health Care Administration Policy-making and Planning, Sterling, Delhi, 1981.

———, Health Care Administration Levels and Aspects, Sterling, Delhi, 1981.

Goel, S.L., Health Care Administration Ecology, Principles and Modern Trends, Sterling, Delhi, 1981.

———, Family Planning Programme and Beyond, New Delhi, Deep & Deep Publications Pvt. Ltd., New Delhi, 1990.

———, International Administration: WHO, South-East Asia Regional Office, Sterling, New Delhi, 1977.

———, Modern Management Techniques, Deep & Deep Publications Pvt. Ltd., New Delhi, 1987.

———, Public Health Administration, Sterline, New Delhi, 1984.

———, Public Personnel Administration, Sterling, New Delhi, 1984.

———, Hospital Administration and Management, Deep & Deep Publications Pvt. Ltd., New Delhi, 1903.

———, Distance Education in 21st Century, Deep & Deep Publications Pvt. Ltd., New Delhi, 2000.

Hanlon, John, Principles of Public Health Administration, C.V. Mobsy, Sthouis, 1969.

ICSSR & ICMR, Health for All-an Alternative Strategy—Report of a Study Group set-up Jointly by ICSSR & ICMR, Pune, Indian Institute of Education, 1981.

Govt. of India, Annual Reports of the Ministry of Health and Family Welfare, Delhi.

———, Committee on Multi-purpose Workers under Health and Family Welfare Programme (Kartar Singh Report), Delhi, Ministry of Health and Family Welfare, Delhi, 1973.

———, Govt. of India, Health in Independent India (G. Borkar Report), Delhi, 1961.

———, Health Survey and Development Committee (Bhore Committee), Delhi, 1946.

———, Lok Sabha Secretariat, Estimates Committees and Public Accounts Committees Reports.

———, Planning Commission, Five Year Plans, New Delhi.

———, Report of Health Survey and Planning Committee, (Mudaliar Committee) Ministry of Health, August-October, 1961.

———, Ministry of Information and Broadcasting, India, 1999, A Refresher Manual, New Delhi, 1999.

———, Initiatives and Best Practices of Government of India for Effective and Responsive Administration, New Delhi, Ministry of Personnel, Public Grievances, and Pensions, 1997.

———, Deptt. of Family Welfare, Reproductive and Child Health (World Bank Component), Vols. I and II, New Delhi, 1997.

———, Report of the Working Group on Health for All by 2000 A.D., New Delhi Ministry of Health and Welfare, 1981.

Gunaratne Herat, V.T., Challenges and Response Health in South-East Asia Region, New Delhi, McGraw Hill, 1977.

Hardon, A., et. al., Monitoring Family Planning and Reproductive Rights, A Manual for Empowerment, London, Zed Books, 1997.
Indian Society of Health Administrators, Bangalore.

Annual Conference Reports
Health for all by 2000 (AD 1980).
The Role of Hospitals in Health Care (1981).
Health Manpower Requirements for 2000 (1982).
Role of the Health Administrator in India (1983).
On Growing Needs of Urban Health Management (1985).
Cost Reduction in Hospitals and Health Care (1986).
Health of the High Risk Groups Mothers, Children and Elderly (1985).
Health of Women and Children for Development (1988).
Health Care for the Villages and Urban Slums (1989-90).
Health of the Youth and the Female Child.
Role of Voluntary Organizations in Health Care in India (1992).

Books
Stress and Health of Executives and Professionals.
Hospital and Health Administration.
Modern Technology for Hospitals and Health Care.
Management for Nursing Administrators.
Community Participation in Health and Family Welfare-Indian Experiences.
Health of the Metropolis-Bangalore-A Guide to Health Planning and Development of Urban Cities in India.
Leadership and Human Resources Development for Health Care.
Managerial Effectiveness for Organizational Excellence.
Computer Applications to Hospitals, Health Care and Medical Education.
Health and Development of the Tribal People in India-A Guide for Professionals and Administrators.
Retirement Planning, Adjustment and Health.
Janovsky, K., Health Policy and Systems Development on Agenda for Research, WHO/SHS/NHP/96.1, Geneva, 1996.
Jesani, Amar & Ganguly, Shilpi, Some Issues in Community Participation in Health Services, FRCH, Mumbai, 1993.
Khandewale, Shreekant V., Health Administration and the Weaker Sections in an Indian Metropolis, Devika Publications, Delhi, 1996.
Klinobbul Krienkrai, Health and Family Welfare Administration in Thailand—A Case Study of Lampang Province (Doctoral Thesis).
Kumar, R., Child Development in India, Ashish, New Delhi, 1988.
———, Environment Pollution and Health Hazards in India, Ashish, New Delhi (Year not mentioned).
———, Youth Health, Problem, Planning and Development, Deep and Deep Publications Pvt. Ltd., New Delhi, 1986.
Lane, S.D., From Population Control to Reproductive Health: An Emerging

Policy Agenda, Social Science and Medicine, 1994.
Lush, L., Integrating Services, from Rhetroic to Action, Development Research Insights, 1997.
Mattoo, P.K., Project Formulation in Developing Countries, Macmillan, Delhi, 1978.
Meher, C. Nanavaty and P.D. Kulkarni, NGO's in the Changing Scenario, New Delhi, Uppal, 1998.
Miller, George E. and Tamas Fulop, Educational Strategies for the Health Professionals, Geneva, WHO, 1974.
Mishra, R.P., Medical Geography of India, NBT, Delhi, 1970.
Murray, C.J.L., Lopez, A.D., The Global Burden of Diseases, WHO, Geneva, Switzerland, 1996.
Myrdal Gunnar, Asian Drama, An Enquiry into the Poverty of Nations, Vol. III, Penguis, London, 1968.
Naik, J.P., An Alternative System of Health Care Service in India Some Proposals, Allied, Bombay, 1988.

National Institute of Health and Family Welfare, New Delhi
Management Training Modules for District Health Offices.
Management Training Modules for Health Offices.
Management Training Modules for Health Assistants (Male and Female).
Management Training Modules for Health Workers (Male and Female).
Management Training Modules for TBA.
Management Training Modules for Health Guide.
Park, J.E. and K. Park (1990), Textbook on Preventive and Social Medicine, Banarasidas Bhanot Publishers, Jabalpur.
Pai Panadiker, V.A., et. al., Organizational Policy for Family Planning, New Delhi, Uppal, 1983.
Pathak, Shankar, Social Welfare, Health and Family Planning in India, Marwah Publications, Delhi, 1979.
Rao, C. Hayavandana, Mysore Gazetteer, Vol. IV, B.R. Publishing Corporation, Delhi, 1984.
Ramanathan, S. (ed.), Landmarks in Karnataka Administration, New Delhi, Uppal, 1998 (Published for Indian Institute of Public Administration, Karnataka, Regional Branch, Bangalore).
Rafei, Dr. Uton M., Primary Health Care in Changing World South-East Asia Regional Perspectives, WHO Regional Office for South-East Asia, Delhi, India, 1993.
Ranga, R.K., Admn. of Family Planning Programmes in India—A Case Study of Haryana (Doctoral Thesis, Panjab University, 1998).
Rao, V.K.R.V., Food, Nutrition and Poverty in India, Vikas, New Delhi, 1982.
Rifikin, S.B., Health Planning and Community Participation, Crown Helm, London, 1985.
Sahni, Ashok, The Third Force in Health Care—Voluntary Sector, Bangalore Indian Society of Health Administrators (1992).

Scott-Samuel A., Total Participation, Total Health, Scottish Academic Press, 1990.

Sarjivi, K.S., Planning India's Health, Orient Longman, Delhi; 1971. Shenoi, P.V. (ed.), Contours of Social and Economic Development Political Issues, Concept, New Delhi, 1997.

Sharma, R.D., Advanced Public Administration, New Delhi, H.K. Publishers, 1994.

Singh, Sarabjit, Management Information System in a Hospital—A Case Study of General Hospital, Chandigarh (Doctoral Thesis, Panjab University, 1991).

Taori, Kamal, People's Participation in Sustainable Human Development (A Unified Approach), New Delhi, Concept, 1998.

Vaeth, R.M., A Theory of Medical Ethics, New York, Basic Books, 1981.

Vettivel, S.K., People's Participation in Social Development, Role of NGO, New Delhi, Vetri Publishers, 1992.

World, Health Organisation Alma Ata Revisited, WHO/SHS/CC/ 94.2, WHO, Geneva, 1994.

Werner, D., Where there is no Doctor?, The Voluntary Health Association of India, Delhi, 1984.

World Bank Financing of Health Services in Developing Countries, Washington, 1987.

World Bank, Development Report, 1993, New York, Oxford University Press.

World Bank, World Development Report, 1997, New York, Oxford University Press, 1997.

World Health Organisation, Annual Report of South-East Asia Regional Office, Delhi, 1997.

———, Bulletin of Regional Health Information, Regional Office for South-East Asia, Delhi, 1980, 1981, 1982, 1983, 1984-85, 1986-87, 1988-90, and 1991-93.

World Health Organization, Collaboration in Health Development in South-East Asia, 1948-88, Fortieth Anniversary Volume (Revised), Delhi, 1992.

———, Community Action for Health, SEA/HSD/185, Regional Office for South-East Asia, Delhi, 1993.

———, Development of Indicator for Monitoring Progress Towards Health for all by the Year 2000, Geneva, 1981.

———, Eighth General Programme of Work—Covering the Period 1990-95, Geneva, 1987.

———, Evaluation of the Strategy for Health for All by the year 2000, Regional Office for South-East Asia, Delhi, 1986.

———, Formulating Strategies for Health for all by the year 2000, Geneva, 1979.

———, Global Strategy for Health for all by the year 2000, Geneva, 1981.

———, Health in Development—Prospects for 21st Century, WHO! DGH/ 94.5, Geneva, 1994.

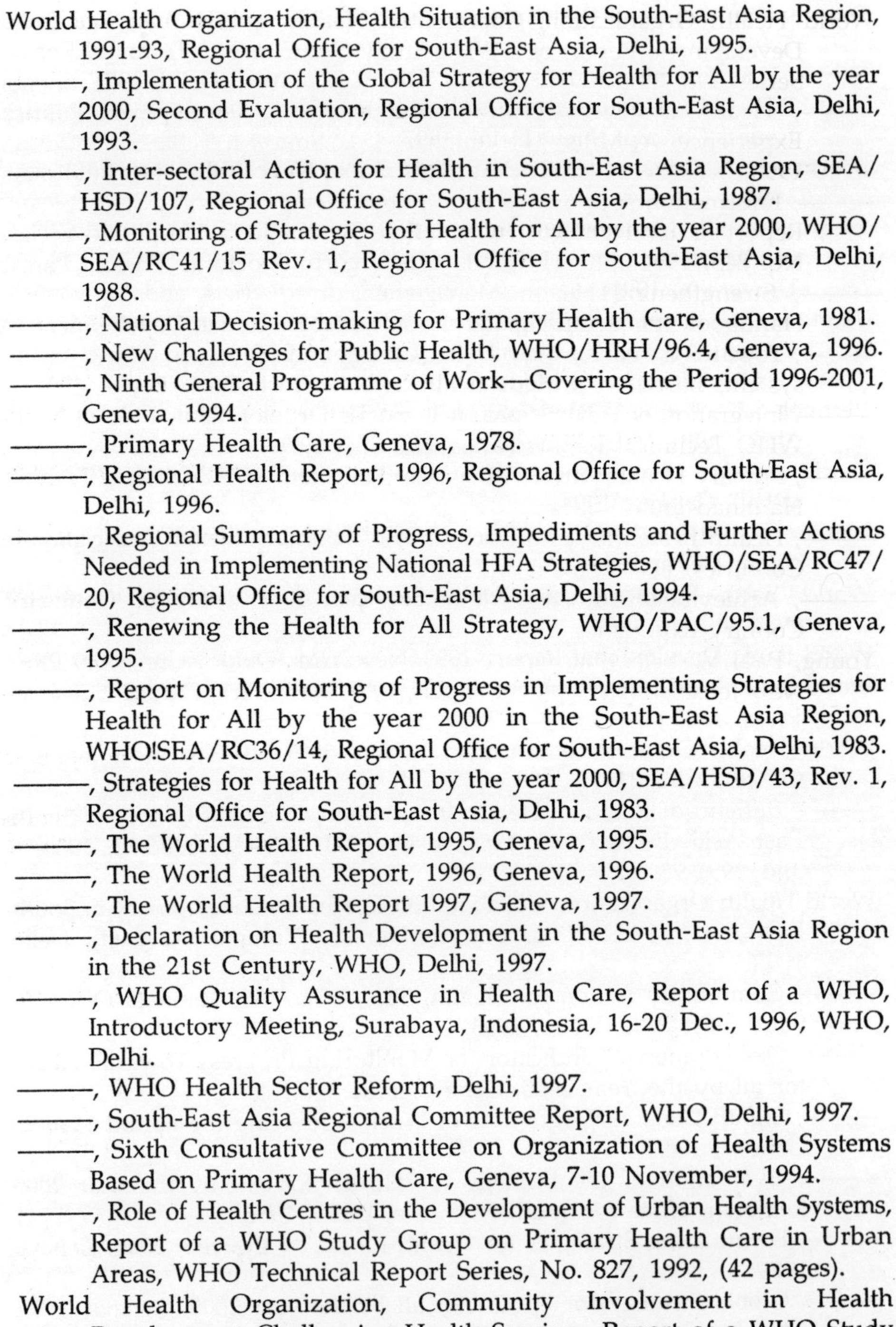

World Health Organization, Health Situation in the South-East Asia Region, 1991-93, Regional Office for South-East Asia, Delhi, 1995.

———, Implementation of the Global Strategy for Health for All by the year 2000, Second Evaluation, Regional Office for South-East Asia, Delhi, 1993.

———, Inter-sectoral Action for Health in South-East Asia Region, SEA/HSD/107, Regional Office for South-East Asia, Delhi, 1987.

———, Monitoring of Strategies for Health for All by the year 2000, WHO/SEA/RC41/15 Rev. 1, Regional Office for South-East Asia, Delhi, 1988.

———, National Decision-making for Primary Health Care, Geneva, 1981.

———, New Challenges for Public Health, WHO/HRH/96.4, Geneva, 1996.

———, Ninth General Programme of Work—Covering the Period 1996-2001, Geneva, 1994.

———, Primary Health Care, Geneva, 1978.

———, Regional Health Report, 1996, Regional Office for South-East Asia, Delhi, 1996.

———, Regional Summary of Progress, Impediments and Further Actions Needed in Implementing National HFA Strategies, WHO/SEA/RC47/20, Regional Office for South-East Asia, Delhi, 1994.

———, Renewing the Health for All Strategy, WHO/PAC/95.1, Geneva, 1995.

———, Report on Monitoring of Progress in Implementing Strategies for Health for All by the year 2000 in the South-East Asia Region, WHO!SEA/RC36/14, Regional Office for South-East Asia, Delhi, 1983.

———, Strategies for Health for All by the year 2000, SEA/HSD/43, Rev. 1, Regional Office for South-East Asia, Delhi, 1983.

———, The World Health Report, 1995, Geneva, 1995.

———, The World Health Report, 1996, Geneva, 1996.

———, The World Health Report 1997, Geneva, 1997.

———, Declaration on Health Development in the South-East Asia Region in the 21st Century, WHO, Delhi, 1997.

———, WHO Quality Assurance in Health Care, Report of a WHO, Introductory Meeting, Surabaya, Indonesia, 16-20 Dec., 1996, WHO, Delhi.

———, WHO Health Sector Reform, Delhi, 1997.

———, South-East Asia Regional Committee Report, WHO, Delhi, 1997.

———, Sixth Consultative Committee on Organization of Health Systems Based on Primary Health Care, Geneva, 7-10 November, 1994.

———, Role of Health Centres in the Development of Urban Health Systems, Report of a WHO Study Group on Primary Health Care in Urban Areas, WHO Technical Report Series, No. 827, 1992, (42 pages).

World Health Organization, Community Involvement in Health Development Challenging Health Services. Report of a WHO Study Group, WHO Technical Report Series, No. 809, 1991 (56 pages).

World Health Organization, Coordinated Health and Human Resources Development. Report of a WHO Study Group, WHO Technical Report Series, No. 801, 1990.

———, Health System Decentralization. Concept, Issues and Country Experience, A. Mills, J.P. Vaughan, D.L. Smith, I. Tabibzadehg, eds., 1990.

———, Information support for New Public Health action at district-level, Report of a WHO Expert Committee, WHO Technical Report Series, No. 845, 1994.

———, Strengthening Health Management in districts and provisions. Handbook for facilitators, A. Cassels and K. Janovsky, 1991.

———, Towards a healthy district, Organizing and managing district health systems based on primary health care, E. Tarimo, 1991.

———, Integration of Health Care Delivery, Report of a WHO Study Group, WHO Technical Report Series, No. 861, 1996.

———, Primary Health Care Reviews, Guidance and Methods, A. El Bindari-Hammad and D.L. Smith, 1992.

———, Health Promotion and Community Action for Health in Developing Countries, H.S. Dhillon and L. Philip, 1994.

———, Achieving Health for All by the year 2000, Midway Reports of Country Experiences, E. Tarimo, A. Creese, eds., (1990).

Young, Paul V., Scientific Social Surveys and Research, Englewood Cliffs, New Jersey, 1966.

Index